Meaningless Suffering

Does suffering have meaning? The leading scholars and practitioners in *Meaningless Suffering* engage with this haunting human question through the lenses of psychoanalytic, phenomenological, and ethical discourse, all the while holding contemporary social concerns in full view.

The authors seek to find ways of speaking about the lived realities and historical moments that make up our social narratives – from the murder of George Floyd to the bird watching incident in Central Park – in order to render visible the entangled forms of the effects of embodiment, ideology, race, social practice, and intersectionality. *Meaningless Suffering* is bookended by powerful pieces by Mari Ruti and Homi K. Bhabha and, in the intervening chapters, the reader traverses the ideas of Augustine, Judith Butler, Fanon, Foucault, Freud, Gendlin, Heidegger, Lacan, Levinas, and Wittgenstein to pass through the realms of classical thought, affect theory, phenomenology, linguistic studies, relational psychoanalysis, somatic studies, intersubjectivity theory, gender studies, critical theory, and philosophical hermeneutics.

This book is essential reading for postgraduate students, scholars, and practitioners working at the intersection of psychoanalysis, race, politics, and culture, as well as students of cultural studies, the humanities, politics, psychology, psychosocial studies, sociology, and social work.

David M. Goodman is the Associate Dean for Strategic Initiatives and External Relations, Director of the Center for Psychological Humanities and Ethics, and an Associate Professor of the Practice in Counseling, Developmental, and Educational Psychology in the Lynch School of Education and Human Development at Boston College, USA. He is also an Associate Professor of the Practice in the Philosophy department in Boston College's Morrissey College of Arts and Sciences.

M. Mookie C. Manalili is a psychotherapist, professor, and researcher with particular interest in suffering, embodiment, meaning-making, narratives, memory, and ethics. He is a psychotherapist in a private group practice, utilising narrative therapy, psychoanalytic approaches, mindfulness traditions, and body-based techniques. He is also Part-Time Faculty at the School of Social Work and Research Consultant for the Morality Lab and the Center for Psychological Humanities and Ethics at Boston College, USA.

Psychology and the Other

Series Editor: David M. Goodman

Associate editors: Matthew Clemente, Brian W. Becker, Donna M. Orange and Eric R. Severson

The *Psychology and the Other* book series highlights creative work at the intersections between psychology and the vast array of disciplines relevant to the human psyche. The interdisciplinary focus of this series brings psychology into conversation with continental philosophy, psychoanalysis, religious studies, anthropology, sociology, and social/critical theory. The cross-fertilization of theory and practice, encompassing such a range of perspectives, encourages the exploration of alternative paradigms and newly articulated vocabularies that speak to human identity, freedom, and suffering. Thus, we are encouraged to reimagine our encounters with difference, our notions of the "other," and what constitutes therapeutic modalities.

The study and practices of mental health practitioners, psychoanalysts, and scholars in the humanities will be sharpened, enhanced, and illuminated by these vibrant conversations, representing pluralistic methods of inquiry, including those typically identified as psychoanalytic, humanistic, qualitative, phenomenological, or existential.

Recent titles in the series include:

Anacarnation and Returning to the Lived Body with Richard Kearney
Brian Treanor and James Taylor

The Psychology and Philosophy of Eugene Gendlin
Making Sense of Contemporary Experience
Edited by Eric R. Severson and Kevin C. Krycka

Levinas for Psychologists
Leswin Laubscher

The Psychosis of Race
A Lacanian Approach to Racism and Racialization
Jack Black

Meaningless Suffering
Traumatic Marginalisation and Ethical Responsibility
Edited by David M. Goodman and M. Mookie C. Manalili

For more information about this series, please visit: https://www.routledge.com/Psychology-and-the-Other/book-series/PSYOTH

Meaningless Suffering

Traumatic Marginalisation and Ethical Responsibility

Edited by
David M. Goodman and M. Mookie C. Manalili

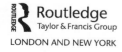

Routledge
Taylor & Francis Group

LONDON AND NEW YORK

First published 2024
by Routledge
4 Park Square, Milton Park, Abingdon, Oxon OX14 4RN

and by Routledge
605 Third Avenue, New York, NY 10158

Routledge is an imprint of the Taylor & Francis Group, an informa business

Designed cover image: Getty

British Library Cataloguing in Publication Data
A catalogue record for this book is available from the British Library

Library of Congress Cataloging-in-Publication Data
A catalog record has been requested for this book

ISBN: 978-1-032-49536-1 (hbk)
ISBN: 978-1-032-49535-4 (pbk)
ISBN: 978-1-003-39432-7 (ebk)

DOI: 10.4324/9781003394327

Typeset in Times New Roman
by Taylor & Francis Books

Contents

This book is dedicated to those dear ones, those whose lives are cut short by the absurdity and alogical nature of suffering in our world. In the wake of our grappling with meaning — may it move us towards, not away, from the unspeakable wound and the suffering Other.

For Philip Cushman, Stephen Gaddis, and Mari Ruti, three people who we lost in these last two years. May their work and passion live on through the voices and moral imaginations of those who have been shaped by their brilliance and love.

Contributors

Mari Ruti (PhD Harvard) is Distinguished Professor at the University of Toronto. She is the author of fourteen books in critical theory, continental philosophy, psychoanalysis, and feminist and queer theory.

Roger Frie is Professor of Education, Simon Fraser University, Affiliate Professor of Psychiatry, University of British Columbia and author most recently of *Edge of Catastrophe: Erich Fromm, Fascism and the Holocaust* (2024).

Lynne Layton is a psychoanalyst, part-time faculty at Harvard Medical School, and a supervisor at the Massachusetts Institute for Psychoanalysis.

Elizabeth Corpt, LICSW, President Emerita, Faculty, Supervising Analyst, Massachusetts Institute for Psychoanalysis, Supervising Faculty, Harvard Medical School, Department of Psychiatry, Editor Emerita, Psychoanalysis, Self and Context. In practice, Arlington, MA.

Lewis R. Gordon is Professor and Head of the Department of Philosophy at UCONN-Storrs. He is the author of many books, including, most recently Fear of Black Consciousness (Farrar, Straus, Giroux, 2022).

John L. Roberts, PhD is Associate Professor at the University of West Georgia. His interests include theoretical and philosophical approaches to psychology, histories of consciousness and subjectivity, and psychoanalysis.

Nahanni Freeman, PhD is a professor of clinical psychology and director of research at George Fox University. Her publications consider intersectionality between science, developmental theories, and theoretical psychology.

Sheila L. Cavanagh is a professor at York University, Toronto, Canada. Her scholarship is in transgender studies, queer theory, and psychoanalytic sociology with a special focus on Bracha L. Ettinger and Jacques Lacan.

Patricia Gherovici, PhD is a psychoanalyst, analytic supervisor, and recipient of the 2020 Sigourney Award . She has authored or edited six books including *Please Select Your Gender* (2010) and *Transgender Psychoanalysis* (2017).

Sam Binkley is Professor of Sociology at Emerson College, Boston. His research examines the social production of subjectivity, identity and personhood through lifestyle literatures and popular texts.

Robin Chalfin is a psychotherapist and clinical supervisor in private practice in Boston, MA, USA. She is the Adjunct Faculty of the Graduate Counseling Psychology Program at Lesley University and serves as a board member and frequent lecturer at the New England Center for Existential Therapy.

Christopher Christian, PhD is the Editor-in-Chief of the journal *Psychoanalytic Psychology*; a supervising and training analyst at the Institute for Psychoanalytic Training and Research (IPTAR), where he is past Dean. He is the co-editor with Patricia Gherovici of *Psychoanalysis in the Barrios: Race, Class, and the Unconscious* (Routledge, 2019).

Karley M. Guterres is a doctoral student in Counseling Psychology at Boston College. Karley has completed fellowships through the Massachusetts Institute for Psychoanalysis, as well as the Albert and Jessie Danielsen Institute at Boston University, and is an affiliate of the Boston College Center for Psychological Humanities and Ethics.

Homi K. Bhabha is the Anne F. Rothenberg Professor of the Humanities in the English and Comparative Literature Departments at Harvard University. He was founding director of the Mahindra Humanities Center at Harvard University from 2011–2019 and director of the Harvard Humanities Center from 2005–2011.

Acknowledgments

The scholars whose work we host in this volume are taking up the most important issues we are facing in our society. We are deeply grateful for their brilliant and powerful voices. Each of the chapters in this volume was originally presented as a conference paper at the Psychology & the Other Conference in 2021. This conference has become, for many of us, a community and space which fosters new and emergent ways of speaking to human identity, potential, and suffering. Our authors speak to these aspects of our human condition on the personal, transgenerational, political, racial, gendered, and economic planes. For their contributions and wisdom, we are truly grateful and excited to share with you all.

Additionally, we'd like to recognize the communities that host and echo these dialogues. We express our gratitude to the folks involved in the Center for Psychological Humanities and Ethics. Thank you to our collaborators at Boston College – Lynch School of Education and Human Development, School of Social Work, School of Theology and Ministry, and Morrissey College of Arts and Sciences (Philosophy and Theology departments). The Society for Theoretical and Philosophical Psychology (Division 24 of the APA) is a kindred organization that has generously supported conversations such as these and has served as an intellectual home. Additionally, we'd like to thank the Albert and Jessie Danielsen Institute at Boston University for their partnership on this venture as we find creative ways of bringing clinicians further into these interdisciplinary dialogues. George Stavros, Steve Sandage, David Rupert, and Lauren Kehoe deserve a specific shout-out.

In terms of editorial support and dialogue about the content of the pages in this volume, we are grateful for those who closely read and engaged the work, giving it greater clarity and depth. These individuals include Sam Aston, Tara Candelmo, Matt Clemente, Ashana Hurd, Julia Goetz, A. Taiga Guterres, Haleigh Karam, Justin Karter, Sophia Shieh, Eric Severson, and Jeff Sugarman. These and other colleagues and friends have helped animate the earnest and passionate pages ahead.

Finally, we'd like to acknowledge and honor Mari Ruti, one of our authors who passed on during the time this volume was being assembled. She was a

plenary speaker at the 2019 conference and her address was enormously impactful. Our words fail to do justice to the depth she invited both in her spoken and written works. Sharing the final sentiments of her obituary…
"Mari approached her illness and treatment with tenacity and determination. She advocated for herself with ferocity, never losing her belief in herself or her instincts. To her last days Mari's courage, incandescent vibrancy, and intellectual rigor was matched only by her kind-heartedness. Mari lived by her theoretical ideals in that she faced the existential crisis of life and treated each new decision as a creative act."

Bringing together a volume with powerful voices such as this can often be an extraordinary labor. However, this occasion felt more like a formative process that took us on an incredible journey. We hope our readers experience this as they work through and grapple with the pages ahead. Perhaps, the question of suffering may be beyond meaning. Yet, perhaps it is this journey to the margins and grappling with responsibility therein that is infinitely meaningful. As our close colleague, A. Taiga Guterres recently exhorted, may we all learn how to pilgrimage into suffering in such a way that lovingly attunes us to one another.

~ David M. Goodman and M. Mookie C. Manalili

Introduction

Problematizing "Meaningful Suffering"

David M. Goodman and M. Mookie C. Manalili

כ לָמָּה יִתֵּן לְ עָמֵ ל אוֹר; וְחַיִּים, לְ מְ רֵ יֽ נָפֶשׁ.
"Why is light given to the toilers,
life to the bitter in spirit?"

(Job 3:20)

Suffering is insufferable. Suffering is excess, a boundary violation, beyond capacities, outside of mastery. Pain hurts, the raw sense data of causal discomfort. Suffering is not the same thing as pain. It is not attributed, clarified, or contained in linearity. The experience of suffering links to registers and constellations of my person, my history, my condition – and beyond my own finitude, towards our world, towards you.

Suffering reduces *and* expands me.

It makes me small, less, and confined without access to ability or identity. It is constriction and prison. It is repetition, cycling and cycling.

Suffering *also* refuses my capacities and ideas, rejects their minuscule registers, and forces enlargement. My story was too small. It renders my story insufficient and calls me into the more-ness of experience and the blinding excess of exposure. It is a refusal of repetition. I can never re-organize in the same way as before. That repetition is unavailable to me now.

It whispers death and chaotically spills into life. Suffering is use-less, for its fullness is beyond use. To make sense of it, to tame it, to orient it to something, some type of explanatory set, is to de-fang suffering's innate absurdity, its moan, its beckon, its evil, its gratuitousness.

Emmanuel Levinas (1988) disputes depictions of suffering quickly made useful and meaningful. In his essay *Useless Suffering*, Levinas represents suffering in the following manner:

> Suffering is, of course, a datum, in consciousness, a certain "psychological content," similar to the lived experience of color, sound, contact, or any other sensation. But in this very 'content' it is an in-spite-of-consciousness, the unassumable.

DOI: 10.4324/9781003394327-1

2 David M. Goodman and M. Mookie C. Manalili

> "Unassumability" that does not result from the excessive intensity of a sensation, from just some quantitative 'too much,' surpassing the measure of our sensibility and our means of grasping and holding; but an excess, an unwelcome superfluity, that is inscribed in a sensorial content, penetrating, as suffering, the dimensions of meaning that seem to open themselves to it, or become grafted onto it... It is not only the consciousness of rejection or a symptom of rejection but this rejection itself: a backward consciousness, 'operating' not as 'grasp' but as revulsion. ... The denial, the refusal of meaning, thrusting itself forward as a sensible quality...
>
> (Ibid., 91–92)

Levinas argues against representationalism, idealism, and psychological interiority that cheapen the "phenomenality" of the other's suffering. Present throughout his larger philosophical project, his primary goal in arguing for its "uselessness" is to protect the ethical bearing of suffering. In foreclosing through the ready mediation of logic, economy, egoism, and knowledge, the call of the suffering-in-the-other is muted, defanged, and domesticated. For Levinas, the "justification of the neighbor's pain" is the "source of all immorality" (Ibid., 98–99).

In this same essay, Levinas points to the collapse of theodicy in Western civilization and problematizes our understanding of suffering's function.[1] Providing theological accounts which rationalize, justify, and defend a meaning for the presence of suffering is simply unethical. For Levinas, the Shoah demands the cessation of this age-old tendency. The excessive nature of gas chambers, extrajudicial killings, natural disasters, untreatable cancer, or the sudden accident of another all scream for suffering to not be reduced into explanation. Rather than grasping ideas, for Levinas, suffering causes a revulsion in consciousness. Indeed, the lived experiences of suffering flood over the abstractions and reductions of thought, and also *is* the spilling over of the ideas.

Nonetheless, in this current world, the temptation of theodicies has simply given way to other versions of explanatory ideologies. These other meaning-making systems seduce us into a premature foreclosure into meaning-making. The echoes from Levinas's exhortation apply even in our secular discourses today: whether it be Progress, Science, Free Market Rationality, Medicine, Common Good, or any other replacement of God. The suffering in the other is justified and is given meaning. There is tremendous peril in our tendency to make the suffering of another useful at the altar of these lesser gods. Levinas warns that this tendency to explain will erode the inter-human order and strip our ethical possibilities with one another.

However, it is difficult terrain to traverse. Levinas is but one voice of many, grappling with this issue. What *is* the relationship between meaning and suffering? Meaning-making is a part of human life, creativity, care, and love. Meaning here also captures the enactment of values, rather than the explanatory set to reduce suffering's implication. Viktor Frankl (1985) reasoned that in and through enacting meaning (even in the midst of suffering), we remain human. In our world with its variegated forms of personal, transgenerational, political, racial, gendered, and economic violence, the chasms between each other might seem infinite. How might we contend with this fraught relationship between meaning and suffering?

This question animates the pages to come. The scholars and practitioners who author these chapters engage with this haunting human inquiry and ancient temptation. They do so through the lenses of psychoanalytic, phenomenological, and ethical discourse, all the while holding contemporary social concerns in full view. This is accomplished through the exegesis of specific events and historical moments. Their analyses lean toward the living texts of the world, where the effects of embodiment, ideologies, race, social practice, and intersectionality can be seen in their entangled forms. Each of these thinkers is aimed at the complicated dynamic of meaning and its relationship to suffering. The authors problematize the meaning-making processes that foreclose experience in the presence of suffering. They take this up through distinct angles and with attention to various psychological, historical, socio-political, and economic practices. The first chapter of the book is a deeply personal account and as the book progresses, the reader will be invited to consider personal and political through various accounts, with the final chapter providing a powerful political account of this intersection between meaning and suffering.

Suffering is meaningless, yet it cannot be left there. There is more at play. It is this play that is at the heart of the volume. The ethical implications could not be more significant.

Note

1 Levinas makes a distinction between suffering-in-the-Other and suffering-in-me. This introduction aims at both forms of suffering, with primacy for the former: "In this perspective, a radical difference develops between **suffering in the Other,** which for me is unpardonable and solicits me and calls me, and **suffering in me,** or my own adventure of suffering, whose constitutional or congenital uselessness can take on a meaning" (Levinas, 1988, 159).

References

Frankl, V. E. (1985). *Man's search for meaning*. Simon and Schuster.
Green, J.P. (2005). *The interlinear Bible: Hebrew-Greek-English*. Hendrickson Academic.
Levinas, E. (1988). Useless suffering. In Robert Bernasconi & David Wood (eds.), *The provocation of Levinas: Rethinking the other*. Routledge.

Chapter I

When the Cure Is that There Is No Cure

Melancholia, Mourning, Creativity

Mari Ruti

This chapter is about melancholia, mourning, and creativity. I draw on the work of Jacques Lacan, Julia Kristeva, and Melanie Klein to develop the idea that creativity, potentially at least, offers an antidote to melancholia as an ontological (existential) predicament. I moreover propose that it may, at least under certain circumstances, do the same even when melancholia is the consequence of more idiosyncratic (unpredictable) traumas. Mourning enters the arc of my argument due to the fact that, as was the case with Freud, Kristeva sees it as a necessary step on the subject's way from melancholia to creativity. In contrast, Klein and Lacan, in their respective ways, appear to consider melancholia *itself* as a springboard of creativity. I am especially interested in the Lacanian credo – paraphrased for the purposes of this chapter – that the only "cure" for our (the subject's) constitutive lack is to recognize that there is no cure for it; the only "cure" for our lack-in-being and the foundational melancholia that this lack gives rise to is to accept that there is no cure for these conditions beyond our capacity to generate objects, ideals, passions, and activities that can, temporarily at least, compensate for them. Creativity, in this sense, is a matter of inserting something meaningful or fulfilling into the void within our being.

At first glance, it may appear callous to propose that there is no cure for our constitutive lack. One of my objectives, then, is to show that, far from being callous, the claim that the only "cure" for this lack is to come to terms with the reality that there is no cure for it is crucial to our ability to lead a rewarding life. Here I need to specify that I do not wish to make this argument about structural traumas such as poverty, racism, sexism, or other social inequalities for the simple reason that, far from being incurable, such problems could be fixed by more just and egalitarian social arrangements. However, I discuss such traumas toward the end of this chapter not only because they are frequently ignored in psychoanalytic accounts of trauma but also because I hope that at least some of what I say about ontological and idiosyncratic injuries may prove valuable while we wait for solutions to structural inequalities – solutions that are maddeningly slow to arrive. My goal is not to be nihilistic but merely to recognize that collective remedies to

DOI: 10.4324/9781003394327-2

structural injustices are unlikely to materialize anytime soon and that many dispossessed individuals are therefore left to their own devices in trying to find ways to cope with their predicament. My point is not to shift the responsibility for solving structural problems from the socio-political and economic collective to individual subjects, as our neoliberal society tends to do, but rather to sidestep the cruelly optimistic mentality that makes it possible for our society to dodge this very responsibility.

Before proceeding, I need to clarify that I use the term *creativity* capaciously, not merely as a matter of high art, brilliant intellectual accomplishments, or lofty ethical ideals, but also as a matter of all activities that contribute to a life that feels meaningful or rewarding to us. As a result, in this chapter, a Nietzschean self-fashioning, of living one's life as poetry – "first of all in the smallest, most everyday matters" (Nietzsch, 1882/1974, 240) – counts as creativity just as much as writing, painting, or composing songs does. Defined in this manner, the contours of creativity are singular, aligned with the inimitability of the person who engages in various sublimatory pursuits.

I

I focus on Lacan, Klein, and Kristeva because all three agree that human beings are not ontologically designed for seamless satisfaction. At most, we experience moments, periods, or spurts of satisfaction (jouissance). Instead of the kind of wholeness and plenitude that we may fantasize about, a buried brokenness of being constitutes the status quo of our lives. Many of us are experts at hiding or ignoring this reality, frequently by filling our lives with so many practical preoccupations that we do not have the time or mental space to pay attention to the ontological void within our being. Nonetheless, there are moments of crises – sudden tears in the normal fabric of our lives – when this void leaps to the forefront of our consciousness, often ushering us to a melancholy crypt of despair that can be difficult to climb out of.

For me, such a moment of crisis arrived when I was diagnosed with metastatic – incurable and therefore terminal – breast cancer. The diagnosis came out of nowhere, like a bolt of lightning, and drastically reconfigured (and disfigured) my life: there was no way to continue living in the way that I had been accustomed to living. If death had until then appeared like a reassuringly obscure event at a hazy, far-off horizon, suddenly it was staring me starkly in the face. It came so close that I could feel its breath on my cheek. "A year, maybe eighteen months," the oncologist told me. The abrupt loss of a future – of what could have been, should have been or might have been – caused the floor to rock back and forth while my stomach did a series of somersaults. I understood why people often throw up when they get dreadful news. My voice was muffled, as was the voice of the doctor speaking to me. It felt like we were speaking underwater while I slowly drowned. It did not feel like the person responding to his questions was me. Numb to the core, I became a spectator of my own life.

I discovered that I was genetically predisposed to the type of cancer I had so that in some ways it had merely been a matter of time before it erupted. The moment I walked out of the hospital, a Heideggerian living-toward-death became the quotidian reality of my life. The occupational hazard of many Lacanians – namely, a keener than usual awareness of the ontological void within our being – reached an unbearable pitch, making my ears ring day and night, especially at night (and it was every night) when I woke up to so much pain that I thought that I would die in the next two minutes.

Still, somehow life limped along. The eighteen months passed. I did not die – yet. And there was a small satisfaction in discovering that I had not been mistaken when, long before falling ill, I had repeatedly claimed that creativity – sublimation broadly understood – may under some circumstances, for some people at least, function as an effective antidote to suffering (see Ruti, 2006, 2009, 2012, 2013, 2018a, 2019). I had never been so naïve as to believe that this reasoning applies to everyone. However, for me personally, creativity – more specifically, writing – had long served as a soothing balm against the grim legacies of poverty and other formative hardships that had threatened to spoil my life even before the utter catastrophe that I was unexpectedly living. For me, it was a tremendous relief to discover that writing did not fail me even in the context of the wreckage that cancer made of my life. I do not dare to generalize about an issue of this magnitude even though I hope that my observations in this chapter strike a chord with at least some readers. All I can say is that, since my diagnosis, the only times I have felt genuinely content and to some extent protected have been when I am writing. I feel that writing turns death into a passive bystander that I can keep at arm's length: if at the hospital I became a spectator of my life, writing turns death into such a spectator.

This feeling may be nothing more mysterious than a matter of being distracted by an activity that causes me to lose track of time – and therefore of death – by facilitating a temporary fall into oblivion. Nevertheless, it emboldens me to articulate one of my arguments as follows: the ontological void – the lack-in-being – that Lacan and Kristeva (and Klein in her own way) theorize is not always the tragedy that one might expect it to be. More specifically, I want to propose that we need this void because we only possess creative capacity – the kind of innovative vitality that can help us cope with life's myriad challenges (in my case, my cancer diagnosis) – insofar as our subjectivity is constituted around it. I in fact want to go as far as to assert that our imaginative powers *increase* when we accept that this void cannot be remedied and begin, instead, to search for ways to forge a liveable life within the lack, break, wound, fissure, or rupture around which our subjective finds its tenuous, ever-shifting parameters. A rupture, after all, is an opening. Admittedly, at times it opens to a disconcerting chasm. But other times, it opens onto potentialities of being that would remain foreclosed if it did not exist, if we were perfectly intact and undamaged creatures.

Let me restate the argument as follows: if we were not fundamentally lacking—if we lacked our constitutive lack – we would not have the creative, innovative capacity to endure the kinds of more contingent lacks (crisis situations, everyday disasters) that most of us, from time to time, are destined to experience. If we had no familiarity – however unconscious – with what it feels like to be lacking, we truly would not know how to react when something went terribly wrong in our lives; we would not know how to even begin to formulate a response to the calamity at hand. I have chosen Lacan, Klein, and Kristeva as my main interlocutors because all three grasp this reality: they share an understanding of the very relationship between constitutive lack, creativity, and our (always fragile) ability to handle contingent traumas that I wish to explore.

Lacan was notoriously more interested in ontological lack than in contingent traumas. However, as a clinician, he could not avoid observing the psychic, affective, and physical effects of idiosyncratic traumas on his patients, with the result that an awareness of suffering beyond existential malaise is at times palpable in his writings even when he does not explicitly name it as such. In addition, Kristeva and Klein frequently *do* name it, as Kristeva does at the beginning of *Black Sun*, where she admits that her topic – melancholia and depression – is deeply personal to her (Kristeva, 1987/1989, 3–5). Not only does Kristeva's text contain compelling accounts of the exertions that her patients make to liberate themselves from melancholia and depression; it also serves as a testimonial to her own efforts to accomplish the same. My argument is profoundly influenced by the fact that she turns to creativity as an antidote that, precariously yet relatively reliably, works for her.

2

In Lacan, we find a lack that constitutes the subject as a socially intelligible but ontologically wounded entity. The sociocultural and linguistic order, the big Other, that surrounds the child from its birth does not leave space for any primordial fusion with its caretaker, instead revealing from the get-go that symbolic castration is the price that the child, and later the adult subject, pays for its viability in this order. The subject may retroactively fantasize about an elementary place of fusion, plenitude, and wholeness, but such a place never existed for the simple reasons that the signifier got there before the child did, pre-empting any possibility of an unmediated relationship to either itself or to its caretakers. The – presumably unconscious – awareness of this reality gives rise to melancholia about a loss that never, in reality, took place but that nevertheless endures as the kind of irrevocable injury that nothing can redeem. Fortunately, this state of affairs also gives rise to desire as an attempt, however incompletely, to address this injury. Creativity – sublimation – then arises as one manifestation of desire, as one means of productively responding to the foundational trauma that haunts the subject.

One can see the trajectory: lack leads to desire, which in turn leads to creativity as a potential antidote to lack (and to the melancholia that this lack begets). No wonder, then, that Kristeva claims that rather than looking for the meaning of the subject's despair, we should reconcile ourselves to the fact that "there is only meaning in despair" (Kristeva, 1978/1989, 5–6): the subject only possesses the capacity to generate meaning of any kind to the extent that lack – and the melancholia that, like a translucent shroud, surrounds this lack – is constitutive of its being. Like Lacan, Kristeva thus draws a connection between the subject's melancholia about its ontological lack and its desire to find ways to heal this lack through the production (creation) of meaning. Even more explicitly than Lacan, she offers creativity as a bridge that, ideally at least, leads from melancholia to meaning. This is why she speculates that there is no imagination – no creative capacity – that is not "overtly or secretly, melancholy" (Kristeva 1987/1989, 6). For her, creativity serves as the sublimatory solution to the subject's fundamental dilemma of not being able to shake its melancholy feeling that it has been deprived of something unfathomably precious.

In Klein, in turn, the beginning of life is characterized by the paranoid-schizoid position: a psychic reality of bits and pieces that does not start to cohere until the child reaches the depressive position, which – despite its connection to melancholia – is a reparative and therefore arguably an intrinsically creative state. The depressive position represents the child's attempt to make up for its – frequently purely imagined but sometimes concretely acted out – aggression, to repair an object that it has destroyed in fantasy, if not in reality. It is through the depressive position that objects lose their quality of being either categorically good or categorically bad and gain the kind of complexity that allows for the coexistence of good and bad qualities in one entity, such as the mother. It is precisely because the child realized that the bad object that it has attacked is also the good object that loves and feeds it that it feels melancholy remorse about the injury it has caused (or believes having caused). The depressive position hence allows the child to begin to integrate objects into multidimensional beings and to take responsibility for how it treats such beings. In short, if the paranoid-schizoid position destroys and shatters, the depressive position repairs and creates.

Lacan, Kristeva, and Klein – in their divergent ways – regard the link between melancholia and creativity (sublimation or reparation, depending on who is speaking) as foundational to human life. Thus far I have referred to the cause of melancholia vaguely, as either an ontological sense of lack or the aggression of the paranoid-schizoid position. Yet all three thinkers use the same term for the object that the subject – we – imagines having lost or injured: the Thing (*das Ding* in German). If for Klein, this primordial object is the mother's body, Lacan and Kristeva conceptualize this originary (non) object more figuratively, as a fantasmatic promise of wholeness that arises retroactively, once our symbolic identity has emerged. As I have noted, in reality, we have lost nothing. Yet the fantasy of the Thing allows us to imagine that one day we may recover what we imagine having lost. However, because the Thing-in-itself is unavailable, the best we can do is to create or discover substitutes for it: objects that we either invent or find in the world and that carry a furtive, cryptic, or shadowy intimation of the Thing's aura can to some extent alleviate our feelings of disappointment, disenchantment, and dislocation.

Real-life objects that give us such an intimation of the missing Thing contain what Lacan calls the *objet a*. The *objet a* – which is yet another product of our fantasy life – can be characterized as a tiny morsel that has become detached from the Thing and that we unconsciously deposit in tangible objects of desire in order to render them desirable. That is, the *objet a* is not an intrinsic – native – component of our object of desire; instead, it is a piece of the Thing that we ourselves fantasmatically place in the object to make this object sparkle with a special iridescence. In this sense, even though we believe that our object is the cause of our desire, in reality, we have, without realizing it, manipulated the situation in such a way that it is the *objet a* – which we ourselves have installed in the object – that mobilizes our desire. One could say that it is fundamental to the structure of desire to be based on fantasy – a fantasy that ultimately has to do with our wanting to fill the lack within our being by inserting into it an object that contains a strong residue of the missing Thing.

Unfortunately, nothing is easier than taking advantage of our yearning for wholeness in order to commercialize our desire, a desire that is driven by our quest for the Thing through various objects that appear to contain the *objet a*. It is easy to craft situations where we chase one enticing object of desire after another because these objects seem to be taking us closer to our goal of regaining the plenitude that we imagine having once possessed. In this scenario, we hope that just around the corner lies in wait an object that will finally offer us definitive satisfaction only to find ourselves perpetually disappointed. This is a perfect example of what Lauren Berlant (2011) calls cruel optimism: we pursue objects that we hope will redeem us but that in the end elude us – thereby causing us to waste precious resources on a mission that will never pay off – and therefore ultimately function as an impediment to our flourishing.

Capitalism thrives on this state of affairs. As Todd McGowan (2016) cogently notes, despite appearances to the contrary, the point of capitalism is not to satisfy us but to dissatisfy us (and to keep dissatisfying us indefinitely). I do not mean that it grants us zero satisfaction. Rather, its genius resides in its ability to offer us just enough satisfaction to make us believe that greater satisfaction is available if we merely keep looking for it. This promise of greater satisfaction entices us to repeatedly return to the stores in the hope that among the seductive, dazzling objects skillfully displayed awaits one that will offer us the satisfaction we seek. However, because our ontological lack is ultimately unfillable, instead of filling it, we merely fill the coffers of the all-too-clever capitalist.

The sparkly avatars of the Thing, the luminous objects on display at department store windows and on our television and computer screens, possess the power to lead even the skeptics among us astray. We may lose our interest in an object almost as soon as we acquire it. Or the object may quickly become outdated, like an iPhone that feels obsolete the minute a newer version is released. Or it may be that at some point a little crack appears on the object's pristine surface so that it no longer satisfies us to the same degree as it initially did. Yet, strangely enough, even after repeated disappointments, many of us do not question the ability of consumer capitalism to eventually provide the fulfillment we are after. It is more likely that we believe that we simply have not yet chanced upon the right object(s).

If the false promises of cruel optimism easily mislead us with inanimate objects, they do so even more effectively with people we desire: there is arguably nothing that promises to return to us the ontological fullness that we yearn for more robustly than the person we love. Indeed, our society explicitly talks about romance as a matter of finding our "missing half." In addition, just as is the case with the enduring appeal of inanimate objects, our romantic disappointments rarely make us question the capacity of love to eventually satisfy us. When love disenchants us, we are more likely to believe that we have not yet found the right person than we are to question the idea that love has the power to heal our wounds, including our previous romantic disillusionments.

3

I have analyzed the complex dynamic of love so frequently in my writings (see Ruti, 2011, 2012, 2013, 2015, 2018a, 2018b) that here I want to focus on the less obvious scenario where we hope that inanimate objects can fill the void within our being. My commentary regarding the ability of consumer capitalism to mislead us should make it clear why many Lacanians shun objects of desire as debilitating fantasy formations. Simply put, the Lacanian credo that the only "cure" for our constitutive lack is to recognize that there is no cure for it should lead us to mistrust the promise of satisfaction that objects offer. This has even prompted some prominent Lacanians (see, for instance, Eisenstein & McGowan, 2012; Edelman, 2004, 2013; McGowan 2013; Žižek, 2009, 2013) to privilege the destructiveness of the drive over the lures of desire. Though I understand the reasons that these critics shun desire and though I often have a great deal of respect for their arguments – especially for McGowan's brilliant analysis of capitalism – I nevertheless believe that there was a reason that Lacan aligned his ethics of psychoanalysis specifically with not yielding on our desire (for a detailed discussion of this theme, see Ruti, 2012, 2015, 2018a).

I concede that no object of desire can return to us the wholeness or definitive satisfaction that we unconsciously desire; I agree that there is no way to heal the lack within our being. Nonetheless, I have a degree of appreciation for the ability of certain objects to capture our interest in a manner that indicates that they have come to house the *objet a*. I am not talking about objects that we might find at Target, though even among those, we could discover some that are surprisingly satisfying. Rather, I am talking about objects that, however partially or fleetingly, offer us genuine satisfaction, that somehow connect us to the "real" of our being. I suppose that I have come to believe that a partial and fleeting satisfaction is better than no satisfaction at all.

I do not see the fact that the satisfaction provided by the glimmer of the *objet a* is fantasmatic as an argument for banning this satisfaction, for what in our lives is not fantasmatic? As far as I can see, fantasy may be the only way that we can ever attain even a little bit of the jouissance of the real. Orgasmic moments of jouissance may feel more "authentic," but they do not last long, nor are they available to all of us. It is, for example, a little-discussed detail that many illnesses for all practical purposes rob people of the capacity to access the real in this manner. Obviously, objects are not accessible to everyone either. Yet there is no reason to assume that all objects in the world are commercial or that every commercial object is to be condemned because it has been manufactured. The conditions in which workers produce objects should be a real political concern – and is certainly an issue that I care about – but I am not sure that the fact that an object has been manufactured *in itself* constitutes a good reason for categorically rejecting it, especially as it is clear that even the staunchest critics of capitalism routinely use objects, such as washing machines, showers, couches, and cars that capitalism makes available. Personally I would take a washing machine over women shredding their fingers on washboards in ice-cold water (which was the reality of my childhood).

Perhaps more to the point, a beautiful view, a rock that I find on the beach, or a flower in a field can function as an object that grants me a special satisfaction, at least for a moment. Sometimes a moment is all I need. Generally speaking, I believe that objects that contain a strong aura of the Thing can connect us to our jouissance in ways that are genuinely gratifying. I am not looking for a purity of satisfaction. I am not looking to heal my wounds or to obtain ontological wholeness. I merely believe that a degree of fulfillment is possible to us as human beings and that sometimes objects can help us attain this fulfillment. In the same way that an object cannot cure my cancer but can lighten the burden of living with it by bringing beauty or joy into my life, some objects have the power to lessen the sting of our ontological lack and of the melancholia that haunts so many of us due to this lack. For this reason, I have never found it useful to disparage all objects even as I remain highly critical of the excesses of consumer capitalism.

As I have started to suggest, there are two ways for objects to appear in our life: we can either invent them or discover them. My writing a book is a matter of inventing an object; it is an act of the kind of creativity that brings me genuine satisfaction and that I discuss in a moment. However, first I want to re-emphasize the possibility that there are times when the simple act of finding a special object in the world, even in the much-maligned marketplace, may enhance the quality of our life – may even contribute to the art of living that I count among the kinds of creative activities that the vast majority of us are capable of. It may be that living with the cloud of death hanging over my head has made me appreciative of tiny objects in ways that I did not used to be, in the same way as it has made me appreciative of tiny everyday experiences, such as watching the sun rise as I work early in the morning, that thrill me.

Here is a simple example. During a recent trip to a small town in the South of France, I bought two silver rings, meant to be worn together, one with a little white pearl and the second with seven narrow bands bunched together to create a wider band. I do not usually wear rings, and rarely buy items during trips, but these rings somehow leapt at me from the display case. The psychoanalyst Marion Milner notes how finding an elegant dress once made her feel recentered and re-empowered after a vexing social interaction that had made her feel personally erased (Milner, 1936, 151–152). I would not go that far. But I cherished the rings, and they quickly became associated with the magical month that I spent in a town that I loved and that gave me a break from the morose realities of being ill. The rings even became associated with the fact that after my trip, I received the first encouraging CT and MRI scans in three and a half years: my cancer had stabilized.

Although I know that there is no direct connection between the rings and the improvement in my cancer, the rings came to represent hope and health. Consequently, when I momentarily thought that I had lost them, I was despondent. I felt that I had lost not only them but also any hope of ever regaining my health. You can therefore imagine my delight when the rings turned up in a small compartment of my bag, where I had slipped them for safekeeping and then forgotten that the compartment existed. Now I only wear them at home, where know that there is no chance of losing them. It is clear that, for me, these rings carry a poignant aura of the Thing. And the fact is that I do not care that I know full well that their appeal is entirely fantasmatic. What does it matter whether my joy is based on fantasy or "reality" – whatever the latter may even mean – as long as it exists? I would rather have a bit of joy than the smugness of theoretical virtuousness (which, truth be told, smacks of a puritanical moralism and righteousness).

Lacan was no stranger to the special delight that objects can provide. In one of my favorite sections of his seminars, he offers an example of an object that grants many people a palpable aura of the Thing: a still life of apples painted by Cézanne. Lacan explains: "Everyone knows that there is a mystery in the way Cézanne paints apples, for the relationship to the real as it is renewed in art at that moment makes the object appear purified; it involves a renewal of its dignity" (Lacan, 1986/1997, 141). By means of the enigmatic purification that art is capable of, apples painted by Cézanne establish a connection to the real – to the locus of jouissance – for those who view them. If there is a mystery in Cézanne's apples, it is not because he paints a perfect replica of an apple but because – by choosing to portray a slightly stylized version of an apple – he is able to capture something of the jouissance of the real in his portraiture of this mundane object. Cézanne is able to bring the viewer so close to the Thing that she is able to feel its aura: it is as if the air between the viewer and the *objet a* (as the emissary of the Thing) embedded in the painting vibrates with this aura. What makes Cézanne an extraordinary painter is that he is able to generate this vibration.

In the same text that contains Lacan's discussion of Cézanne, Lacan defines sublimation as a matter of raising a mundane object to "the dignity of the Thing" (Lacan, 1986/1997, 121). It is therefore not a coincidence that he claims that an apple painted by Cézanne renews its dignity: due to his unusual skill, Cézanne raises an ordinary apple to the dignity of the Thing. Lacan concedes that the effect is imaginary, that even Cézanne cannot grant us direct access to the Thing-in-itself. Yet his talent as a painter allows him to conjure up an evocative trace of this Thing. Cézanne's genius as a painter resides in his ability to instill the mystery of the *objet a* in an entirely banal object. For many people who view Cézanne's paintings, they appear to contain something inscrutable beyond the objects that they depict. There is a tone, timbre, or resonance to his art that is highly distinctive yet elusive. Lacan implies that what we sense is the dignity of the Thing that arises to the surface in Cézanne's art.

Recall that I said that there are two ways to obtain objects that bring satisfaction: we can create or discover them. For those who view Cézanne's paintings, they are objects that they have discovered in the world in the same way that I discovered my rings in the south of France. However, for Cézanne himself they were objects that he created. My sense is that when it comes to the degree of satisfaction, of jouissance, granted by an object, the ability to create it may be more powerful than merely finding it. Moreover, although it may at first glance appear that the creative solution to attaining satisfaction – and therefore at least momentarily silencing the ache within our being – is reserved for the select few who possess a special talent, my inclination is to insist that this is not necessarily true. Even though most of us do not possess Cézanne's aptitude, we may nonetheless be able to create objects that allow us to activate the dignity of the Thing, even if merely momentarily: books, songs, ceramics, clothes, jewelry, paintings, bridges, buildings, gardens, flowerbeds, delicious food, tasty bread, and a large array of objects of daily use.

The satisfaction that we procure from such activities is not negligible. The special objects that we create (or even merely discover) hold a unique significance for us, functioning as stand-ins for the Thing; they resonate on the frequency of the Thing, thereby allowing us to perceive its sublime residue. That is, our ability to raise mundane objects to the dignity of the Thing saturates ordinary objects with its radiance. And if certain objects possess a greater power to galvanize us than others, it is because such objects impart more of the Thing's aura. As fantasmatic as their effervesce may be, we experience it as "real," as a source of authentic jouissance. This is why we are not mistaken when we privilege such objects over others that fail to have a comparable impact even though by so doing we by necessity render ourselves vulnerable to the possibility that our object could get displaced, damaged, or destroyed – that we might end up having the mourn the loss of our object. This is the price we pay for reaching for a morsel of sublimity within the weave of our everyday life.

Lacan offers an example of an everyday creative act by describing a decorative string fashioned out of empty matchboxes that a friend of his had strung around his mantlepiece. In this string, boxes are connected to each other by inserting the inner compartment of a box some way into the slightly larger outer shell of the next one and by repeating the action enough times to create a long sequence. This is an instance of creativity on a much more humble scale than Cézanne's paintings, yet Lacan insists that there is something about his friend's contraption that reveals a trace of the Thing's dignity. More specifically, he claims that his friend's string of matchboxes is "not simply an object," but "in its truly imposing multiplicity" approximates the Thing (Lacan, 1986/1997, 114). Lacan goes as far as to state that rather than being merely an assemblage of ordinary matchboxes, the collection illuminates the trace of the Thing that "subsists" in the matchbox (Lacan, 1986/1997, 114): it makes the sublime appear in the most commonplace of objects. In this sense, sublimation is not merely a matter of artistic innovation, but also, on a much more basic level, of inducing the Thing to materialize within the mundane weave of everyday life.

The string of matchboxes is Lacan's way of explaining how ordinary objects become invested with a special meaning. The example demonstrates "the transformation of an object into a thing, the sudden elevation of the matchbox to a dignity that it did not possess before" (Lacan, 1986/1997, 117). Yet, as Lacan continues, "it is a thing that is not, of course, the Thing" (Lacan, 1986/1997, 118). The object – in this case, the matchbox – elevated to the nobility of the Thing is still a substitute in the sense that it can never give us the Thing-in-itself. Yet an object that contains even a small trace of the Thing acquires "a dignity that it did not possess before." It may be a mere ricochet of the Thing, yet it still comes closer to the Thing than other objects; it grants us a tiny portion of jouissance that connects us to the luster of the Thing.

4

I have valorized the power of sublimation, claiming that there is something about objects that appear to contain the *objet a*, whether we have created or discovered such objects, that helps us cope with the ontological lack within our being. However – and here we reach the gist of my argument – we are only able to take advantage of this sublimatory solution to the extent that we abandon the notion that we may one day be able to recover the Thing-in-itself. That is, we have to accept the Lacanian credo that I have already evoked a couple of times, namely that the only "cure" for our foundational lack is that there is no cure for it. I have attempted to show that discarding the ideal of a definitive cure makes it possible for us to obtain the kind of partial (yet "real") satisfaction that clinging to this ideal would impede. In more philosophical terms, one could say that exchanging the ideal of transcendence beyond the world for an ideal of transcendence *within* the world renders a degree of fulfillment obtainable.

Let me restate my argument as follows: accepting the reality that there is no cure for our existential malaise keeps us from wasting our life in chasing the untenable goal of healing our lack. That is, accepting the lack of a definitive cure allows us to direct our attention to endeavors over which we have some control; it frees us to pursue modalities of living that are both realistically attainable and potentially even rewarding – gratifying despite being imperfect. Unfortunately, because the mundane objects that contain the *objet a* are by necessity mere pale imitations of the Thing-in-itself, it can take prolonged mourning to reconcile ourselves to the reality that these imitations, these faint echoes of the Thing, are the only portion of the Thing that will ever be available to us. Yet I believe that those of us who have managed to make peace with this reality possess the best chances for fashioning a life that feels both rewarding and dynamic.

Kristeva, who is profoundly interested in psychic rebirth, argues along related lines when she notes that sublimation is an attempt to "secure an uncertain but adequate hold over the Thing" (Kristeva, 1987/1989, 14). Like Lacan, Kristeva believes that sublimation can offer an effective "'container' for the lost Thing" (Kristeva, 1987/1989, 14). Looking back at the earliest stages of life, she follows Lacan in proposing that "lack is necessary for the *sign* to emerge" (Kristeva, 1987/1989, 23). In other words, the child, in order to find its way from the oceanic semiotic – which, for Kristeva, is loosely equivalent to the Lacanian real – to the symbolic order, produces vocalizations that are the symbolic equivalents of what it is lacking, namely the Thing. It is as if the child said to itself – and I quote Kristeva speaking in the voice of the child – "No, I haven't lost; I evoke, I signify through the artifice of signs and for myself what has been parted from me" (Kristeva, 1987/1989, 23). This is a situation where the child enfolds traces of the Thing into its incipient artifice of signs in order to hold onto a residue of the Thing at the very moment when it is forced to relinquish it.

Kristeva specifies that the signifier's triumph over the lost Thing, over the subject's constitutive lack, is always precarious, flimsy at best. It is demolished whenever the subject falls into melancholic paralysis, which not only entails the inability to use the signifier in an innovative manner but also, in extreme cases, to use it at all. In such instances, the subject becomes aphasic, apathetic, exhausted, and even agoraphobic. It seeks solace in the silent and solitary crypt of its melancholia.

On the flipside, Kristeva believes that whenever the subject is able to find its way out of its crypt of melancholia and begin to mourn the loss of the Thing – or the loss of some real-life object, ideal, or person that it may have experienced – it can resort to the signifier as an antidote to the Thing's ability to pull it into a pit of despair. As Kristeva proposes: "Sublimation weaves a *hypersign* around and with the depressive void. This is *allegory*, as lavishness of that which *no longer is*, but which regains for myself a higher meaning because I am able to remake nothingness" (Kristeva, 1987/1989, 99). Humans are unique among animals not only in the sense that they are haunted by a sense of inner nothingness but also in the sense that they are able to "remake" this nothingness: in the place of nothingness, they can place words, images, and other creations. In sum, according to Kristeva, humans can transcend their grief of being separated from the Thing by working through their melancholia to the point of becoming interested in the life of signs. In this manner, Kristeva concludes, "beauty emerges as the admirable face of loss" (Kristeva, 1987/1989, 99).

The danger of falling back into the crypt of melancholia, where fantasies of being reunited with the Thing dominate, is ever-present, which is why the signifier's power to connect us to meaning – to our ability "to remake nothingness" – can never be guaranteed. This is why many creative individuals like to begin a new project the moment they have completed the previous one: this ensures that melancholia does not get a chance to defeat the signifier's power to fend off its seductive stasis. Creative individuals know that if creativity keeps melancholia at bay, ceasing creativity can all too easily provide an opening for melancholia to slip past their defenses.

It is not for nothing that in the western world, there has always been a close link between creativity and depression. If my analysis is right, this link makes perfect sense: when the creator temporarily stops creating, she leaves the door open for melancholia; conversely, if she is caught in the grip of melancholia, she is unlikely to be able to create. For many of us, there are periods when the signifier fails at the task of connecting us to meaning. During such periods, we yield to silence and relative immobility. We retreat into our vault of melancholia, unable to mourn, with the consequence that making our way back to the world of signification can feel utterly impossible. In such situations, taking a shower can feel like a daunting act. The hope –

Kristeva's hope, the hope of psychoanalysis, my hope – is that somehow we will eventually manage to grab hold of the signifier in order to pull ourselves out of the swamp of melancholy stupor.

I hope that my account of how the trace of the lost Thing finds its way into our attempts to generate meaning makes it easier to understand why, for both Lacan and Kristeva, creativity in the sense of being able to play with signifiers, to create new forms of signification (of meaning), can only emerge when the signifier is animated by the drive energies of the real, by jouissance. That is, the dynamic that I have explored in the context of mundane objects, such as my silver rings or the string of matchboxes that Lacan describes, applies to signification as well: when little bits of the Thing get taken up – activated – by the signifier, it becomes revitalized, just like objects that contain an aura of the Thing become special, vibrant entities for us.

Another way to express the matter is to suggest that language that feels alive or innovative contains an undercurrent of drive energies that both Lacan and Kristeva associate with the Thing, Lacan with the real and Kristeva with the semiotic as the terrains within which the Thing finds its fantasy-generating power. These drive energies give our language the distinctive cadence that each of us possesses when we speak or write. There is a rhythm, an idiosyncratic sonic quality, to language that runs underneath our sentences that distinguishes our way of using language from the ways in which others use it. Arguably, one index of creativity is the degree to which jouissance is able to animate our language so that we do not end up speaking or writing in a monotonous, lifeless – that is to say, boring – manner.

The drives are frequently destructive: jouissance can wreak a lot of havoc. When Lacan and Kristeva – and also Klein, whom I will get to in a moment – talk about the drives, ultimately they are talking about the death drive. As Lacan explains in his seminar on James Joyce (Lacan, 2005/2016), creative language often destroys language in order to rebuild it anew. In extreme cases, such as the writings of Joyce, the annihilation of language is drastic, but so is its innovative reconstitution. Likewise, Kristeva (1974/1983) ties poetic, creative forms of language not merely to the commingling of the signifier and jouissance but also to the manner in which writers, in admitting jouissance into their sentences, perform a highly violent act. This is what a lot of experimental writing (and also painting, such as surrealism) is all about: language gets mangled to the point that it becomes malleable and therefore available for radical forms of manipulation. Though this interests me theoretically, what interests me even more is the manner in which jouissance infuses everyday life with its unruly yet vitalizing energy.

Transporting the theoretical insight about the manner in which art, when it manages to be creative, takes place at the intersection of the signifier and jouissance to broader real-life concerns may at first glance seem like a stretch. But I hope that, upon reflection, you agree that the more we are able to allow jouissance to fill our being, to inhabit the nooks and corners of our psyche, affects, and body, the more alive – singular, unique, and creative – we feel. Of course, when we open ourselves to the disruptiveness of jouissance, we may also appear extremely odd. The more jouissance dominates our being, the less we are able to meet the normative definition of what it means to be a socially intelligible subject. For this reason, it can feel risky to invite jouissance to infiltrate our self. Yet doing so may be the price of releasing our singularity.

This is why Slavoj Žižek (2007) goes as far as to suggest that we should learn to enjoy our symptom. After all, the symptom, however painful or bizarre, is the site of our singularity in the sense that it represents the node where the symbolic, imaginary, and real components of our being intersect and intermingle in ways that give rise to our unique psychic, affective, and bodily makeup. Lacan calls this node the sinthome. The details of the sinthome – our most fundamental symptom – reside beyond the parameters of this chapter, but I am tempted to say that if we have a soul, it is in the sinthome that we should look for it.

My psychoanalytic version of the soul is far from the harmonious entity that spirituality has traditionally offered us as a form of solace. This is because there is nothing soothing about the sinthome. Our sinthome-soul is a contorted, deformed, derailed, and uncanny entity. I am not even sure why I want to call it the soul. Perhaps this seemingly odd impulse is explained by the fact that there is something about the concept of the soul that has historically singularized us. I remain invested in the notion that there is great value in considering individuals as singular entities. If I regard the sinthome as a psychoanalytic version of the soul, it is because I want to communicate that what is most singular about us – most characteristically "us" about us – is not necessarily always beautiful. Instead, it can be extremely uncomfortable both to ourselves and to those around us. Yet it is only within the folds of such singularity that we might expect to find creativity in the sense that I comprehend it instead of a purely manic, and hence ultimately ineffective, defense against loss and melancholia.

5

How does Melanie Klein fit into all this? Surprisingly well. To begin with, Klein has what Amy Allen calls a "realistic" view of the human subject in the sense that she places the death drive at the center of her theory. Klein states: "The repeated attempts that have been made to improve humanity – in particular to make it more peaceful – have failed, because nobody has understood the full depth and vigor of the instincts of aggression innate in each individual" (Klein, 1975, 257). Lacan would not use the term *instincts* because of their biologistic connotation, preferring to talk about the drives instead, but he – as well as Kristeva, I believe – would agree that aggression, the death drive, is a core component of subjectivity and that a psychoanalysis that does not recognize this ceases to be analysis proper and becomes "mere psychology." Klein, in fact, explicitly argues that psychoanalysis has been the only western discourse to have taken seriously the foundational role that aggression plays in human life, including child development.

In Kleinian theory, the main task that the child faces is to move from the aggression that is fueled by fear and anxiety and that characterizes the paranoid-schizoid position – in which the child both lashes out at others and, in a paranoid manner, expects retaliation – to the depressive position, where it begins to integrate objects into complex entities in the manner that I described earlier. This is when the child begins to repair relational ties that the paranoid-schizoid position has severed. The child's perception that it has hurt the other, for instance its caretaker, by its aggression, and its consequent guilt and depression about its own aggression, drive it toward reparation. As I have noted, reparation, in turn, is arguably a form of creativity.

One could say that any act of reparation is one of creativity: whether it is a matter of repairing a broken plate or a broken interpersonal tie, some creative labor goes into the process. Some reparative acts are obviously more intricate and demand a greater degree of active effort than others. But the point is that the moment the child reaches the depressive position, creativity is built into the fabric of its everyday life, especially into its object relations. Moreover, this dynamic is not limited to children but encompasses the adult subject as well because Klein does not believe that either the paranoid-schizoid position or the depressive position are ever fully overcome. This is why she does not talk about developmental stages but rather positions. These two positions – the paranoid-schizoid and depressive positions – remain a part of the adult subject's psychic makeup and the subject tends to circle in and out of them repeatedly throughout its life.

Those who are unfamiliar with Kleinian theory may find it confusing that, for Klein, the depressive position is a desirable goal that the child, and also the adult subject, attempts to reach. It is counterintuitive to view depression as a psychic or affective state worth pursuing. But, for Klein, the guilt and anxiety that we feel when we find ourselves in the depressive position, afraid that we have injured someone we love, generate the impulse to repair that drives creativity. If Kristeva claims that creativity can only emerge when the paralysis of melancholia is overcome and we are able to begin the process of mourning, Klein appears to believe that our ability to dwell within our depression, to remain in our melancholy crypt, gives rise to the creative act of reparation.

For Kristeva, the transition from melancholia to mourning is essential because mourning implies movement. It entails our ability to gradually distance ourselves from the object that we have lost; it entails a gradual severing of psychic and affective ties that, though slow, eventually ushers us to a state of mind where we are able to find new objects of desire and love. This was also Freud's (1917) original interpretation of mourning and melancholia in the essay by the same name – an interpretation that led him to regard melancholia as a pathological state. However, in his reassessment of the theme

(Freud, 1923), he revised his view in ways that implied that our character is on some level a function of our melancholy relationship to the losses we have endured—that who we, on the most fundamental level, are represents a layered sedimentation of object losses that we have not been able to entirely overcome. Already in his initial analysis of mourning and melancholia, he wondered why a person had to be ill to possess a clear understanding of the human predicament. His revision of his earlier account resuscitated this question. Why, indeed, is it that self-understanding requires such a deep familiarity with the more shadowy side of life?

In the present context, what is important is that both Freud and Kristeva believe that the transition from melancholia to mourning gradually allows us to transcend our loss and to rebuild our life with new objects. It is true that, for both Freud and Kristeva, the lost object is incorporated into our psyche and therefore remains forever alive and consequential to us. However, in the external world, the object is reluctantly relinquished. Although, as we saw earlier, Kristeva admits that on some level our refusal to accept the loss that we have suffered and our subsequent attempt to enfold traces of our lost object into our sentences is a precondition of our creative power, ultimately, for her, renouncing the lost object – which is accomplished by moving from melancholia to mourning – is the price we pay for our psychic and affective rebirth and the creativity that accompanies this rebirth.

One way to resolve the apparent contradiction in Kristeva's theory is to recall that when she talks about enfolding traces of the lost object into our sentences, she is referring specifically to the Thing as a fantasy object. In contrast, when she asks us to renounce our lost object in favor of new objects of desire, she is referring to real-life objects. A second way to resolve this contradiction is to resort to Freud's account of character formation by concluding that it is possible, even necessary, to cherish a residue of the lost object within our inner life even as we allow ourselves to move toward new objects. That is, a psychic and affective faithfulness to lost objects should not be viewed as antithetical to our ability to invest ourselves in new objects. This may explain why Klein seems to suggest that there is something generative about allowing ourselves to inhabit the static place of melancholia – of depressive repair – for longer than our society, in its pursuit of productivity and cheerfulness, deems desirable. There is something to be said for allowing ourselves the time and space to mourn properly so that the objects that we have lost genuinely become incorporated into our psychic and affective lives before we begin to look for ways to rebuild our lives.

6

At this juncture, it is important to do what is too rarely done in contemporary theoretical discussions of trauma, namely to distinguish between three different genres of injury: ontological, structural, and idiosyncratic. The fact that few critics think in terms of these distinctions creates many of the most vicious – yet completely unnecessary – ideological battles among critics who in principle could row in the same direction. Rather, many critics get caught up in defensive postures where their main goal seems to be to prove that critics whose vocabulary of traumatization differs from their own are politically objectionable. Instead of attacking the real enemy – for instance, the neoliberal capitalist establishment that strives to deny that trauma even exists by advocating positive thinking as a remedy to all of our problems, thereby placing the responsibility for improving our lot solely on our personal ability to think ourselves out of pain – critics who all in their own ways would like to create a more egalitarian society keep tearing each other apart. In this context, the so-called "narcissism of small differences" creates divisions that are unfortunately far from being small: it splits the left, making it laughably easy for the right to defeat us. What, exactly, is the point of the infighting when the solution is as simple as admitting that there are various forms of trauma that interact and frequently intersect in interesting ways—ways that it would serve us well to better understand instead of trying to show that our particular approach to trauma is the most virtuous of all.

Perhaps I do not see the point of the ideological rifts between, say, Lacanians (who focus on ontological lack), affect theorists (who focus on structural injuries), and relational analysts (who focus mostly on idiosyncratic wounds) because I have experienced all three of these forms of trauma and therefore recognize their simultaneity as a cruel potentiality. As a human being, I am an ontologically lacking entity who sometimes – against my own better judgment – hankers for a sense of wholeness. As someone who spent the better part of her life working inhumane hours to dig herself out of poverty, I understand something about the psychic, affective, and physical legacies of structural injuries even in situations when such injuries have in principle been transcended. And I am not so senile as to have forgotten what it was like to be so poor that dinner could not be assumed. Finally, as someone who, after a genuinely sucky childhood and decades of trying to prove myself to a father who saw it as his mission to convince me that I would "never amount to anything," now lives with terminal cancer – with mastectomy scars where my breasts used to be, insane pain in my bones, the realization that I will never be kissed again, and the constant awareness that my "life" is merely a kind of antechamber of death – I also know something about idiosyncratic wounds that fall on you because of the cards that you were dealt by destiny (for lack of a better word). Sticking to the western world, besides terminal illnesses, idiosyncratic wounds include dreadful childhoods, alcoholic parents, stints at a mental hospital, debilitating accidents, and countless other unpredictable everyday disasters.

One of the many things I have learned the hard way is that destiny does not give a damn about whether you have already endured what you yourself consider as your fair share of hardship. It does not spare you from incurable cancer just because you grew up poor with an abusive father. If anything, the former probably has something to do with the latter. It seems to me that destiny likes to repeatedly pile layer upon layer of misery on some of us while letting others off fairly easily. That said, I have also learned that appearances can be deceptive, which means that these days, when I look at people on the street, I assume that many of them suffer in ways that I cannot see. I know how easy it is to fool people. For example, my mother does not know that I have terminal cancer because I know that this information would crush her. I do not tell her because I want her to live the rest of her life, which has been full of suffering, with as little pain as possible. So when she asks me to lift something heavy, I nod and smile even when the opioids have worn off and the pain is unbearable.

Even if many of us suffer in ways both visible and invisible, we certainly do not suffer equally. Suffering is unfairly distributed. Yet there seems something strange about the idea that there are right or wrong ways to suffer. It is obvious that Lacan, Kristeva, and Klein for the most part remain on the level of ontological loss: the loss of the Thing (or, for Klein, the mother) as the foundational fact of subject formation that turns lack, injury, and disorientation into the subject's existential condition. However, this does not mean that they would deny the reality of structural or idiosyncratic traumas. Indeed, as analysts they must have seen plenty of such traumas. As for us who are analyzing trauma in the twenty-first century, there is no excuse for confusing existential injury with more structural or idiosyncratic traumas that result from the ways in which precariousness – human vulnerability – is unevenly distributed across individuals and groups.

On the one hand, all of us are creatures of lack by virtue of being human; on the other, many of us also belabor under the unbearable weight of additional traumas that have to do either with structural social inequalities or with the idiosyncratic arc of our lives. Some structural injuries are visible; others remain invisible and clandestine. Either way, they must be carefully distinguished from ontological lack because, as I noted at the beginning of this chapter, they could be cured by more egalitarian social arrangements. This is why I would never be so naïve (or arrogant) as to suggest that creativity, even broadly understood, should be considered as the first line of defense against them. In the case of structural traumas, political solutions should clearly be our priority.

That said, I believe that there are *certain* circumstances where creativity as a form of sublimatory inventiveness could help alleviate the pain of even those who suffer from structural traumas. In addition, I believe that it is possible that creativity could be an effective counterforce against some idiosyncratic traumas. At least, I have personally experienced it as such. A great deal depends on the specifics of the situation. Saying this does not suggest that I want to cancel political efforts to rectify structural traumas or practical efforts to address idiosyncratic traumas, such as better health care – far from it. I am merely saying that while we wait for our efforts to bear fruit – while we wait for the more egalitarian society that we would like to see come into being or when the health care system keeps failing us, as it seems to do on a regular basis—there may be some solace in dipping into the reservoir of our sublimatory resources.

One reason I believe this to be true is the following: due to the slowness with which structural inequalities are being addressed and the difficulty of adequately responding to idiosyncratic injuries, these two genres of traumatization, though in principle different from ontological lack, can over time come to *feel* ontological in the sense that they become embedded within our being, plaited into our psychic, affective, and physical constitution. In other words, even though I would never posit that structural inequalities do not have a cure or that idiosyncratic injuries cannot be alleviated by practical measures, it feels that we need to take into account the possibility that over time, while we wait for collective remedies and concrete solutions, these ailments can begin to feel just as intractable as ontological lack. When that happens, creativity can serve as a potential antidote to despair.

Creativity should not be seen as an alternative to political and practical efforts but merely as a supplement to such efforts – as a temporary placeholder for the sturdier remedies and solutions we hope to achieve. The more temporary this placeholder, the better. It would be important to defend against the possibility of our neoliberal society striving to turn it into a permanent solution, thereby evading responsibility for structural and concrete solutions, as it tends to do. However, denying the potential of creative activities, which could be as simple as painting a rundown apartment or setting up a community garden in a poor neighborhood, to provide solace on grounds of ideological purity would be a mistake for the simple reason that whatever can be done to diminish people's suffering in the here and now is valuable and does not in principle need to interfere with our pursuit of long-term solutions. If anything, it may give us the boost of vitality that we need in order to keep agitating for the political and practical results we wish to achieve; it may provide a degree of immunity against the exhaustion that we can all too easily feel when we are up against bureaucratic institution that deliberately place obstacles in our way.

When I say that the distinction between ontological, structural, and idiosyncratic injuries may in some cases begin to blur, I do not mean that their acuteness becomes analogous, for I have always believed that, compared to structural traumas such as racism or idiosyncratic traumas such as violent childhoods, the severity of ontological lack is negligible. I am hence by no means suggesting that refuges stuck at border crossings; people struggling to put food on the table; indigenous and trans women confronting violence or murder; or Black people enduring daily racist aggression, police brutality, the prison-industrial complex, or even death, should take up painting to soften their suffering. Such a suggestion would be absurd. At the same time, I do not think that political and practical activities on the one hand and creative activities on the other are mutually exclusive or antithetical to each other. If anything, creativity may help us bring about a more egalitarian world by enabling us to first envision its details. As José Muñoz (2009) suggested in his analysis of utopian thinking, without the ability to imagine a better world, it is impossible for us to ask for it; it has to exist as a concept in our minds before it can become a reality.

This is how imaginative activity may, in some instances, merge with political and practical goals. It may even become a component of what Kristeva (1997/2002) calls *intimate revolt*: the attempt to refashion the world through psychic, affective, and concrete acts of reinvention. Such an image of revolt as a matter of gradual revision, modification, and amendment may not entail the same bold robustness as our usual understanding of radical revolutionary change. However, as Maggie Nelson (2016), among others, reminds us, our standard vision of revolutionary activity may to some extent be outdated and possibly even overly masculinist in painting a portrait of robust heroism. At the very least, rethinking resistance in terms of small acts of everyday defiance – of intimate revolt – rather than in terms of grand, radical revolutionary gestures may allow us to add new items to our toolbox of resistance. Moreover, there is once again no need to see these two ways of going about social change as being antithetical to each other. Perhaps they could even complement each other in the manner that I alluded to a moment ago when I made a case for the revitalizing potential of creative activity: intimate revolt – small acts of defiance that result in psychic, affective, and physical rebirth – could re-energize the lives of people in ways that would allow them to imagine, and perhaps even to undertake, the kinds of bolder gestures of resistance that revolutionary thinkers and activists are calling for.

Many of us get worn out by our quotidian struggles. We need moments of respite. We need to slow down, and at times even to opt-out of the performance principle of our neoliberal society, which demands impossible levels of speed, exertion, attention, and accomplishment at the same time as it urges us to keep smiling (to adhere to its creed of positive thinking). Reaching for the replenishing resources of intimate revolt over the more rigorous alternative of a full-blown revolution makes a great deal of sense, practically speaking. Perhaps this is what neoliberal capitalism counts on. Perhaps its performance principle is on some level an instrument for suppressing our revolutionary inclinations. However, our recognition of this insidious strategy does not unfortunately change the exhausted parameters of our lived reality.

I speak solely for myself when I say that I am too tired for a revolution. I have spent the last four years fighting a medical establishment that denies me potentially effective treatments on the basis of the idea that I do not deserve them because I am going to die anyway – so why waste the money? – and that more or less explicitly wants me dead so that I cease to be a burden on the system. Because of this dispiriting predicament and the fact that, with the exception of a blissful hiatus of about five years before falling ill, my entire life consisted of relentless struggle, I do not have it in me to become a revolutionary subject. The best I can aspire to is to be the kind of creative subject who is capable of continual renewal, of tiny acts of opting out and of choosing differently. This, currently, is my version of self-fashioning. It is born of the recognition that there are, after all, limits to human resilience.

7

Much of my commentary in this chapter reflects my current personal predicament. Even the chapter's core idea – that the only "cure" for ontological and certain types of idiosyncratic losses is to recognize that there is no cure for them – arises from the fact that I am living with an incurable illness. On a more positive note, creativity, especially writing, has long served as a genuine source of solace for me.

I have good reasons to feel terrified. Writing is among the few activities that allow me to temporarily push my terror aside. As a result, although, as I have emphasized, I would never want to suggest that creativity offers an antidote to all genres of trauma, let alone that we fail as human beings when we are unable to translate our suffering into some kind of creative transformation, I have learned that, for me personally, it generates enough distance between my subjectivity and my suffering to allow me to feel that my suffering is merely one component of my being rather than my entire reality. This distance collapses every time the bubble of creativity bursts: the doorbell rings, the phone rings, the world makes its "ringy" demands. In the same way that waking up in the morning (every morning) makes me realize that I am living my biggest nightmare, the illusion that my subjectivity does not coincide with my suffering shatters at the slightest interruption. But while it lasts, the illusion – the distance between my subjectivity and my suffering – is where I find a measure of peace.

As Nietzsche (1873/1984) observes, a person who is never able to forget becomes so oversaturated by memories that he becomes like an overagitated insomniac who, despite all his excess energy, cannot get anything done – cannot focus on anything. Writing, for me, allows for the kind of forgetting that allows me to defeat my over-agitation so that I can proceed with the task at hand. Likewise, Lacan's claim that there is no cure for ontological lack has helped me better cope with my predicament. Even though incurable cancer is not identical with ontological lack, it comes close in being irreversible. As a result, Lacan's stance has allowed me to accept that although my life will remain irrevocably marred, damaged, imperfect, and defective – even though I live "castration" as a concrete reality in the sense that even my body is no longer intact – it nevertheless remains worth living.

The morning when I started to draft this chapter – when I was trying to balance the desire to write with the necessity of doctors' appointments – I startled myself by thinking, "I need to schedule time for dying." I stopped in my tracks and said out loud to myself, "Are you insane?" Yet upon reflection, I was forced to admit that my unconscious had produced was a fairly realistic plan of action. I countered it by thinking, "But I'm too busy to die. I can't schedule this death because I have too many books and essays to write, including one on mourning, melancholia, and creativity." Before cancer, writing had fairly reliably compensated for the structural and idiosyncratic damages of my life – poverty and an abusive childhood, respectively – whereas during cancer it has kept me afloat in the fantasmatic sense (which nevertheless feels entirely real to me) of giving me an unshakeable faith in the notion that I have too many pages to write to be ready to die.

Those who, like me, find in creative activity a bulwark against their trauma know that the process has to be constantly renewed. Psychic rebirth is not a task that we can ever be done with. In addition, it rarely happens in a linear fashion but tends to proceed haltingly and obliquely, frequently with considerable backsliding. New traumas can reactivate old ones. And old ones can blindside us when we least expect them to. Yet it is more or less the only thing that those of us who are "wired" to seek consolation in it have left to hang onto.

I am a lover of the ocean, always seeking its majestic yet soothing company. But under my current circumstances, I find that a metaphoric ocean of sorrow – like the Lacanian real or the Kristevan semiotic (both of which have a tenuous relationship to Freud's "oceanic feeling") – keeps trying to pull me into its melancholy depths. This ocean would have swallowed me a long time ago if I had not found a way to attach myself to the signifier, which functions like a hook attached to a slimy brick in the seawall that separates the ocean from dry land. I cling to this hook. It is the only thing that keeps the crashing waves from suffocating me.

I choose that word *suffocating* carefully. It hearkens back to my childhood when my father tried to suffocate me on a regular basis. In his defense, he might have thought he was playing when he threw a thick wooly blanket over my head and pinned me to the floor, but I – tiny, helpless, and screaming for my life – thought that I was being murdered. Afterward, I cried hysterically for hours. Even now that my father is dead, I cannot forgive him for this. Everything else – the endless verbal putdowns, the accusations of utter stupidity and worthlessness, the piercing declarations of ugliness – I can write off as resulting from his own horrible childhood. But not the sadistic torture of his own daughter. Not his inability to recognize that if she was screaming bloody hell, fought like a wild cat, and spent the rest of the day crying, she was probably not enjoying his game.

The word *suffocation* also connects me to the here and now when my own body is trying to suffocate me by generating countless little lesions in my lungs that could at any point grow to the point that I can no longer breathe. Intuitively, I see a connection between the past and the present: I see a connection between how, since early childhood, I have been fearfully watching over my shoulder, afraid of a blanket suddenly being thrown over my head, too afraid to relax my body or to breathe deeply, and the cancer that is now assaulting my body. I keep thinking that have *no* positive memories of my father. I keep thinking that forgiveness – especially the forgiveness that women are expected to extend to the violent men in their lives – is overrated. I would rather focus my energies on hanging onto the hook in the seawall – the signifier – for as long as possible.

Those suffering from melancholia try to swim in the ocean of sorrow – indefinitely until exhaustion gets the better of them. In contrast, those who have started to surmount their melancholia, who have started to move toward mourning, have, like me, found a hook in the seawall to attach themselves to so that the ocean can no longer sweep them backward. And maybe one day they find enough strength to climb over the seawall and start walking on the beach, not away from the ocean, not forgetting its melancholy pull, but alongside it, aware of its sublimity. Maybe they start to build sandcastles – temporary creations that will be washed away by the high tide. However, such rudimentary creations can be the starting point for more permanent ones.

And maybe, just maybe, one day someone will show up on the beach and extend their hand in healing friendship. The fact is that I would not be here, finishing this chapter, if this had not happened to me. First one person. Then another. And another. Dozens of them. They raised money, a *lot* of money so that I could get treated at a private facility when the public system declared me "too close to death" to help me. They created a protective circle of friendship around me so that I was never emotionally alone even when, by choice, I was physically alone. These friends have given me unqualified love, scintillating conversations, shoulders to cry on, reasons to laugh, drives through the countryside, trips to foreign lands, walks on pretty beaches, and delicious meals. Some have even chosen to write books with me. Like writing, they have given me periods when I have been able to forget that I am ill. They have given me the gift of (more) life – literally. There can never be any question of reciprocity. The only thing I can do is to try to honor the gift by writing as long as I can.

References

Berlant, L. (2011). *Cruel optimism*. Duke University Press.

Berlant, L., & Edelman, L. (2013). *Sex, or the unbearable*. Duke University Press.

Edelman, L. (2004). *No future: Queer theory and the death drive*. Duke University Press.

Eisenstein, P., & McGowan, T. (2012). *Rupture: On the emergence of the political*. Northwestern University Press.

Freud, S. (1917). Mourning and melancholia. In J. Strachey (Ed.), *The standard edition of the complete psychological works of Sigmund Freud*, vol. XIV (pp. 237–258). Vintage.

Freud, S. (1923). The ego and the id. In J. Strachey (Ed.), *The standard edition of the complete psychological works of Sigmund Freud*, vol. XIX (pp 1–66). Vintage.

Klein, M. (1975). *Love, guilt, and reparation and other works 1921–1945*. The Free Press.

Kristeva, J. (1983). *Revolution in poetic language* (L. Roudiez, Trans.). Columbia University Press. (Original work published 1974.)

Kristeva, J. (1989). *Black sun: Depression and melancholia* (L. Roudiez, Trans.). Columbia University Press. (Original work published 1987.)

Kristeva, J. (2002). *Intimate revolt: The powers and limits of psychoanalysis* (J. Herman, Trans.). Columbia University Press. (Original work published 1997.)

Lacan, J. (1997). *The seminar of Jacques Lacan (1959–1960): The ethics of psychoanalysis* (D. Porter, Trans.). Norton. (Original work published 1986.)

Lacan, J. (2016). *The seminar of Jacques Lacan (1975–1976): The sinthome* (A. R. Price, Trans.). Polity. (Original work published 2005.)

McGowan, T. (2013). *Enjoying what we don't have: The political project of psychoanalysis*. University of Nebraska Press.

McGowan, T. (2016). *Capitalism and desire: The psychic cost of free markets*. Columbia University Press.

Muñoz, J. (2009). *Cruising utopia: The then and there of queer futurity*. NYU Press.

Nelson, M. (2016). *The argonauts*. Graywolf.

Nietzsche, F. (1974). *The gay science* (W. Kaufmann, Trans.). Vintage. (Original work published 1882.)

Nietzsche, F. (1984). *Untimely meditations* (J. R. Hollingdale, Trans.). Cambridge University Press. (Original work published 1873.)

Ruti, M. (2006). *Reinventing the soul: Posthumanist theory and psychic life*. Other Press.

Ruti, M. (2009). *A world of fragile things: Psychoanalysis and the art of living*. SUNY Press.

Ruti, M. (2011). *The summons of love*. Columbia University Press.

Ruti, M. (2012). *The singularity of being: Lacan and the immortal within*. Fordham University Press.

Ruti, M. (2013). *The call of character: Living a life worth living*. Columbia University Press.

Ruti, M. (2015). *Between Lacan and Levinas: Self, other, ethics*. Bloomsbury Press.

Ruti, M. (2018a). *Distillations: Theory, ethics, affect*. Bloomsbury Press.

Ruti, M. (2018b). *Penis envy and other bad feelings: The emotional costs of everyday life*. Columbia University Press.

Žižek, S. (2007). *Enjoy your symptom!: Jacques Lacan in Hollywood and out*. Routledge.

Žižek, S. (2009). *The plague of fantasies*. Verso.

Žižek, S. (2013). *Less than nothing: Hegel and the shadow of dialectical materialism*. Verso.

Chapter 2

Open Wounds of Racial Terror

The Elaine Race Massacre

Roger Frie

Histories of racial violence cast long shadows. As Brian Stevenson, Director of the Equal Justice Initiative has said, "We need truth and reconciliation in this country, but you have to tell the truth before you get to reconciliation" (cited in Bonds Staples, 2018). Telling the truth involves confronting and disclosing the realities of racial terror, past and present. But it's hard to do when historical truths are purposefully silenced by a majority that seeks to ignore its perpetrator past and deny its historical responsibilities in the present.

The Elaine Race Massacre occurred just over one hundred years ago on the banks of the Mississippi River, in Phillips County, located on the isolated Arkansas Delta region. It is one of the worst acts of racial violence in American history, yet has the distinction of being one of the least known. There is perhaps a tortured logic at work: the greater the crime, the greater the silence. When silence about a mass racial crime is able to stretch over a century, talk of dissociation and denial hardly seems sufficient. It points us in the direction of profound structural and systemic inequalities that support and maintain a narrative grounded in white supremacy.

When we confront the dark past and recognize the traumas that have followed from a history of deep and abiding injustice, we begin to shed light on the challenges of historical responsibility. The process of attending to the injuries that follow from historical trauma, while simultaneously recognizing our own implication in the system that has caused and sustained them, is complex. It requires us to acknowledge the limits of what we know and to reflect on our own subject positions. Where do we stand in relation to the suffering in our midst and how might we benefit from social systems that keep reconciliation at bay? As a privileged white male academic and clinician, I recognize that there is much I fail to see and understand by virtue of my place in society. But these limits do not relinquish me of a responsibility to engage with the perpetrator past and to speak out. On the contrary, they compel me to move out of my comfort zone and look for counter-narratives that challenge the assumptions I hold.

DOI: 10.4324/9781003394327-3

We have an ethical obligation to address violent and traumatic histories, even if they happen before we are born. If we are able to listen for and recognize voices that have been silenced, we may even take an initial step towards repair. As a historian and psychoanalyst, I research and write about the perpetration of mass racial violence and its effects, not least in the context of my own German family history (Frie 2017, 2019). Indeed, I believe that there is much to be gained from treading on unfamiliar ground. It is this belief that led me to travel to the Arkansas Delta in the fall of 2019, to the location of the killing fields, to speak to descendants of the victims and perpetrators and to directly engage with what I knew only from afar. I was unprepared for what I saw and heard. The extent of the massacre, the horrendous crimes that were committed, along with the utter lack of justice for the victims and their families, is difficult to bear.

The divided community of Phillips County today has been inalterably shaped by its history of racial violence and poverty. For those who directly experience society's injustices the massive crime of the past continues to be felt. The organized racial terror campaigns and mass lynching that marked the late nineteenth century and continued well into the second half of the twentieth century may have ended, but the oppression experienced in their wake is an ongoing form of trauma that connects the past with the present. The long shadow cast by the Elaine Massacre will not fade away.

The silence that followed the massacre, and the fact that not a single white perpetrator was ever brought to trial for his crimes, is akin to an open, festering wound. The work of memory demands that we witness what took place and find words for what has so long remained unspoken. Acts of memorialization can serve to identify and strengthen the obligations of memory. But the passage of time, the pervasiveness of the silence and the depth of the suffering mean that the challenges are enormous. Because the Elaine Massacre remains little known, this chapter will begin by focusing on the events themselves in order to reveal the systemic and structural racism that enabled the violence to unfold, unhindered. I then turn to the act of silencing, memorialization and the challenge and obligation of memory.

Prologue

Over the course of my research, I was privileged to speak numerous times with a descendant of the massacre, Sheila Walker, before her death earlier this year after a long fight with cancer. I want to begin by sharing some of Sheila's story. Sheila was seven years old when she moved to Chicago with her mother and sister from a small town in Arkansas where she grew up. It was the mid-1950s and they were following the path so many African Americans took before them to escape the racial violence and injustices of the Jim Crow South. An early memory from Sheila's first year in Chicago stands out for her. It was of adults speaking in hushed voices in an adjoining room. She could make out just a single name: Emmett Till. Sheila sensed something was wrong by the sound of her mother's voice, but it took several more days before she discovered what the name meant.

The racial terror that led to the so-called Great Migration was also the cause of Emmett Till's heinous murder. Emmett was only fourteen years old, a young Chicago boy visiting his relatives in Mississippi. When his savagely mutilated body was finally returned to his mother, she was adamant that her son be on full view so that a nation might know the brutal reality of lynching. Emmett's body lay in an open casket for five days. At least 50,000 people lined up to pay their respects and acknowledge the grievous crime that had been committed on an innocent child. The murderers, two white men from a small Mississippi Delta town, escaped justice.

Although it was many years ago, Sheila remembers the day her mother visited the casket very clearly. Her mother's reaction on coming home reso-nated with meaning. As Sheila tells it: "She just took us in her arms and wept... I remember looking down at my left hand and thinking that just because of my skin color I could also be killed." It was that moment, Sheila says, that "I began to recognize how segregation and racism affected me."

What Sheila did not know as a child, and would learn only much later in life, was that Emmett Till's brutal murder touched on the unspoken history of racial trauma in her own family. Sheila's family members were survivors of the Elaine race massacre that resulted in the murder of hundreds of innocent African American men, women and children during a single, fateful week in September, 1919.

The Road to Slaughter

I had travelled to Phillips County to better understand the legacy of the racial terror that shaped the region and continues to shape the United States today. According to the Equal Justice Initiative, Phillips County has the ignominious distinction of having the highest recorded number of lynchings of all the southern counties.[1] Phillips County stretches for some fifty miles along the Mississippi River, from the county seat of Helena in the north to a series of ever smaller settlements in the south. The entire county sits opposite the State of Mississippi, separated by the river, but connected by a long history slavery, share cropping and white supremacy.

The entry of the United States into World War I in 1917 was seen by many African Americans as an opportunity to fight for the equality they continued to be denied. They fought courageously and were awarded for their bravery, despite the discrimination and segregation they experienced in the military. But, any hopes that gains on the battlefield would translate into changes back home were quickly dashed (see Williams, 2010). White Amer-icans feared that returning black soldiers could use their military training to demand equality and better labor conditions. In the summer and fall of 1919, vicious anti-black race riots (akin to the pogroms in Europe) erupted in twenty-six cities throughout the country. The worst violence occurred in the Arkansas Delta at the end of the so-called Red Summer, named for all the blood that was spilled.

In Phillips County an estimated 1,000 local African American soldiers returned home, veterans who brought with them the experience of a different life outside the Delta, and a firm belief that conditions in the south needed to change (Stockley, 2001). Sharecroppers, emboldened by returning soldiers, looked for ways to assert their rights and many turned to the Progressive Farmers and Household Union of America. What they were not prepared for, indeed, what they could not imagine was the kind of backlash they would face for attempting to organize.

Throughout the cotton growing regions, white land owners had used a system of debt peonage to keep sharecroppers bound to the land in forced labor, unable to assert their rights or leave in search of better conditions. Debt servitude was really only slavery by another name. Although debt peonage had been outlawed by federal statute in 1867, it became an accepted part of southern life (Blackmon, 2008). With the active support of state and county governments, southern landowners maximized profits while asserting absolute control. Harsh penalties, beatings, and murder were met out with chilling frequency. Lynching and racial terror were the tools of white southern power.

The Conflagration

It began on the night of September 30, 1919, when a union meeting was called at the Hoop Spur church, three miles north of the small town of Elaine.[2] Black families had gathered to hear speeches. Knowing of the threat posed by the landowners, they posted guards outside to watch for trouble. Sheila Walker's great-grandmother, Sallie Giles, her teenage grandmother, Annie, and her two great-uncles, Milligan and Albert, were among those in attendance. Gun fire suddenly broke out as men working on behalf of the planters peppered the church with bullets. Shots were returned by the guards. In the mêlée, a special agent of the Missouri Pacific Railroad was killed (McWhirter, 2011, 216–217 and Whitaker, 2008, 83–84). Inside the church, pandemonium broke out. Sheila's family members dove for cover, desperately trying to shield themselves and the other children from the hail of bullets. After a pause in the shooting, they fled into the darkness through broken windows and doors.

News of the killing travelled fast. The story told was that black union organizers had shot a white man. In the dead of night, the Phillips County sheriff set about deputizing a posse of white men (Whitaker, 2008, 85, 93). Early on the morning of October 1, the posse arrived at Hoop Spur and the indiscriminate shooting of black people began. Sharecroppers were murdered in the fields, in their homes, or as they ran for cover. Sallie and Annie hid in fear for their lives as they witnessed the killings. Milligan, who was only fifteen, was shot in the face and the bullet lodged in the back of his neck. Albert, the older brother, was pursued and shot five times. One of the bullets went clear through his skull.

Newspaper headlines and telegrams across the region spoke of a "Negro Uprising," fanning the flames of white hatred and insecurity. As the day progressed, armed white men from nearby towns and counties and from the neighbouring states of Mississippi and Tennessee poured into the area, ready to unleash "white justice." As the armed white men began to drive south on the road to from Helena to Elaine, they shot men, women, and children in the fields where they worked. According to a *Memphis Press* reporter who traveled with one group, the fields were soon emptied and men began shooting at the dead bodies that now littered the edge of the road, using them as target practice to unleash their rage (Whitaker, 2008, 98).

At noon on October 1, the mayor of Elaine contacted the Arkansas Governor, Charles Brough, to request troops to put down "race riots in Elaine" (Stockley, 2001, 3). Brough wasted no time in sending a telegram to U.S. war secretary, Newton Backer:

> Race riots in Elaine, Phillips County, this state. Four white said to be killed. Negroes said to be massing for attack. Request commanding general Camp Pike be authorized to send such United States troops as may be necessary and called for by me.
>
> (cited in Stockley, 2001, 3)

Brough's request was immediately granted. Early on October 2, Governor Brough led nearly 600 federal troops into the town of Elaine (Woodruff, 2003, 86). The killings that began with the white posse on October 1 were now taken over by the military. Many were battle hardened troops freshly returned from Europe and among their number was a twelve-gun machine-gun battalion that saw action in the Second Battle of the Marne (Woodruff, 2003, 86).

Descent into Barbarism

The military commander, Colonel Jenks, set up machine-gun posts in Hoop Spur and Elaine and ordered his troops to shoot any blacks that refused to disarm or who posed a threat. The killings and barbarities that began on October 1 continued unabated throughout the following days. The difference was that now the might of the U.S. military was on display.

The troops were sent out to search the fields around Hoop Spur. In one instance a squad of troops surrounded some fifty blacks hiding in a bayou and opened fire. Afterwards, only fifteen were reported arrested. In another instance four black men who were seen trying to move towards the river and shot down by machine gun. When the bodies were found, two of their number turned out to be veterans who were still wearing their khaki uniforms (Whitaker, 2008, 122). Only a short time before they had fought a common European enemy.

Troops were also sent to the large Lambrook plantation. While some soldiers shot at sharecroppers, others took the lead in interrogations (Stockley, 2001, 43). In his autobiography, *All Out of Step*, the plantation owner and heir to the Listerine fortune, Gerard Lambrook, recounts the military's interrogation of a black union leader devolved into torture, then murder:

> Troopers brought him to our company store and tied him with stout cord to one of the wooden columns on the other porch. He had been extremely insolent, and the troopers, stung by the loss of two of their men that day in the woods, had pressed him with questions. He continued his arrogance, and one white man, hoping to make him speak up, poured a can of kerosene over him. As he was clearly unwilling to talk, a man suddenly tossed a lighted match at him. The colored man went up like a torch and, in a moment of supreme agony, burst his bounds. Before he could get but a few feet he was riddled with bullets. The superintendent told me with some pleasure that they had to use a fire hose to put him out.
>
> (Lambert, 1956, 77)

Nor was this kind of barbarism isolated in nature. In 1925, a white Arkansas itinerate journalist, Louis Sharpe Dunaway, published a book called *What a Preacher Saw Through a Keyhole in Arkansas*, for which he had interviewed witnesses of the massacre. Although Dunaway, like Lambert, was clearly racist, he was nevertheless averse to the behaviour of the troops, describing them as having gone on a "march of death" where they "committed one murder after another with all the calm and deliberation in the world." (cited in Whitaker, 2008, 118). Of the nearly 600 soldiers, there were some who tended to injured sharecroppers like Milligan and Albert Giles, who were transferred to a hospital before being imprisoned. But as historians have begun to show, it is hard to doubt the accumulation of evidence for the atrocities committed by the military (Stockley and Whayne, 2002, 280–281).

It took until October 7 for the killing to stop. A report was issued that day by the Camp Pike troops to the War Department in Washington, stating that "order restored and the work of troop completed" (Whitaker, 2008, 123). By the time it was over, the massacre that began at the Hoop Spur church just north of Elaine had engulfed virtually all of Phillips County, reaching up and down a fifty-mile length of the Mississippi River.

The guiding rationale, it seemed, was to ensure the completion of the cotton harvest. Prices were high and there was significant money to be made.

Working closely with the landowners, Colonel Jenks issued a public announcement to share croppers:

> No innocent Negro has been arrested.... All you have to do is remain at work just as if nothing had happened. Phillips county has always been a peaceful, law-abiding community, and normal conditions must be restored right away. Stop talking! Stay at home – Go to work – don't worry!
>
> (cited in Stockley, 2001, 81)

The military worked hand-in-hand with the white establishment and on October 10, 1919, Governor Charles Brough wrote a personal note of thanks the Newton Baker, the Secretary of War in Washington:

> I wish to take this, my earliest opportunity, to express the gratitude of the State of Arkansas for your prompt action in permitting Federal troops to go to the scene of the recent race disturbances in Phillips County.... These brave soldiers, armed with high powered rifles and machine guns, were tireless in their apprehension of the leaders of the race disturbances and in the suppression of mob violence. I am gratified to be able to inform you, Mr. Secretary, that the white citizens of Phillips County ... co-operated to the fullest extent to prevent mob violence, and at the same time run down bad negroes who were responsible for the outbreak.
>
> (Desmarais, 1974, 189)

In fact, it was the military's liberal use of machine gun weaponry that contributed to the high number of deaths. The exact number is unknown. Estimates vary widely. Sharpe Dunaway, who by the time of his death was referred to as "the best-known newspaper man in Arkansas" offered an unsubstantiated total of "856 negroes ... killed" (Dunoway, 1925, 109). By contrast, the Equal Justice Initiative has recently concluded that there were 234 deaths. What is not in doubt is the sheer scale of the vicious, wanton violence that took place. Not a single white was ever brought to trial for their murderous actions. And to this day, no official governmental investigation of the massacre has ever been carried out.

Rule of Silence

The silence that ensued after the massacre was like an icy covering that refused to melt. It was the silence of white complicity encompassing not just Phillips County, the state of Arkansas and its southern neighbours. It was a national silence, borne without shame.

In Phillips County the status quo of white supremacy continued, unabated, spurred on by a specious narrative: an attempted black uprising had been heroically quelled, tragically costing the lives of five brave white men. The narrative was supported by a steady string of reports that were issued from Helena. On October 3, the Gazette, Arkansas's leading newspaper, baldly stated that "Negroes Plan to Kill All Whites" (NYTimes, October 3, 1919).[3] On October 6, *The New York Times* ran a front-page article with the headline: "Planned Massacre of Whites Today: Negroes Seized in Arkansas Riots Confess to Widespread Plot." Drawing on reports from Helena, the article told readers that:

> Bands of negroes in southern Phillips County, of which this city is the seat of government, had planned a general slaughter of white people in this locality tomorrow… . Confessions made by some of the captured negroes and other information indicated a widespread plot… . This report and evidence found locally lead authorities here to believe the contemplated uprising was of more than a local nature.
>
> (*NYTimes*, October 6, 1919)[4]

These reports, like the nationally circulated newspaper articles in which they appeared, were aimed at fanning white fears and rage about the danger posed by African Americans, a racist trope still used to this day. The way in which the national media covered the massacre shows that it was a tool of white supremacy, a phenomenon that we continue to observe.

Over time, the events in Phillips County became known as a black riot that had been heroically foiled by the swift actions of courageous white men. The narrative of a riot was buttressed by mass arrests and convictions that were based on confessions obtained through torture. The fact that the massacre was actually lynching on a mass scale made no difference. Many whites felt neither guilt nor shame, and those who did, hid their participation. The silence of the perpetrators reinforced the silencing of the victims.

In the black community, there were fearful whispers, but silence was essential to ensure safety. Those who could, moved away from the site of the massacre. Black communities became still more cautious, and distrust of white authority continued to harden. Yet stories of the massacre never entirely disappeared. They continued to be shared between family members over time, cautionary tales, half spoken and halting. Memory fragments that were passed down from one generation to the next.

The suffering and trauma endured by Sheila Walker's family led them to move to the town of Hot Springs, Arkansas, where Sheila was born. When Sheila was a child, she often visited with her uncle Jim, whom she remembers fondly as a kind and gentle man. It was only decades later that she learned that Uncle Jim, as she knew him, was Milligan Giles, the fifteen-year-old boy who almost died in the massacre. After being arrested, Milligan had been given a sentence of twenty-one years but he was eventually released. His brother, Albert Giles, was a member of the Elaine 12, who were convicted of murder and given the death sentence. A white jury had taken less than five minutes to decide on their guilty verdicts. In the years that followed, the fearless anti-lynching efforts of Ida Wells-Barnett and the legal campaign of Scipio Jones eventually led to the supreme court ruling on due process, securing the release of the Elaine 12 and setting the groundwork for a nascent civil rights movement.

But while the massacre may have ended, the racial terror did not. Just two years later, in 1921, Will Turner, a nineteen-year-old resident of Helena was accused of assaulting a white woman, a familiar and specious narrative that was used as a pretense for murder. A group of "thirty armed men" took Turner from the deputies who arrested him and shot him repeatedly. When Turner's body was returned to Helena it was set on fire by a crowd in front of the courthouse. According to one local newspaper "a great time is reported to have been had by almost the entire white population of Helena" (Snell Griffith, 2021). Turner's brutal murder was followed by the lynching of Owen Flemming in 1927, which occurred only five miles south of Elaine. As the civil rights attorney, Grif Stockley (2009) points out, it became a mantra that Phillips County had never had a lynching and never would. This capacity to deny reality has remained a feature of Arkansas race relations into the present.

Sheila Walker was in her twenties when she first learned of the massacre. It was the early 1970s and she was visiting with her grandmother, Annie Giles in Arkansas. In the course of spending time together, her grandmother shared stories of the past. As Sheila tells it, Annie began to describe events that happened to her when she was a teenager and living in Hoop Spur. She recounted going to the Hoop Spur church with her mother and brothers to attend a union meeting. Annie continued, but there was a quiver in her voice: "I knew that something was going to happen in that church – and then they started shooting. People were dying in front of me. I grabbed some children and got out of the church through the back." Reliving this memory caused Annie to collapse in tears and she was unable to finish the story. After that, each time Sheila asked her grandmother what happened, Annie would break down, unable to continue. It was not until many years later, when she was approaching fifty, that Sheila's own mother, Sara Black, helped her to connect the dots, telling her that Annie Giles was probably talking about the "Elaine Riot."

The survivors of the massacre, along with their descendants, had powerful reasons for remaining silent. But the rule of silence among the perpetrators and bystanders was, if anything, even stronger. After the massacre, white residents of Phillips County did not to talk about what happened. Their silence encompassed churches, newspapers, schools, and the judicial system. It is a silence that has been difficult to break.

Arriving in Elaine

The Hoop Spur church, where the massacre began, no longer exists and its location is unmarked today. The share cropper's cabins, like the cane breaks in which they sought refuge, are nowhere to be seen. A century has passed and so much has changed. And yet, as I drove through the cotton fields toward Elaine, it felt like the past was all around me, closing in like a dense fog and increasing my sense of discomfort.

When I arrived on Main Street in Elaine it was eerily quiet. The only cars I saw were two police cruisers, parked neatly in front of the local police station, located in the center of the block. At first glance the station appeared to be the only occupied building. I walked slowly up one side of the street and then back down the other, trying to take in what I saw.

The town of Elaine is even smaller today than it was a hundred years ago. There are about 500 people living there now and the buildings on Main Street, where the white posse and army once gathered, are almost entirely empty. Some store fronts are shuttered and others sit in a dilapidated state, abandoned or left to ruin. It is a similar story in many small rural towns.

Beyond the police station, and the many small churches, I spot few signs of life. At some point a white person appears, seemingly out of nowhere, and asks in a pointed manner if I need any help. They repeat the question, in firmer tone, clearly unsatisfied with the answer I provide. It didn't feel like simple curiosity. More like the kind of suspicion that is reserved for outsiders, with a clear but unspoken message: "What happened here was long ago, it doesn't concern you. Move along." The presence of the so many confederate flags on buildings in and around Elaine gave the comments added meaning. The atmosphere was stifling, ominous. The fear expressed by some in the black community is not difficult to understand.

African Americans comprise more than sixty percent of Philips County, yet the median household income of black families is only half that of whites. The wealth divide is especially evident in rural towns like Elaine, where sixty-five percent of African Americans live under the poverty line, compared to just thirteen percent of whites. Schools remain segregated in all but name: public schools are virtually all black. White children attend private academies set up in the wake of desegregation. In Elaine the black community lives on one side and the white community on the other. In Helena the racial segregation is similar. The one place where black and white seem to interact on a daily basis is the local Walmart, which today is the sole retail outlet for the entire area. Like everyone else, I eventually headed to the Walmart to get food, and the level of forced proximity of the black and white communities in that enclosed space was quite stunningly different from what I had seen or experienced elsewhere.

When you are somewhere unfamiliar it's easy to misinterpret what you see and hear. The rural South is a place that is often misunderstood, especially by those who visit from the North. Its brutally violent history and continuing racial tensions can loom large in the minds of visitors. Like Canadians who wish to believe that racism is something that exists only south of the border, many Northerners like to think that "race" is a uniquely southern problem. We all have our preconceptions, some more convenient than others. Yet I couldn't shake the disquiet I felt and my interaction on Main Street didn't help.

The sensations I experienced were familiar to me. Dark histories cast long shadows wherever they exist. Legacies of perpetration can be surprisingly similar, even when they are separated by geography, culture and language. What does it mean to inherit a perpetrator past that still haunts the present? I think back to the discomfort I felt when I visited Bergen Belsen for the first time, located an hour away from the German city in which my parents grew up and where most of my family continues to live today. Or the smaller concentration subcamp only a short distance from my mother's home, which provided limitless labour for the Nazi armaments industry in which my grandfather was employed. Or the numbness I experienced when I was first learned of the unspoken history of the man I had known and loved as a child, the grandfather who turned out to be a Nazi party member and supporter of Hitler and his regime. A silenced history that had been passed down to me by succeeding generations of my family.

Much has changed in Germany, yet the remnants of that dark past are given renewed voice by the rise of the new right-wing political movements and by Germans who increasingly want nothing to do with the obligations their history bestows on them. I hear similar themes in the comments made by white residents in Elaine. The former mayor of the town believes that discussion of a massacre is "somebody trying to make something out of nothing much to talk about." He acknowledges that violence occurred, but questions the severity. According to the mayor's father-in-law only "about 25 people" were killed (cited in Nasir, 2019). The owner of Elaine's hardware store seems to agree. It bothers him that experts can shape a narrative and say "this absolutely happened" (cited in Edwards, 2018). He doubts the high death toll and wonders how events that took place one hundred years ago can still be relevant. Yet he is also quick to add that his own family members helped black farmers escape the violence.[5] In a manner akin to German descendants, he feels that his own family history and struggles are ignored. There are many in the white community who deny the facts of history, or who continue to insist it remains irrelevant, a construction of a woke, liberal culture.

The Challenge and Obligation of Memory

In the face of such wilful denial, it can be hard to know how to move forward. In her important book, *On the Courthouse Lawn*, Sherrilyn Ifill argues that

> Lynching is local. No presidential apology or Senate resolution can heal communities where violent pogroms or lynchings take place. No 'national conversation' can take the place of locally based dialogue in which members of a discrete community come together to talk about how specific instances of racial violence affected their communities.
>
> (Ifill, 2018, 127)

According to Ifill, memorialization needs to be combined with concerted local efforts to repair in the form of education programs, investigations into the past, markers on crimes sites, public apologies or financial compensation for victims and their descendants. The goals are clear, but so is the intransigence of most of the white community and its unwillingness to address the perpetrator past – or present.

As Sheila Walker put it to me, the Elaine Massacre is "a wound that never healed." Its traumas continue to be felt and the inequality and distrust it has sown runs deep. The challenge of addressing the past is exacerbated by the segregation and economic distress that affects much of the black community today, not only in Elaine, but throughout Phillips County. Openly remembering the victims of racial violence disrupts the status quote and the historical white ownership of public spaces. When a memorial is established, it can be a tangible reminder of the violence and criminal actions that took place. But it is at best an initial step on the long road to reconciliation, which must address not only the past, but the deep injustices and inequality that exist in the present.

The challenge of memorialization has become particularly relevant in the past several years. In September 2019, exactly 100 years after the catastrophe, a privately funded memorial to the victims of the Elaine massacre was established in Helena, across from the court house where sixty-five African American men were tried with prison sentences ranging from one to twenty-one years and where the Elaine 12 were given death sentences. The memorial came about through the combined effort of a group of prominent descendants of victims and perpetrators, many of whom live outside the area. Their willingness to speak out, to find words to fill the silence has created a shared opportunity for remembering. As Kyle Miller has noted, "Memorials matter… . If anything, this will cause a conversation. It's going to get people to start communicating about the massacre, what it was, what it represented. That's important" (cited in Clancy, 2019). It offers a small spark of hope and suggests that historical awareness can evolve over time, even when the process is grindingly slow.

In the wake of the memorial, opportunities for dialogue between descendants of the victims and perpetrators have emerged. The relationship between Sheila Walker and Chester Johnson, a grandson of one of the perpetrators, has become an example for engagement and reconciliation (Johnson, 2020). David Solomon, son of a long-standing, prominent Jewish family in Helena and a beneficiary of the white establishment, provided the funds for the memorial. Like so many others, he grew up without knowledge of the massacre or the support that his own family members provided.

As important as these steps have been, it's an open question whether the memorial can spur meaningful change. The memorial's presence in Helena has been contested. Many of the region's white residents have chosen to ignore the monument while members of the black community in Elaine have expressed a belief that it should have been built there, or that the money used for the memorial could have been better spent. When I asked some of the memorial's committee members why it was not constructed in Elaine, a common response was the fear that it would be destroyed. A recent fire at the planned site of an Elaine memorial museum on Elaine's Main Street, and the destruction of a tree planted at the former location of the Hoop Spur church, would seem to bear this out.

The impulse to silence and deny the history of perpetration is strong. In Arkansas, as elsewhere, Republican-controlled state houses are legislating what schools can teach about the past. Not only has the Elaine Massacre been absent from local school curricula in Phillips County and in Arkansas as a whole, it has until now been absent from curricula across the country. Without a vocabulary for remembering, without a willingness to address the dark past and the wounds that remain unhealed, without an awareness of the structural and systemic basis of racism, it is difficult to have meaningful engagement. As the philosopher, David L. Smith, has remarked:

> To combat dehumanization, it's vital to get to know our past in all of its horror and tragedy, because doing so punctures the self-serving illusion of American exceptionalism. A public that is educated about its own dark history will not only have to admit that they – that is, we – are capable of the very worst, but also will become more open to recognizing the persistence and rebirth of dehumanizing attitudes in the present.
>
> (Smith, 2020, 33)

The work of historical memory and responsibility needs to be both personal and collective in scope. It requires members of the majority like myself to examine the historical responsibilities we bear; it asks us to listen for untold stories and be willing to face our own complicity in systemic silencing. A willed and wilful ignorance must not be allowed to stand in the place of informed understanding. As a German-Canadian who lives in Vancouver, I may be distant from the events of the Elaine massacre I described in this chapter. But each of us, no matter what our location, needs only to look around us to see similar wounds resulting from silenced histories of racial trauma and violence. I want to conclude by drawing on two such examples that were especially present during my research and writing of this chapter.

I live in Vancouver, Canada, in a multi-ethnic country that is widely recognized for its liberal values and its embrace of multiculturalism, particularly when compared with its southern neighbour. What is less known, not least among majority Canadians themselves, is that the country has a 200-year history of slavery and that anti-Black racism today continues to challenge the notion of a cohesive and just society (Frie, 2020; Maynard, 2017). This struggle to know and remember is similarly evident in Canada's long history of subjugating Indigenous peoples. The reality of what today is justly called the "Indigenous genocide" continues to be, quite literally, unearthed. In the summer of 2021, approximately 1,000 unmarked graves of Indigenous children were uncovered adjacent to so-called Indian Residential Schools across western Canada. One such school was located only an hour from where I grew up. I spent my childhood in ignorance of its existence and of the violence and abuse that took place there. Schools in name only, they were actually government funded institutions of assimilation whose express purpose was to extinguish Indigenous life and culture. How might my ignorance have reflected and also contributed to the general indifference among majority Canadians and the Canadian media at the time? In the years ahead, there is an expectation that a great many more unmarked graves of young children will be located. For Indigenous peoples these gruesome "discoveries" have not come as a surprise. They have long grieved the thousands of children who were forcibly taken away to residential schools and never returned.

I finished writing this chapter while I was completing a visiting professorship in Berlin. This provided me with yet another direct opportunity to reflect on how silencing can exist side-by-side with attempts to address and disclose the traumatic perpetrator past. Embedded in the sidewalks of my single residential block in central Berlin were over forty stumbling stones, each one containing the name of a person who was killed by the Nazi terror. These individual plaques are affixed to cobblestones and placed in front of the victim's last known residence. In Berlin today there are over 5,000 such stumbling stones. This is a notable achievement, and for many observers, myself included, the stumbling stones are a particularly compelling form of memorialization. Despite this important step, however, there are tens of thousands more victims of Berlin's pre-war Jewish community who were forcibly deported and killed in the Holocaust and whose names are not yet remembered in this way.

There is also another side to the challenge of memorialization. While it is vitally necessary to commemorate the victims, the struggle to know and remember the Holocaust in German families often suggests (Frie, 2017, 2018) that the role of the perpetrators, their supporters, and the bystanders who willingly looked away is easily cast aside and forgotten. The historian Eelco Runia has captured the dilemma of memorialization and responsibility when he states: "The more we commemorate what we did, the more we transform ourselves into people who did not do it" (Runia, 2007, 320). As a German descendant whose own grandfather was a member of the Nazi party, a story long covered over in silence, the stumbling stones bring the complexity of memory of bear. Each time I look down at a stumbling stone I try to acknowledge the person who died, reflect on what their life may have been like, and think about the tragedy and trauma that they and their family were forced to endure. Then I try to turn my attention to the perpetrators, supporters, and bystanders. How many of them lived on my residential block in Berlin, and in the very same building as each of the victims who are commemorated on a stumbling stone? Has their direct or indirect role in the genocide been identified and acknowledged? For German descendants like myself, asking these questions is not easy because it inevitably implicates our own family members. But nor is it idle chatter. It speaks to the dangers that a bystander culture can pose in the face of racial oppression. Addressing perpetrator histories openly and honestly is about engaging the racial terrors of the past and the moral obligations of memory in order to take a stand on the injustices of the present.

As these examples from Vancouver and Berlin, and as my discussion of the Elaine massacre seeks to show, the process of uncovering silenced histories is far from straightforward. It took nearly a century for the first mass graves of the 1921 Tulsa massacre to be exposed. How much longer will it take to reveal the extent of the horrors in Elaine? It's hard to talk about reconciliation when these massive crimes have yet to be addressed, when the names of the victims remain unknown, when descendants of the perpetrators refuse the face the past, and when racial discrimination and oppression continues, unabated. But silenced historical traumas don't go away, they wait to be seen and heard. Knowing and engaging these histories is an initial and necessary step in the long road toward responsibility and repair.

Notes

1 According to Equal Justice Initiative (2017), there were at least 245 lynchings recorded in Phillips County during this period. EJI refers to the murder of African Americans in the Elaine Massacre as lynchings. As I will discuss below, the exact number killed in the massacre has long been a point of discussion, since exact figures remain unknown. For more information see: https://eji.org.
2 A "spur" is a section of railway that usually extends off a main railroad track to allow for the loading and unloading of train cars.
3 *The New York Times Index, October-November-December, 1919*, Volume 7, No. 4 (New York: New York Times Co., 1919), 261.
4 *The New York Times*, October 6, 1919. https://timesmachine.nytimes.com/timesmachine/1919/10/06/118161202.html?pageNumber=1.
5 See Stoppford (2020, chapter 5), "Elaine, Arkansas: The multigenerational legacy of white supremacy" for important and revealing interviews with descendants of victims of the Elaine Massacre.

References

Blackmon, D. B. (2008). *Slavery by Another Name: The Re-enslavement of Black Americans from the Civil War to World War II*. Anchor Books.

Bonds Staples, G. (2018, December 10). Pushing America to face its racist past. *The Atlanta Journal-Constitution*. http://ajc.com.

Clancy, S. (2019, September 29). Marking a Tragedy: Memorial to those who died in the Elaine Massacre enmeshed in controversy. *Arkansas Democrat Gazette*. https://www.arkansasonline.com/news/2019/sep/29/marking-a-tragedy-20190929/?features-style.

Desmarais, R. H. (1974). Military Intelligence Reports on Arkansas Riots: 1919–1920. *The Arkansas Historical Quarterly*, 33, 189.

Dunoway, L. S. (1925). *What a Preacher Saw Through a Key-Hole in Arkansas*. Parke-Harper Pub. Co.

Edwards, B. (2018, April 23). Divided Town Struggles to Remember What Really Happened During 1919 Arkansas Killings, *Montgomery Advisor*. https://www.montgomeryadvertiser.com/story/news/2018/04/23/tragedy-narrative-elaine-arkansas-phillips-eji-lynching-memorial-museum-peace-justice-montgomery/522362002/.

Equal Justice Initiative (2017). *Lynching in America: Confronting the Legacy of Racial Terror*, 3rd Edition. Equal Justice Initiative.

Frie, R. (2017). *Not in my Family: German Memory and Responsibility after the Holocaust*. Oxford University Press.

Frie, R. (2019). History's ethical demand: Memory, denial and responsibility in the wake of the Holocaust. *Psychoanalytic Dialogues, 29*, 122–142.

Frie, R. (2020). Recognizing white racism in Canada. *Psychoanalysis, Self and Context*, 15, 276–280.

Frie, R. Ed. (2018). *History Flows Through Us: Germany, the Holocaust and the Importance of Empathy*. Routledge.

Ifill, S. (2018). *On the Courthouse Lawn: Confronting the Legacy of Lynching in the 21st Century* (2nd ed.). Beacon Press.

Johnson, C. (2020). *Damaged Heritage: The Elaine Race Massacre and A Story of Reconciliation*. Pegasus Books.

Lambert, G. B. (1956). *All Out of Step: A Personal Chronicle*. Doubleday.

Maynard, R. (2017). *Policing Black Lives: State Violence in Canada from Slavery to the Present*. Fernwood Press.

McWhirter, C. (2011). *Red Summer: The Summer of 1919 and the Awakening of Black American*. Henry Holt Company.

Nasir, N. (2019, July 25). In a Small Arkansas Town, Echoes of a Century-Old Massacre. *AP News*. https://apnews.com/1718cdcb42c54771b4079ece2ab9b559.

Runia, E. (2007). Burying the dead, creating the past. *History and Theory*, 46, 313–325.

Smith, D. L. (2020). *On Inhumanity: Dehumanization and How to Resist It*. Oxford University Press.

Snell Griffith, N. (2021). William Turner (Lynching of). https://encyclopediaofarkansas.net/entries/william-turner-8269/.

Stockley, G. (2001). *Blood in Their Eyes: The Elain Race Massacres of 1919*. The University of Arkansas Press.

Stockley, G. and Jeannie M. Whayne (2002). Federal Troops and the Elaine Massacre: A Colloquy. *The Arkansas Historical Quarterly*, 61, 280–281.

Stoppford, A. (2020). *Trauma and Repair: Confronting Segregation and Violence in America*. Rowman and Littlefield.

Whitaker, R. (2008). *On the Laps of Gods: The Red Summer of 1919 and the Struggle for Justice That Remade a Nation*. Three Rivers Press.

Williams, C.L. (2010). *Torchbearers of Democracy: African-American Soldiers in the World War I Era*. University of North Carolina Press.

Woodruff, N. E. (2003). *The American Congo: The African American Freedom Struggle in the Delta*. Harvard University Press.

Chapter 3

Reparation

Discussion of Roger Frie's "Open Wounds of Racial Terror: The Elaine Race Massacre"

Lynne Layton

I offer this response in appreciation not only for Roger's stirring chapter on the silenced history of what happened in 1919 in Elaine, Arkansas, but for what Roger's work in general has brought into the field of psychoanalytic psychology: a plea to confront histories of perpetration and implication, to tell the truth about these histories, and to take responsibility for them. As Roger says about the Elaine events, a 100-year history of silence calls for more than talk of dissociation and denial but rather demands that white people look at the US history of systemic racism, anti-Black racism, and White Supremacy. Heeding Bryan Stevenson's (2015) challenge to white people that we "get proximate," Roger goes to Arkansas, arguing that "there is much to be gained from treading on unfamiliar ground." Amen.

In these brief remarks, I want to elaborate on two themes. First, I want to talk about truth-telling and some of what might be involved in the process of hearing and seeing silenced stories. This is something the clinical field knows a lot about. But white clinicians have not been adequately trained to be able to hear the culturally silenced stories of oppressed groups. Second, I want to look at how those of us who are, in Michael Rothberg's (2019) terms, "implicated subjects," might think about what we need to do to make reparation and build a culture of repair. Roger begins with a quote by Bryan Stevenson: "you have to tell the truth before you get to reconciliation." My second set of remarks reaches beyond truth-telling and puts a slight twist on Stevenson's words: as Dr. David Ragland (2018–2019), leader of the Grassroots Reparations Campaign with which I have worked for the past four years has forcefully argued, the midpoint between truth-telling and reconciliation is reparations. No repair, no reconciliation.

So, first, how to listen to history. As we are learning all too clearly, *again*, key to both listening and to having a sense of what needs to be repaired is discerning what social forces control the historical narrative and to what psychosocial ends control of the narrative is sought. In an episode of *The Ezra Klein Show* (2021), Ibram X. Kendi spoke to the current right-wing fervor against schools teaching the 1619 Project and whatever it is this group thinks of as critical race theory. These curricula, they scream out, are

DOI: 10.4324/9781003394327-4

teaching white kids to hate themselves and hate the US. As Roger's paper tells us, projection and projective identification are the key defenses perpetrators used and continue to use to claim victimhood and blame the victims. Kendi argues that the desperate attempt to control what kids in school learn suggests that defenders of White Supremacy are actually anxious that they are losing control of the narrative. But, in US history, we find that just about every time anxious feelings emerge in the white public sphere, violence against Blacks ensues (Anderson, 2016).

Given my understanding, following Gramsci (1971), Stuart Hall (1980, 1982), and others, that history always involves a struggle over meaning between dominant and subordinate forces, and given that white people are positioned systemically in a superior position to Black people in the US, I think that white people need to develop the capacity for the kind of double consciousness called for by Black philosopher George Yancy (2012) in *Look! A White*: that is, to listen to narratives, critically, both as dominant race/class forces intend us to hear them, and, simultaneously, as subordinated groups are likely to hear and experience them (see also, Jacobs, 2016).

Roger argues that the work of historical memory and responsibility has to happen on both a personal and a collective level, and recent experiences have convinced me that this is painfully true. On the personal level, I have constantly been shocked into awareness of how I hear things in cross-racial meetings as a White person and sometimes miss completely how what has been said is landing on Black, Indigenous, and People of Color (BIPoC) participants. I then often end up unconsciously practicing what DiAngelo (2018) calls white solidarity, tacitly or openly supporting the white person. What I'm suggesting here is that this is in part because I've embedded myself in one version of history and power relations, the dominant version.

When I think of the collective-level need to practice double consciousness, what comes to mind is a Gil Scott-Heron (1970) spoken word poem called "Whitey on the Moon" that I first heard in an episode of the television show Lovecraft Country (Green and Sackheim, 2020). In alternating lines, Scott-Heron's poem contrasts "facts on the ground," the conditions of poverty in which many Black people in the US lived in the late 1960s, with the enormously expensive "achievement" that their labor in part funded and from which they derived no benefit: Whitey on the Moon.

In a documentary about the 1969 Harlem Cultural Festival (Thompson, 2021), Black audience members were asked how they felt about the 1969 moon landing. Like Scott-Heron, they felt that it was scandalous given the poverty levels in the US. I was a politically active teenager in 1969, protesting the Vietnam War and fighting for women's rights; and yet, embedded in white dominance and its self-congratulatory narratives, I would not have been able to hear that poem the way I painfully hear it now: as calling out the violent effects of White Supremacist, anti-Black policy choices, as deconstructing any pretense to white innocence, and as demanding repair.

I agree with Roger that 100 years of silence about the Elaine massacre makes talk of denial and dissociation insufficient, but I do think that part of the work of dismantling systemic racism is truly to understand how White Supremacy is lived at an individual level. And one way it is lived is by refusing to let uncomfortable histories disrupt the dominant narrative. Today, in progressive white circles and especially in dominant liberal media, you can hear even the most critical white voices enact the kind of unconscious slippage that disavows racism and keeps dominant narratives in place: for example, the Big Lie is constantly put forth as merely being about a stolen election. But the Big Lie is that the election was stolen by Black and Brown people and that is why it is they, not white people, who have become the targets of so-called "election integrity" laws. Within our own psychology and psychoanalytic institutions, I have witnessed an insistent pressure to appropriate and dilute antiracism work in order to bolster a multicultural ideology that celebrates difference and consistently refuses to acknowledge how the operation of power relations maintains a racist status quo.

And now to talk a bit about repair. Here, again, which historical narrative White people can hear is crucial to how we make sense of what it might mean to take responsibility as implicated subjects. Rothberg's (2019) concept of implicated subjects moves us beyond the split categories of perpetrator and victim, and beyond even the triad of perpetrator/victim/bystander, to address how those of us who are neither victims nor perpetrators of atrocities like slavery, for example, are yet implicated in the history of slavery and in perpetuating its afterlives. In their paper on the psychological case for reparations, Nichols and Connolly (2020) describe how white denial of moral injury, that is, the white refusal to acknowledge the crime of slavery, manifests in a doubling down on violence against any Black efforts at liberation (see also Connolly et al., 2021, 2022). One thing that strikes me about the Elaine massacre, the correct way to name what the dominant white narrative has called a "race riot," is that it is a link in the long historical chain of racial capitalism. The history of that massacre teaches us not to consider in isolation class and race but rather to look at them intersectionally. The massacres of Red Summer and those that took place in 1921 in places like Tulsa were not only anti-Black but anti-worker, aimed at efforts to keep Blacks from unionizing and accumulating wealth. As Roger notes of the Elaine massacre, white perpetrators were in part motivated by protecting the completion of the cotton harvest against Black attempts to unionize. A narrative ploy that seems always to work in the US is to condemn such actions as "socialist" or "communist." But understanding the racial capitalism narrative as historical fact means that any adequate repair must aim at erasing the racial wealth gap in the US. Reparations are not only a debt owed for a history of slavery, but also for the afterlives of slavery, the way the disavowal of the crime issues in repeated criminal acts of anti-Blackness. Roger reports that sixty-five percent of African Americans in Phillips County live under the poverty line versus thirteen percent of Whites, and that the median household income of Black families is only half that of White families. Muñoz et. al.'s (2015) report to the Federal Reserve Bank of Boston found that the average net wealth of a white family in Boston was $247,500 in comparison to $8 for a Black family.

Roger notes that there was controversy in the Black community surrounding the monument erected to memorialize the Elaine massacre. Some of the controversy concerned the feeling that memorials do not address or repair the current conditions of systemic racism. In her book, *Trauma and Repair*, Annie Stopford (2020) reports that David Solomon, the key figure behind the monument erected in Helena, had asked a Black pastor to organize other pastors to get behind the effort, but the pastor decided not to collaborate because he thought reparation efforts should address the current conditions of no fresh food, poverty, unequal education, etc. Such controversy has haunted reparations movements repeatedly through their history: who gets to decide what is reparative? The white people paying reparations? Or the affected parties themselves? It has to be the affected parties.

What constitutes repair? Roger quotes Sherilyn Ifill, who basically describes the five dimensions of reparations called for in a UN Report on reparations (United Nations, 2005). Economic compensation is one, but another, satisfaction, does include memorials, and most African-American groups working on reparations do call for memorialization as a corrective to denied histories. Memorials are a part of the truth-telling process, as are apologies. Indeed, the National African American Reparations Commission (NAARC), a major Black-led reparations organization, asked its white fund-raising arm, Fund for Reparations Now!, to devote its first fundraising project to building the Elaine Legacy Center – in Elaine. Recall that part of the controversy was that the monument was put in Helena and not in Elaine. NAARC is working with families in Elaine to uncover the histories, build the museum, and contribute to other reparations efforts asked for by descendants of the massacre and Elaine community members.

Another of the five dimensions of reparations in the UN report is "rehabilitation," by which is meant repair of psychological and physical harm experienced by African Americans as a result of slavery and its afterlives. Repair work for white clinicians might begin with listening to the stories of BIPoC clinicians who have been harmed by our institutions – and then asking what kinds of actions would constitute repair.

During a Reconstructionist Jewish teach-in on reparations, lawyer and journalist Eric Greene (2021) asserted that the US population is not only addicted to amnesia about history but also allergic to accountability. The fifth UN dimension on reparations is the guarantee of non-repeat. As a psychoanalyst, I am quite attuned to the power of repetition compulsions: individual, relational, and historical. So, the guarantee of non-repeat stands out to me as a crucial element of reparations: systems of racism have to be dismantled, and we white people, as implicated subjects, have to be involved, at both a personal and a collective level, in dismantling them. To return to Stevenson's admonition to "get proximate," I end by calling on all of us implicated subjects to get involved in reparations work at whatever level you wish: grassroots, local, state, federal. The call to white clinicians and educators is to do whatever we can to guarantee non-repeat.

References

Anderson, C. (2016) *White Rage. The Unspoken Truth of our Racial Divide.* Bloomsbury Publishing.

Connolly, M., Gobodo-Madikizela, P., Layton, L., Nichols, B. (2021, April 22) What's repaired in reparations. A conversation among psychoanalytic and social activists. *Couched* (podcast hosted by Billie Pivnick and Romy Reading). https://couchedp odcast.org/whats-repaired-in-reparations-a-conversation-among-psychoanalytic-a nd-social-activists/.

Connolly, M., Gobodo-Madikizela, P., Layton, L., Nichols, B., Pivnick, B., and Reading, R. (2022) What's repaired in reparations: A conversation among psychoanalytic and social activists. *Psychoanalytic Dialogues* 32(1), pp. 3–16.

DiAngelo, R. (2018) *White Fragility.* Beacon Press.

Gramsci, A. (1971) *Selections from the Prison Notebooks*, edited by Q. Hoare and G. Nowell Smith. International Publishers.

Green, M. (Creator) and Sackheim, D. (Dir.) (2020, August 23) Whitey's On the Moon, Episode 2, Lovecraft Country, HBO.

Greene, E. (2021, August 8) Teshuvah on stolen land. A Reconstructionist Day of Learning on Reparations to Begin the Month of Elul, online presentation.

Hall, S. (1980) Encoding/decoding. In S. Hall, D. Hobson, A. Lowe and P. Willis (eds.) *Culture, Media, Language. Working Papers in Cultural Studies, 1972–1979.* Hutchinson, pp. 128–138.

Hall, S. (1982) The rediscovery of "ideology": Return of the repressed in media studies. In M. Gurevitch, T. Bennett, J. Curran and J. Woollacott (eds.) *Culture, Society and the Media.* Methuen, pp. 56–90.

Jacobs, L. (2016) Dialogue and double consciousness: Lessons in power and humility. *Gestalt Review* 22(2), pp. 147–161.

Klein, E. (2021, July 16) Ibram X. Kendi on what conservatives – and liberals – get wrong about antiracism. The Ezra Klein Show.

Muñoz, A., Kim, M., Chang, M., Jackson, R.O., Hamilton, D., and Darity Jr., W.A. (2015), March 25) The Color of Wealth in Boston. https://www.bostonfed.org/p ublications/one-time-pubs/color-of-wealth.aspx.

Nichols, B. and Connolly, M. (2020) Transforming ghosts into ancestors. Unsilencing the psychological case for reparations to descendants of American slavery. https://ifp e.wordpress.com/2020/05/14/transforming-ghosts-into-ancestors-un-silencing-the-p sychological-case-for-reparations-to-descendants-of-american-slavery/.

Ragland, D. (2018–2019) The midpoint between truth and reconciliation is reparations. *Fellowship*, 82(1–12), p. 4.

Rothberg, M. (2019) *The Implicated Subject: Beyond Victims and Perpetrators*. Stanford University Press.

Scott-Heron, G. (1970) *Whitey on the moon. Small Talk at 125th and Lenox*. Flying Dutchman.

Stevenson, B. (2015) *Just Mercy: A Story of Justice and Redemption*. Scribe Publications.

Stopford, A. (2020) *Trauma and Repair. Confronting Segregation and Violence in America*. Lexington Books.

Thompson, Ahmir (Questlove) (Dir.) (2021) Summer of Soul (...Or, When the Revolution Could Not Be Televised). Searchlight Pictures and Hulu.

United Nations (2005) UN General Assembly Resolution 60/147, Basic Principles and Guidelines on the Right to a Remedy and Reparation for Victims of Gross *Violations of International Human Rights Law and Serious Violations of International Humanitarian Law*. United Nations Basic Principles and Guidelines on the Right to a Remedy and Reparation for Victims of Gross Violations of International Human Rights Law and Serious Violations of International Humanitarian Law. https://en.wikipedia.org/wiki/UN_General_Assembly_Resolution_60/147.

Yancy, G. (2012) *Look, A White! Philosophical Essays on Whiteness*. Temple University Press.

Chapter 4

Ethical Labor

A Step Toward Reparations Within Psychoanalysis

Elizabeth Corpt

In this chapter I put forth the idea of ethical labor (Corpt, 2020) in psycho-analysis to both reorient our thinking in this increasingly diverse and chan-ging world and as a step toward reparation for our field's overall blindness to the larger social context. During the early process of writing this chapter, I was alerted to the recent publication of a paper by Donald Moss (2021) in the *Journal of the American Psychoanalytic Association*: a paper called "On Having Whiteness". Moss's paper immediately captured my attention as it was articulating the very problem I set out to address. So, I will begin here.

Moss's provocative lightning rod of a paper was reportedly making its way across social media and causing somewhat of a stir. This kind of response is exceptionally unusual for any piece of psychoanalytic writing. Moss, a well-respected and already well-published relational psychoanalyst, was not new or strange to the larger psychoanalytic community, so what was causing the stir? Was it because he was directly challenging Whiteness? Apparently so. Moss's words drew harsh pushback on Fox News. Any white supremacist who was paying attention would certainly have taken notice. Clearly, he hit a nerve. In the US, psychoanalysis, regrettably, offers little and gets little response from the public at large. Moss provided us some free if fleeting publicity, but of a rather complicated sort.

For those who are not familiar with this text, Moss puts forth the following:

> Whiteness as a condition one first acquires and then *has* – a malignant, parasitic-like condition to which "white" people have a particular sus-ceptibility. The condition is foundational, generating characteristic ways of being in one's body, in one's mind, and in one's world. Parasitic Whiteness renders its hosts' appetites voracious, insatiable, and perverse. These deformed appetites particularly target nonwhite people. Once established, these appetites are nearly impossible to eliminate.
>
> (Moss, 2021, 355)

DOI: 10.4324/9781003394327-5

Prior to accessing the actual paper, I listened to an impassioned YouTube pushback response by the philosopher and psychoanalyst, Jon Mills (2021). Mills was protesting the rejection of his letter to the editor of JAPA as well as rebuking Moss for having played into identity politics in what Mills saw as Moss's racist-encouraging and split-promoting rhetoric. Mills critiqued JAPA for having tarnished psychoanalysis and the reputation of a peer reviewed journal by publishing a piece that allegedly, according to Mills, did not go through the traditional peer-review process. All this unfolded as my co-editor and I were in the process of orchestrating the traditional peer review process of another provocative psychoanalytic article addressing unconscious defensive structures of Whites and Whiteness. This piece, by a new BIPOC contributor, was a welcome challenge to our primarily white journal.

To be fair, Moss says outright, "This is not a traditionally organized text. No clear path links my argument to that of my predecessors. This formal peculiarity might be the product of my effort to braid together two incompatible voices…both inside and outside the affliction" (Moss, 2020, 355). He was presenting himself to us as both inside and outside: as one who is guilty, perverse, and responsible for perpetrating the very affliction he is also observing and critiquing. This intrigued me. This is most certainly the exception within psychoanalysis: an analyst's full-on public exposé and critique of rather profound flaws in his own identity. Some colleagues were wondering if he had he gone off the deep end. Clearly, he was calling out whites in general, but by his referring to himself as an insider, not merely an outside neutral analyzer of someone else's pathology, he was also calling out overwhelmingly white psychoanalysis.

Do we, in an overwhelmingly white field, need jarring out of our carefully peer-reviewed ideas? According to the American Psychoanalytic Association's statistics, of its 3,000 members, around twenty are Black (Powell, 2020). The ratios at independent psychoanalytic institutes are likely similar or, in some cases, possibly worse. This tells us something significant. In the world of psychoanalysis, BIPOC clinicians seem to not have felt invited or welcomed. I agree with Moss that something is terribly wrong here; something insidious, perpetuating, and inhospitable. And, clearly, we need to be jarred and disrupted.

Moss jars us out of our conception of ourselves as good, well-intentioned, empathic, self-reflective, and well-analyzed healers who hold knowledge about the depth, workings, and ways of the human mind. To become an analyst, we are each required to delve deeply into the workings of our own minds as part of our belonging to this elite discipline. Had racism, classism, or sexism been lurking there, surely, we would have discovered it, articulated it, analyzed it, and worked it through, right? If only this were the case. If we fail to hold this knowledge with humility, we can easily be seduced into a God-like stance. We can deceive ourselves into thinking we've covered most, if not all, of our bases. But, as we know, unconscious defenses are skilled at hiding what we do not want to know, or know, but do not want to acknowledge.

Eyal Rozmarin, a relational analyst, has something important to say about this. He states:

> ...as psychoanalysts, we are not well-equipped to address what happens at the level of the social. This is because psychoanalysis – with few exceptions, at least until recently – has had great difficulty considering its obvious embeddedness in given social, historical, and political orders. The social is so glaringly absent in most psychoanalytic thought as to suggest that it is repressed. We might say that the social is the unconscious of the unconscious of psychoanalysis.
>
> (Rozmarin, 2017, 459)

This bears repeating...*the social is the unconscious of the unconscious of psychoanalysis.* So where do we start in confronting this? To confront this, we must be willing to locate ourselves within a broader context.

As a psychoanalyst, as a white psychoanalyst, and as a white psychoanalyst from a working- class familial background, I have always experienced myself as somewhat on the periphery of my field because of the social/cultural aspects of my background. I grew up in Detroit, a city long immersed in complex race relations. Only recently have I come to learn of Detroit's deep and painful history of slavery (Mills, 2017). Many Blacks and Native Americans were enslaved by early wealthy fur traders How could I not have been taught this history? The race riots in the late 1960s, and the fire-red sky viewed from the safety of the suburbs – a result of my parents' white flight from the city – were rife with the afterbirth of what Moss refers to as white parasites and the ghosts of slavery. With a clear sense that something was amiss, I chose sociology as my major. I then moved on to clinical social work, and then to psychoanalytic training, undergirded by a growing interest in philosophy. In various ways, I've managed and chosen to position myself as inside while holding on to a position and a view from the outside. I cannot help but to feel called upon to research, study, reflect upon, and act upon what I see and experience as the disavowal of a serious study of racism along with other isms within psychoanalysis. I felt compelled to write about my own lived experience of classism in relation to my psychoanalytic training (Corpt, 2013). How else could I have authentically approached my life as an analyst? After all, I now find myself in what Dews and Law (1995) refer to by the title of their book on working class academics, *This Fine Place So Far from Home.* And I am personally aware – in body and mind – of the cost of this shift and jump in class position.

In my approaching the writing this or any paper, I fully expect the eventual return of my own ghosts of classism and make allowances for the extra amount of effort it would require to push back against these voices saying: "who do you think you are? You don't belong here". I say this out of an obligation to locate myself, as myself, as my vulnerable and socially contextualized self, because only in doing so, can I attempt to empathize with people of color who struggle with their version of what W.E.B. Du Bois (1903) referred to as "double consciousness". We are all ethically obligated to locate ourselves in relation to those with power and those without. This reflective exercise seems crucial both to us as individuals and to us as a field. Without it, we set ourselves up to repeat history. The major tenet of psychoanalysis is, after all, the belief that unconscious experience, including social unconscious experience, if not formulated, articulated, digested, and ultimately, deeply understood – in other words, brought to consciousness and held there to inform thought and action – simply awaits repetition.

So, what do we do about what lurks unconsciously in the unconscious of psychoanalysis? This is the place where deep history holds, not only decades of social unrest, political domination, violence, colonization, oppression, racism, anti-Semitism, class struggle, and enslavement – all of which have shaped, impacted, and traumatized individual minds and bodies throughout time and human history – but an accompanying deep history of universalizing intellectual and psychoanalytic thought. Psychoanalysis, throughout its own evolution, has brought numerous generative ideas to the table to help us understand the nature of human suffering and the ways to alleviate it: This evolution continues today. We have incorporated, built upon, and, to some extent, moved beyond Freud, Klein, and Lacan into contemporary extensions of these ideas, including attachment theory, infant studies, intersubjectivity, relationality, and the more recent focus, over the last decade, on the social, cultural, political context. Lynne Layton's (2006) overarching concept of normative unconscious processes highlights the interplay between psyche and culture. Many Relational psychoanalytic theorists have gone on to build upon and expand this ground (Altman, 2006; Aron, 2016; Aron & Starr, 2013; Benjamin, 2021; Gaztambide, 2019; Grand, 2014; Gump, 2010; Harris, 2019; Knoblauch, 2020; Leary, 2012; Orange, 2020; Straker, 2011; Suchet, 2007), etc. But, according to Celia Brickman (2018), in its early days, psychoanalysis did significant damage by participating in the splitting of the world into the primitive and the civilized. Brickman's (2018) brilliant book, *Race in Psychoanalysis: Aboriginal Populations in the Mind*, examines psychoanalysis from Freud to the present. After walking us through the horrors of the evolutionary triumphalism of white-skinned Europeans, and Freud's reliance on some of these anthropological conceptions of primitivity to undergird his ideas about the deep structure of the mind, she concludes:

> Over the last decade of the twentieth century and the first decades of the twenty-first, the authoritarian tendencies of the traditional structures of psychoanalysis, like the colonial influences of early anthropology with

which they are linked, have increasingly come under question, and alternative forms of conceiving both the analytic encounter and the knowledge it generates have been taking shape... American psychoanalysis has not been subject to a postcolonial critique from within its ranks.

(Brickman, 2018, 225)

As an overwhelmingly white profession, psychoanalysis has managed to avoid interrogating its role. Only recently, has the work of Fanon (1952/2008) entered some of our syllabi and our theorizing. A growing number of psychoanalytic practitioners (Aron, 2016; August, 2016; Brothers, 2016; Corpt, 2016; Emanuel, 2016; Orange, 2016; Layton, 2016; Salberg, 2016; Saporta, 2016; Smothers, 2016) have begun to address the ethical turn in psychoanalysis via their participation in the bi-annual Psychology and the Other conference (Goodman and Severson, 2016): Goodman and Severson see their mission as promoting "ethics as first psychology" (Levinas, 1989). Further change in psychoanalysis, however, is wholly dependent upon the persistent voices of BIPOC practitioners, the ever-widening scope of analysts and analysands, and our willingness to be open to new ideas.

One of the primary reparative goals of individual psychoanalytic work is to help the suffering patient come to terms with the impact of painful and traumatizing past events. All of this is meant to free up the present from simply being a repeat the past, but more importantly, to open the present to new future possibilities. Can we, as a field, do this for ourselves and by ourselves? I am a firm believer in deep reflection and self-analysis. I am, however, not at all convinced that, if left on our own, we can do this work, particularly when the suffering caused by injuries of the past is being disproportionately born by only some in the field, and not by all.

The American philosopher, Lewis Gordon (2016), writes the following:

Where a discipline treats itself as the world, as all of reality, and its methods as "complete," its practitioners forget it's a human-created practice. ...They turn their discipline inward into itself as the world and treat it as closed. In the human sciences, the result is asserting as problems those who do not "fit" the dictates of the discipline.

(Gordon, 2016, 21)

If this is the case, then we are facing an ethical crisis. We faced a similar crisis regarding homosexuality until it was finally de-pathologized in 1973. Only years later were gay applicants finally welcomed into the field.

As I see it, the overarching ethical challenge is this; It is for us to use the valuable knowledge we have accrued – knowledge helpful to our suffering patients – while simultaneously opening ourselves up to exploring and interrogating the very limits, constraints, and injurious aspects of that very knowledge. A view from outside the field can only but help us. Beyond this, I believe it is also imperative for us to acknowledge and own the injuries we have caused and continue to cause. This will require the exercise of ethical labor; of our pushing ourselves beyond ourselves.

For psychoanalysis, I am suggesting an expanded way to think about ethics. We are all familiar with the various code of professional ethics. These codes of ethics are meant to pull us in and scaffold us by requiring us to abide by a communally accepted code of behaviors or ways of thinking. We need these, but they are not adequate. What I am suggesting is a kind of ethics that works to push us out, beyond our siloes, into a liberatory reach and stretch, to a place from which we can freely engage with and learn from others. From this place, we are called to review, rethink, reform, reaffirm, and/or refresh our ideas as we engage with and wrestle with the ideas of others. This activated and liberating ethics requires an ongoing exercise of labor intent on opening us up, disquieting us, rendering us vulnerable, interrupting us, and, at times, shaking us to our core. The intention of this labor is not to undo the lines and frames of our thinking, nor to cause chaos, or madness, but rather, to help us question the underlying assumptions of those lines and frames; to keep them fresh, updated, breathing, flexible, and reflective of who we strive to be.

The literary critic and cultural historian, Geoffrey Galt Harpham, someone who writes extensively about ethics, sees "dynamic engagement with otherness as a key to the kingdom of ethics: where such engagement is, there is ethics" (Harpham, 1999, x). Harpham goes on to say:

> ethics exerts whatever force it does by virtue of its singular capacity to adhere to, affiliate with, bury itself in, provoke, or dislodge other discourses. Ethics…realizes its full creative potentiality not in "itself," but as a kind of X-factor, a bracingly alien incitement to inquiry and discrimination.
>
> (Harpham, 1999, xiii)

In other words, only by opening our thinking to other disciplines, other voices, and other perspectives, can we keep psychoanalysis relevant to this increasingly multi-cultural and complex world.

For a discipline whose modus operandi demands privacy, confidentiality, and reserve, this labor presents us with a unique challenge. Our general tendency is to gravitate inward. Let me try to explain the dilemma we face, but from within the perspective of the consulting room.

Psychoanalysts and psychotherapists learn to wait for a patient to speak their concerns before responding; otherwise, one cannot know how best to be of help. Even across theoretical differences, this work involves two persons engaged in an extended deep dialogue over time. In general, a good analyst remains silent only when there is good reason to do so. Like Freud, we are present, and actively involved, if not in words, then in thought and feeling. Unlike Freud, we tend to no longer think of an interpretation as *the* truth delivered from the pristine and well-analyzed superiority of the analyst's mind, but as part of an emergent process. Complex truths and understandings emerge out of two minds, deeply engaged with each other, and mutually influencing each other, around addressing the suffering of one.

There is no limit to what I can learn in following my patient's words, rhythms, silences, and unconscious communications. I find myself, however, increasingly questioning the commonly held belief that hearing from the patient and staying close to the patient's experience will teach me all I need to know about helping my patient. What if my patient carries unformulated social, cultural, historical, or intergenerational traumas which, by their very nature, cannot yet be formulated, thought, or spoken? Although I always prefer to stay close to my patient's subjective reality, and respect my patient's sense of timing, I simply do not think this is enough anymore. In fact, I think there are aspects of my maintaining this belief in waiting to be taught, or waiting to learn, which could harbor within it my own prejudices, blind spots, dissociations, or erasures. My maintaining this kind of silence could be experienced by my patient as an expression of my elitism, white privilege, indifference, ignorance, and inhospitality.

If we are to move beyond our blind spots regarding "the social unconscious", then we must be willing to perform the ethical labor of educating ourselves, not only about our own dissociated histories and the ways we are implicated in the injuries of others, but to educate ourselves regarding the lives and histories of those different from ourselves. As an analyst, at the very least, I need to contemplate how these differences may live in me and between me and my patient in the consulting room. I need to be ready and willing to communicate or signal my openness, respect, and curiosity about my patient's lived experience and cultural history and how it may differ from mine. And should my patient's personal or historic human-to-human trauma history be one in which dissociation, erasure, disavowal, and shame, figure large, then I must consider whether my patient may, or may not, feel silenced by my whiteness. The possible power relations at work in the room may simply and understandably inhibit my patient from speaking. I may need to be the one to first inquire and signal my openness.

This all falls within the realm of empathic inquiry; what every good therapist practices. But it's the erasure of the social that concerns me. I am not suggesting we usurp or intrude upon our patient's narratives, listen any less intently, or take on the role of teaching the patient who they are. Rather, we need to create a receptive space within ourselves from which we can signal a welcoming curiosity. We need to be mindful and watchful for signs of the strain of double consciousness, disavowal, dissociation, and the overall burdensome way those who are oppressed need to work, not only to know and manage themselves in our presence, but to know and manage the unconscious oppressor.

This raises other important questions for us to consider. How do we, as psychoanalysts, move out from within our own siloed existences? How do any of us, really? Are we not ethically responsible for the limitations of our ideas as well as the useful and positive influence of our ideas? Likewise, are we not ethically responsible for the impact of our blind spots, injuries, and erasures, and whatever they have communicated about our values? Is the upholding of the ethics of a discipline the responsibility of the individuals within that discipline or of the collective, or both? Furthermore, is there an overarching ethics that sits above whatever singular codes of ethics keeps a field's practice habits constructive and cohesive? And if the collective falls short in thinking about ethics, who is to blame? And what constitutes adequate reparation for any wrongs committed.

Let us return to Harpham's notion: to "engage Otherness is the key to the kingdom of ethics" (Harpham, 1999). Although this idea holds within it a profound rightness, we know engaging with otherness can be strenuous, and disorienting. To deepen our understanding of the depth of such a challenge, I turn to the philosopher, Emmanuel Levinas. Donna Orange, psychoanalyst and philosopher, was the first to introduce Levinas and several other Western philosophers to psychoanalysis. Orange's project has been to deepen the connection of psychoanalysis to other ethical and humanistic enterprises and "to induce both curiosity and a sense of feeling more at home and competent in the world of ideas" (Orange, 2010, 2). I turn to Levinas now precisely because I find his writings, and the effort they demand of the reader, unique in their capacity to upend and broaden assumptions about the nature of human subjectivity and human-to-human relating. In fact, to my mind, engaging with these ideas enacts the very disruption and disquiet that Levinas (1981) is asking us to endure when facing alterity and the other.

Levinas, a Lithuanian Jew and former student of Heidegger, suffered the profound loss of family members in the Holocaust, and spent years in a Nazi work camp. He made it his project to interrogate and articulate the essence of what he saw as the philosophical origins of subjectivity, and the extent to which our very subjectivity can only be born out of our infinite responsibility to the other; the other who is beyond me, above me, and takes me hostage. Levinas (1969) uses the simple metaphor of opening the door to explain what he means. For Levinas, this humble hospitable gesture, accompanied with the words "après vous" – after you – is the linguistic acknowledgement of the other's overarching command that I care for him above me; an infinite command not demanded, but proclaimed, by the other's very existence. For Levinas, "to perceive that we come after an other whoever he may be – that is ethics" (Levinas, 1999, 167).

Levinas's radical assertions, which can only be given scant review here, call for the exercise of a kind of labor. This is a specific kind of labor involving a reach beyond one's involvement in one's everyday Being; what Levinas means by the tasks and responsibilities of one's everyday existence. According to Levinas, only by embracing this overarching ethical demand, the "otherwise than being", and in suffering the other's existence – their alterity – can we, as human beings, hope to refrain from collapsing into a totalizing stance in which we risk, reducing the other to the same, thereby killing or abandoning of the other. Levinas says the following:

> As if, unknown by the other, whom already, in the nakedness of its face, it concerns, it "regarded me" before its confrontation with me, before being the death that scares me, myself, in the face. The death of the other man puts me on the spot, calls me into question, as if I, by my possible indifference, became the accomplice of that death, invisible to the other who is exposed to it; and as if, even before being condemned to it myself, I had to answer for that death of the other, and not leave the other alone to his deathly solitude. It is precisely in that recalling of me to my responsibility by the face that summons me, that demands me, that requires me-it is in that calling into question-that the other is my neighbor.
>
> (Levinas, 1999, 24–25)

There is a profound sense of urgency, disruption, vulnerability, and disquiet at work here. Levinas issues an unrelenting call for us to be ready, and willing, and brave enough to act on the behalf of the other. This requires a kind of dedicated attention that has the potential to shakes one's boundaries and assumptions. But what or who can provide the impetus for us to choose to exercise such ethical labor? From where will such willingness come? From empathy, education, consciousness raising, reparative guilt, or shame?

Although Levinas focuses us primarily on the other, he also leaves room for us to consider the other within. This brings us full circle, back to the realm of psychoanalysis, unconscious experience, and the unconscious of the unconscious of psychoanalysis; all we tend to disavow, dissociate, repress, suppress, project, and split off; in other words, the feeding ground for murderous hatred and Othering.

Moss's (2021) controversial paper was accompanied by a paper by Dorothy Evans Holmes (2021). Holmes, a well-respected Black analyst, chairs the Holmes Commission of the American Psychoanalytic Association, APsaA's organizational response to the murder of George Floyd. Holmes and her commission members function as the persistent voice of the other within American psychoanalysis. Holmes, in a more traditional and nuanced way, considers racism as "a disavowed marauding presence in the white psyche, a pathological formation that weakens psychic structures and creates a vulnerability to acting out that is hateful, discombobulated, and destructive" (Holmes, 2021, 237). In her description of what racism creates, Holmes is not quite as jarring to white sensibility as Moss, although she is no less strident in the measure she takes of this kind of Whiteness. Holmes, rather benevolently, I think, turns to the metaphor of ghosts – the ghosts of racism – those whom we defend, protect, and maintain our attachments to through the disavowal of our hatred of otherness and the simultaneous disavowal of our own inner otherness. Holmes borrows the metaphor of ghosts from the psychoanalyst Hans Loewald. Loewald wrote of ghostly presences made up of the destructive split off parts of the unconscious which, through the process of analysis, could be tamed and transformed into useful ancestors (Loewald, 1960, 29). For Holmes, protection of our ghosts takes place through a "whiteout" (Holmes, 2021, 240): Holmes's play on the use of Wite-out correctional fluid used to cover up what cannot be seen. Holmes goes on to say: "whites need their racial ghosts in order to maintain their unbridled access to hate, which, when it erupts, or when someone confronts them with it, is quickly disavowed" (Holmes, 2021, 244). Such disavowal provides what Holmes sees as a "license to hate on the basis of one's unexamined whiteness as an entitlement" (Holmes, 2021, 245). According to Holmes, to do otherwise, to face our whiteness and our racism, is to face inevitable loss and the mourning of our entitlements. Psychoanalysis, according to Holmes, has so far failed by offering "no theories or recommended treatments – on racial ghosts, that is, on race as aspects of all of us that are split off" (Holmes, 2021, 238).

I experienced my own "whiteout" when I came to the case examples in Holmes's paper. In anticipation of reading the article, I assumed that all three cases would address Black-White issues as their primary focus. Only one case concerned itself specifically with the patient's transference feelings about his Black nanny onto Holmes's. In her two remaining case examples, Holmes's identity as a Black psychoanalyst – as an interested, curious, skilled, and open subject in the room who happened to be Black – served as a kind of secondary catalyst for her two white patients and the eventual realizations and explorations of their disavowed white race anxieties and conflicts. Upon reflection, I realized that I had unconsciously expected Holmes, in her Blackness, to work for me by laying out Black-White scenarios to help teach me about race. As though the only race scenario from which I could learn would be a Black-White scenario. As if only Blackness holds race. I was shocked at my own white-out. And of the many times I have failed to consider the presence of and impact of race while sitting with my white patients. Holmes asks, "would a typical white therapist have expressed any curiosity about race or ethnicity or found access to such work (Holmes, 2021, 248).

Clearly, it seems to me, we, who are white, are rightfully being called to account for what we have failed to do ourselves. We have off-loaded the work of thinking about race and the complexity of our own race and its implications and deeply troubled history onto the shoulders of people of color.

Adrienne Harris refers to this as a "blank psychic space" which she defines as follows: "Deeper than depression, deeper than rage, there is a blankness, a place where there is not sufficient structure for mourning, where the psyche gives way" (Harris, 2019, 8).

Some years back, following a conference in which the presenter was calling into question the overarching emphasis placed on unconscious experience in psychoanalysis, I engaged a colleague in conversation over the coffee break. With near panic on his face, he said something like: "If we don't have the unconscious, then what do we have left?!" I was stunned. I knew enough to keep my thoughts private. I had to protect my insider position with respect to this colleague – someone very much an insider. I was, at that point in my career, a passing outsider – a younger analyst from a working-class familial background - with my own insider status to protect. I was not yet sturdy enough or ready to fully "out" myself, as painful as that is to now admit. Such are the workings of shame and vulnerability when confronted with power, prestige, the status quo, and a desire to belong.

What "we have left", beyond and beside unconscious processes, are the rigors, demands, and horrors of consciousness from which we, as humans, tend to retreat. What is consciously unbearable, sinks into unconsciousness. We are naturally wired for this, however, if certain psychological defenses are systemically condoned and encouraged by certain groups, as Moss and Holmes are clearly suggesting, then we have a problem. The unbearableness of our common human frailty and vulnerability needs to be faced by all of us, and not, disproportionately by some. This is the territory we as psychoanalysts need to consider, engage with, and address, and not only in the privacy of our consulting rooms.

The publicly televised killing of George Floyd, a present-day lynching, was a shock to many across the country and around the world, but not to people of color. There is a long history of lynching in this country: lynching without consequence. But this time, this public killing of a person of color had a different impact. Many were jarred awake by this event; it was a Levinasian "instant" (Levinas, 2001 104) – the kind of instant that grips you and calls you into an inescapable ethical awareness of our infinite responsibility to the other. Prior to this, a very small handful of progressive psychoanalytic institutes had begun implementing anti-racism, diversity, and inclusion initiatives. This event only further deepened their commitment to address systemic racism as an important aspect of their ethical mandate. Charla Malamed, a young professional aspiring to become an analyst, and curious about the overall response and sensitivity of various analytic institutes to race-related issues, independently conducted an informal poll of analytic institutes. Identifying themselves as someone interested in training, Malamed queried some thirty-nine analytic institutes across the country. Many were part of the

American Psychoanalytic Association, and some were independent institutes. Their questions were quite straight forward:

Does your institute have a published statement on Racial Justice?

If so, please send to me.

If not, why not?

Do you offer tuition scholarships/financial aid?

Do you offer aid specifically dedicated to BIPoC/under-represented populations?

What are the eligibility requirements?

Do you have more than 4 BIPoC faculty/supervisors who are currently active at your

institute?

Does your institute have an active racial/social justice task force/committee?

(Malamed, 2021)

A few APsaA-affiliated institutes provided links to the APsaA website and its Anti-Racism statement, but few had moved beyond this to show any evidence of their further institute work on the matter. A handful responded with suspicion by suggesting a formal request be submitted to the institutional review board before these questions could be answered. A couple of institutes responded by indicating an earnest wish to begin addressing these concerns: some having made some inroads into policy and training changes meant to encourage more candidates of color, etc. According to Malamed, (2021) a majority did not respond at all.

In 1995, Tony Morrison wrote an essay on Racism and Fascism in which she said the following: "Let's be reminded that before there is a final solution, there must be a first solution, a second one, even a third. The move toward a final solution is not a jump. It takes one step, then another, then another" (Morrison, 2019, 14). Morrison goes on to list ten quite chilling and disturbingly banal steps involved in stripping of the other of their humanity. I want to bring our attention to her number ten: "Maintain, at all costs, silence" (Morrison, 2019, 15).

It is profoundly unethical for anyone or any discipline to be silent on the matter of racism: a slow moving and silent form of fascism that implicates us all. How can we, as a discipline, speak and act against racism? I agree with Annie Lee Jones that it will take more than adding a few BIPOC authored papers to the syllabi or a few Black faculty to the training program roster, rather, it starts by "conceptualizing psychoanalytic training so that the lack of diversity is considered unethical and not good practice" (Jones, 2015, 724). Amen to that. But to get to that point will require the expenditure of ethical labor on everyone's part, not just on the part of the suffering few. It will require overwhelmingly white psychoanalysis to look within for signs of unconscious racism, classism, sexism – the ghosts of racism that do their mischief in whites - and outward, to a conscious study of the history of race, culture, philosophy, sociology, post-colonial studies. And we could clearly benefit from more than a Euro-centric perspective. If we are to keep ourselves alive and relevant, we need to embrace disruption, interruption, and expansion of our ideas and perspectives beyond silos.

In conclusion, I want to say a few more words about another way to think about labor; labor as in giving birth. Recently I have begun studying Hannah Arendt's concept of natality as a bulwark against totalitarianism; a "new beginning" (Arendt, 1998, 9) that has the capacity to "set something in motion" (Arendt, 1998, 177). It seems to me there may be a bridge here and a sense of hope. The work of psychoanalysis is about offering a chance at a new beginning and setting something in motion towards something better, less painful, and free from the unconscious repetition of the past. I particularly appreciate Rosalyn Diprose's and Ewa Plonowska Ziarek's comprehensive read of Arendt's conceptualization of natality. They see her as, not only emphasizing a new beginning, but, in addition, calling our attention to the importance of the "human agent as a perennial beginner, who, by acting and speaking, can begin something new in history" (Diprose and Ziarek, 2018, 4), and the importance of "being-with a plurality of distinct others" (Diprose and Ziarek, 2018, 5). So, in this spirit, I call upon us to engage our differences and embrace disruption, so we can dare to begin something new.

References

Altman, N. (2006) Black and white thinking: A psychoanalyst reconsiders race. In R. Moodley & S. Palmer (Eds.). *Race, Culture, and Psychotherapy: Critical Perspectives in Multicultural Practice*. Routledge.

Aron, L. (2016) *Mutual vulnerability: an ethic of clinical practice*. In D. Goodman and E. Severson (Eds.). *The Ethical Turn: Otherness and Subjectivity in Contemporary Psychoanalysis*, Routledge, pp.19–41.

Aron, L. & Starr, K. (2013) *A Psychotherapy for the People: Toward a Progressive Psychoanalysis*. Routledge.

Arendt, H. (1998) *The human condition*. University of Chicago Press.

August, P. (2016) *What fascinates: re-reading Winnicott reading Blanchot*. In D. Goodman and E. Severson (Eds.). *The Ethical Turn: Otherness and Subjectivity in Contemporary Psychoanalysis*, Routledge, pp. 286–293).

Benjamin, J. (2021) Acknowledgment, Harming, and Political Trauma: Reflections After the Plague Year. *Psychoanalytic Perspectives*, 18, pp. 401–412.

Brickman, C. (2018). *Race in Psychoanalysis: Aboriginal Populations of the Mind*. Routledge.

Brothers, D. (2016) "Screams and shouts": trauma, uncertainty, and the ethical turn. In D. Goodman and E. Severson (Eds.). *The Ethical Turn: Otherness and Subjectivity in Contemporary Psychoanalysis*, Routledge, pp. 117–124.

Corpt, E. (2013). Peasant in the analyst's chair: reflections, personal and otherwise on class and the forming of an analytic identity. *International Journal. of Psychoanalytic Self Psychology*, 8, pp. 52–67.

Corpt, E. (2016) The Complications of Caring and the Ethical Turn in Psychoanalysis. . In D. Goodman and E. Severson (Eds.). *The Ethical Turn: Otherness and Subjectivity in Contemporary Psychoanalysis*, Routledge, pp. 109–116.

Corpt, E. (2020) Ethical labor: the ground between experience near and experience distant: discussion of Cushman's two world's or one. *Psychoanalysis, Self, and Context*, 3, pp. 227–229.

Dews, C.L. & Law, C.L. (1995) *This Fine Place So Far From Home: Voices of Academics from the Working Class*. Temple University Press.

Diprose, R. & Ziarek, E.P. (2018) *Arendt, Natality, and Biopolitics: Toward Democratic Plurality and Reproductive Justice*. Edinburgh University Press.

Du Bois, W.E.B. (1903) *The Souls of Black Folks, Essays and Sketches*. A.C. McClurg.

Emanuel, C. (2016) *The disabled: the most othered others*. In D. Goodman and E. Severson (Eds.). *The Ethical Turn: Otherness and Subjectivity in Contemporary Psychoanalysis*, Routledge, pp. 270–285.

Fanon, F. (1952) *Black skin, White masks*. Grove Press.

Gaztambide, D. (2019) *A People's History of Psychoanalysis*. Lexington Books.

Goodman, D. & Severson, E. (2016) Introduction: ethics as first psychology. In D. Goodman and E. Severson (Eds.). *The Ethical Turn: Otherness and Subjectivity in Contemporary Psychoanalysis*, Routledge, pp. 1–18.

Gordon, L.R. (2016) *Disciplinary Decadence: Living Thought in Trying Times*. Routledge.

Grand, S. (2014) Skin memories: On race, love, and loss. *Psychoanalysis, Culture & Society*, 19(3), pp. 232–249. https:doi.org/10,1057.pcs.2014.24.

Gump, J. (2010) Reality matters: The shadow of trauma on African American subjectivity. *Psychoanalytic Psychology*, 27, pp. 42–54.

Harpham, G.G. (1999) *Shadows of Ethics: Criticism and the Just Society*. Duke University Press.

Harris, A. (2019) The perverse pact: racism and white privilege. *American Imago*, 76 (3), pp. 309–333. doi:10.1.1353/aim.2019.0026.

Holmes, D.E. (2021) "I do not have a racist bone in my body": Psychoanalytic perspectives on what is lost and not mourned in our culture's persistent racism. *Journal of the American Psychoanalytic Association*, 69(2), pp. 337–358.

Jones, A.L. (2015) A psychoanalytic reader's commentary: on erasure and negation as a barrier to the future. *Psychoanalytic Dialogues*, 25, pp.719–724.

Knoblauch, S.H. (2020) Fanon's vision of embodied racism for psychoanalytic theory and practice. *Psychoanalytic Dialogues*, 30, pp. 299–316.

Layton, L. (2006) Racial identities, racial enactments, and normative unconscious processes. *Psychoanalytic. Quarterly*, 75, pp. 237–269.

Layton, L. (2016) *Yale or jail: class struggles in neoliberal times.* In D. Goodman and E. Severson (Eds.). *The Ethical Turn: Otherness and Subjectivity in Contemporary Psychoanalysis,* Routledge, pp. 75–93.

Leary, K. (2012) Race as an adaptive challenge: working with diversity in the clinical consulting room. *Psychoanalytic Psychology,* 29(3), pp. 279–291.

Levinas, E. (1969) *Totality and Infinity: An Essay on Exteriority.* Duquesne University Press.

Levinas, E. (1981) *Otherwise Than Being: Or Beyond Essence.* Duquesne University Press.

Levinas, E. (1989) *Ethics as first philosophy. In S. Hand (Ed.) The Levinas Reader.* Blackwell.

Levinas, E. (1999) *Alterity and Transcendence.* Columbia University Press.

Levinas, E. (2001) *Existence and Existents.* Duquesne University Press.

Levinas, E. (2003) *Humanism of the other* (trans. N. Poller). University of Illinois Press.

Loewald, H.W. (1960). On the therapeutic action of psychoanalysis. *International Journal of Psychoanalysis,* 41, pp. 16–33.

Malamed, C.R. (2022). Does your institute have an anti-racism commitment?: Interrogating anti-racism commitments in psychoanalytic institutes. *Psychoanalysis, Culture, and Society* 27, pp. 375–385. https://doi.org/10.1057/s41282-022-00285-1.

Mills, T. (2017) *The Dawn of Detroit: A Chronicle of Slavery and Freedom in the City of the Straits.* The New Press.

Mills, J. (2021, July 16) The scandal in whiteness theory in psychoanalysis [Video]. www.youtube.com/watch?v=GlkM29qaig4.

Morrison, T. (2019) *Mouth full of blood: Essays, speeches, meditations.* Vintage.

Moss, D. (2021). On having whiteness. *Journal of the American Psychoanalytic Association,* 69 (2) 355–371.

Orange, D.M. (2010). *Thinking for Clinicians: Philosophical Resources for Contemporary Psychoanalysis and the Humanistic Psychotherapies.* New York: Routledge.

Orange, D.M. (2016). *Is ethics masochism? or infinite ethical responsibility and finite human capacity.* In D. Goodman and E. Severson (Eds.). *The Ethical Turn: Otherness and Subjectivity in Contemporary Psychoanalysis,* Routledge, pp. 57–74.

Powell, D. (2020). Race, African Americans and psychoanalysis: Collective silence in the therapeutic situation. *Journal of the American Psychoanalytic Association,* 66 (6).

Orange, D.M. (2020) *Psychoanalysis, History, and Radical Ethics.* Routledge.

Rozmarin, E. (2017) The social is the unconscious of the unconscious of psychoanalysis. *Contemporary Psychoanalysis,* 53(4), pp. 459–469.

Salberg, J. (2016). Gender and the Jew: the other within. In D. Goodman and E. Severson (Eds.). *The Ethical Turn: Otherness and Subjectivity in Contemporary Psychoanalysis,* Routledge, pp. 164–177.

Saporta, J. (2016) Changing the subject by addressing the other: Mikhail Bakhtin and psychoanalytic therapy. In D. Goodman and E. Severson (Eds.). *The Ethical Turn: Otherness and Subjectivity in Contemporary Psychoanalysis,* Routledge, pp. 209–231.

Smothers, B. (2016) Creativity and Hospitality: negotiating who or what is known in psychoanalytic psychotherapy. In D. Goodman and E. Severson (Eds.). *The Ethical*

Turn: Otherness and Subjectivity in Contemporary Psychoanalysis, Routledge, pp. 253–269.

Straker, G. (2011) Unsettling whiteness. *Psychoanalysis, Culture & Society*, 16(1), pp. 11–26. http://doi.org/10.1057/pcs.2010.

Suchet, M. (2007) Unraveling whiteness. Psychoanalytic Dialogues, 17(6), pp. 867–886. https://doi.org.proxy2.library.illinois.edu/10/1080/10481880701703730.

Chapter 5

Some Fanonian Insights on Racism's Challenges to Psychoanalytical Practice

Lewis R. Gordon

This chapter addresses a set of themes that have been under investigation in African diasporic thought on the human sciences for more than a century (see Firmin 1885; Gordon, 2008), though for the sake of brevity I will highlight ideas from one because of his now universal recognition among practitioners – Frantz Fanon – and place him in conversation with some important recent critical discussions of racism's challenges for a rigorous and ethically-attuned understanding of psychoanalytical practice.

Fanon's impetus for writing *Peau noir, masques blancs* (*Black Skin, White Masks*, 1952) was an observation from his experience as a medical intern in Lyon, France. A healthy person, Fanon observed, suffers in an unhealthy society. To align that person with that society would, in effect, be to render her, him, or them unhealthy. What else should we call a person who is at home in dehumanizing environments?

Fanon noticed that many "clients" of color who consulted him suffered from how they were being treated in the colonial, racist, and sexist society in which they were condemned to live. They were, as W.E.B. Du Bois succinctly formulated it half a century earlier in *The Souls of Black Folk* (1903), constructed as "problems." But are they properly problems when they are angry or dejected at dehumanization? Consider, for example, that drapetomania (the "illness" of enslaved people desiring freedom), "diagnosed" by the physician Samuel A. Cartwright in 1851, was once influential in US psychiatry (Greenberg, 2013). Should Fanon's psychiatric efforts, legitimately understood in his times, have been devoted to producing happy slaves and masters or enforcers at home with technologies of colonization and enslavement?

This raises a serious problem for those who are at home in racist societies. If white society, for example, is unhealthy because of the whiteness it cultivates, then the narcissistic rage against efforts to transform it – efforts ranging from the neoconservative and neoliberal hoopla stirred up against critical race theory to Black Studies, Ethnic Studies, wokeness, and the many community-oriented projects ranging from Black Lives Matter to the countless civic organizations against class, gender, racial, and LGBTQI+

DOI: 10.4324/9781003394327-6

discrimination and exploitation – are clearly symptomatic of efforts to maintain it.

Fanon's initial formal psychiatric training was in positivist approaches to clinical therapy and forensic psychiatry. He was critical of his professors' reduction of mental illness to neurological dysfunction or damage. His accepted dissertation, which focused on Friedreich's ataxia, demonstrated the distinction, but his initial one, which was originally entitled "Essai sur la désalienation du Noir" (but renamed "Peau noir, masques blanc" at the encouragement of Éditions du Seuil's editor Francis Jeanson in agreement with Fanon's brother Joby Fanon's (2014) recommendation of "Essai sur la désalienation du Noir et du Blanc"), revealed his commitment to psychoanalysis and explored problems of colonized human science as sociogenetically produced. He later elaborated the constructive side of his critique in his research with the great Catalan psychiatrist François Tosquelles in his postdoctoral studies in institutional therapy at Saint-Alban-sur-Limagnole.

I bring this up because of the similarities of Fanon's approach and relational psychoanalysis, which is the framework from which Elizabeth Corpt offered her reflections in her insightful paper, "Ethical Labor: A Step Toward Reparations Within Psychoanalysis," at the Psychology and the Other conference in Boston in 2021. Similar to what Corpt recommended in that splendid plenary lecture, Fanon conducted a decolonizing critique of Lacanian psychoanalysis in which he demonstrated how, despite its semiological virtues, it fails to account for convergences of antiblackness and gender through ignoring the wider social-historical colonial context of their production. Corpt joined Fanon in reminding fellow therapists and theorists of human science that psychoanalysis also involves meta-psychoanalysis, and this critical social question – sociogenetic elements – are crucial features of metacritical reflection on therapeutic practices. Fanon added the observation that a core element of many forms of mental illness, versus neurological illness, is narcissistic disorder, whether of the sadistic or abject kinds. In the social-historical context of Euromodern societies, Fanon regarded whiteness and its assertions of "supremacy" as exemplars of narcissistic disorder made normative and ordinary.

I should like to stress that Fanon did not consider narcissism in and of itself a bad thing. He famously stated in *Peau noir, masques blancs* that he embraced his narcissistic quest for his humanity. He meant by this that humanity, as an expression of human beings, is in practice human reality disclosing itself through its reflections. It is a movement from zoological being to symbolic, social reality in which living requires, fundamentally, meaning. A perversion of this phenomenon is a flight from the social dimensions of meaning into the self at the expense of others, of a bloated inwardness at the price of outward relations that include care, empathy, and other forms of affective expressions of social life.

Fanon observed, aside from narcissistic disorder, another peculiar problem at the heart of racism. It is not, as commonly thought, a fear of the Other, because implicit in the Other is a Self that returns its gaze. It is actually an effort to place a category of people outside of the framework of Self/Other relations. It is an effort to eliminate sociality and, by extension, ethical life in relation to such people by forcing them outside of normative relations. Ethics, as it turns out, is reserved for those inside of the Self/Other relationship. This enables the identification of a peculiar twist in the kind of narcissistic disorder racism manifests, for it is not about an individual white, for example, but about a judgment ascribed and supported across people designated white. In other words, racists and the institutions that support them – racism – produce a performative contradiction of an antisocial sociality in which there is a segregated world of "us" in which the racially degraded are not really a "them." There is the logic of a bifurcated world of contraries in which one group represents universal presence and the rest (not properly "others") exemplify universal absence. Interaction is thus forbidden in that world because it produces contradictions; it communicates the falseness of that world through any moment of symbolic invasion – even where that could take the form of a look, a touch, or a word.

Concretely, Fanon's point is already there in the title of his classic 1952 text. It could easily be misinterpreted – as it has over many years – as black people wearing white masks, often of assimilation. What Fanon was arguing, however, is that antiblack racist and white supremacist societies seal black people into their skins and mandate white people to wear white masks. The sealed skin is a lie, since it hides the humanity of the people. The white masks are lies because they also hide the humanity of the people. The lie to black people is that they are not human. The lie to white people is that they are, by virtue of being white, superior to all other human beings. What would that be but gods? There are thus pleasing falsehoods (for whites) that hide displeasing truths (for blacks). The displeasing truth is that, as Fanon put it, they live in societies attempting the murder of humanity.

Fanon is aware that blacks among themselves and whites among themselves are fully aware of their humanity. But antiblack racism and white supremacy makes the former have to struggle against dehumanization when in the presence of whites and the latter often put on masks to lie to black people that they are superior to them. Those white masks of lies are also, at times, what some black people come to believe white people actually are, and those blacks attempt to acquire those masks. But the central point is that many whites invest in those masks when they think of themselves in relation to nonwhite people, especially blacks.

A defense mechanism against facing this displeasing phenomenon is to leap into the arms of nonrelational notions of identity and self. An asocial "truth" offers solace. This delusional refuge takes many forms, including conceptual frameworks or practices to support it. Among them is the transformation of terms that identify such flight and bearers of such masks into slurs. I have already identified such in the attacks against critical race theory and being woke, but one that has much valence beyond rightwing and fascist forces is "identity politics."

Turning terms into slurs is an effort to eliminate relations. Slurs are calls – perhaps urgings or threats through ridicule – for members of an "insider group" not to listen to outsiders and get in line with familiar practices of delegitimation and exclusion. The implications of these slurs are more insidious than they may at first appear. They boil down to this. Don't listen to those (non)people and whatever discourse that may facilitate their appearance or voice. In her lecture, Corpt touched upon this dynamic through her invocation of Toni Morrison's (1995, 384) observation that racism and fascism depend on the maintenance of "… at all cost, silence." Along a process of chipping away at the humanity of the outside group, there is the concluding complicity of an absence of addressing what is going on. A form of insidious silence becomes as banal as quietly taking out waste. This phenomenon is, by the way, was observed by Steve Bantu Biko in South Africa in *I Write What I Like* (1978), and by many, mostly women intellectuals over the ages. As Christine de Pizan made clear in *Le Livre de la Cité des Dames* (*The Book of the City of Ladies*, 1405) and *Le tresor de la cité des dames de degré en degré* (*The Treasure of the City of Ladies*, 1405), silence maintains systems of lies. Speech facilitates appearance, and it is a primary way through which the power of appearance emerges in political life. As oppression involves acts and institutions of disempowering a people, the consequence of silence is the logical conclusion of disempowerment: disappearance.

Clinical practitioners of psychoanalysis may wish to rethink various theoretical underpinnings of therapy in terms of challenges such as those posed by Fanon and François Tosquelles, wherein, as Camille Robcis (2021) explains, the problem of "concentrationism" emerges from depersonalization and isolation from social reality. This problem can occur not only at the level of the patient as an "object" of therapeutic practice but also at the methodological levels of disciplinary practice. Where a human science fails to consider the possibility of its role in attempted legitimization of authoritarianism, colonialism, fascism, racism, and sexism, it contributes, through an absence of critical reflection, to the cultivation of oppression. For Fanon, this meant that colonialism was more than a material practice; it was also way of producing problematic forms of knowledge, which includes problematic understandings of normality in which the problem status of a patient is presumed an ontogenic reality on one hand, a phylogenic one on the other, with ignored sociogenetic factors (Fanon, 1952; Bulhan, 1985; Gordon, 2015). In my work (for example, Gordon 2006, 2021), I call this phenomenon of a presumed intrinsic legitimacy of the discipline and its practices *disciplinary decadence*. For brevity's sake, disciplinary decadence involves the ontologizing of one's discipline and the fetishizing of its methodological framework. The effect is the treatment of the discipline as though created by a god. This leads to theodicean rationalizations and defensiveness of the discipline, and it also leads to insularity into which the practitioners treat the discipline as reality instead of a point from which to reach for reality and, by extension, others. Reaching for reality involves considering the communicative and ethical practices of what I call *teleological suspensions of disciplinarity*. This involves the constant realization of one's discipline's not being absolute but, instead, a doorway into what transcends it. It thus entails being willing to go beyond one's discipline for the sake of reality. This willingness affects its methodological assumptions. Instead of treating methods as absolute or complete, the practitioner treats them as a relational practice that could encounter their limitations. Placed in the context of human science, this involves a willingness to admit that there are times when people's failure to fit into the methodological framework of a discipline may be a sign of the discipline's limitations instead of the people. A practitioner who fails to consider this is compelled to cry: "What's wrong with these people!"

In the context of psychoanalysis, a critique of disciplinary decadence occasions a teleological suspension of psychoanalysis. A teleological suspension of psychoanalysis involves psychoanalysts being willing, paradoxically, to go beyond psychoanalysis for the sake of its commitments to making conscious what has been rendered unconscious. There is an ironic plea not only for ethics but also rigor. As the psychoanalyst must also undergo psychoanalysis – indeed, often in real clinical time to avoid projection – so, too, must the discipline and its framework. Indeed, I use the word "discipline" in a reserved way here, since I agree with Barnaby Barratt in his *"Rediscovering Psychoanalysis" Trilogy* (2013, 2016, 2019), that psychoanalysis must transcend orthodoxy, which means it must always be self-critical and, thus, engage in practices of what Sonia Dayan-Herzbrun calls "undisciplining," in her article "To Undiscipline Knowledge: Toward a New Geography of Reason" (2021), through the relational learning of ongoing, decolonizing practice of growth via communication. In short, disciplinary "purity" – a feature of neat, "clean" orthodoxy – is patently an aspiration that would mark the death knell of psychoanalysis.

The ethical dimension of taking such critically reflective paths takes many forms. Corpt, for example, appealed to Emmanuel Levinas for insights on ethics. The Levinasian arguments, although important in the specific I-Thou relationships of which Martin Buber also wrote in *Ich und Du* (*I and Thou*, 1923), faces some problems here, however. I have already hinted at one in pointing to Fanon's observation about racism as not ultimately about the Other (although there are *others* involved) but, instead, about the elimination of the self/other relationship regarding certain groups of people while maintaining it among the subject's "in group" and, thus, also ethics. This observation makes racism, although having ethical implications, a fundamentally political problem requiring political solutions, for what maintains the separations of groups are institutions of power that limit the options of a group to transform how its members are affected by the dominating or hegemonic group. The Levinasian model is locked primarily in a liberal framework, which prioritizes *ethical* over *political* forms of responsibility. The problem is that racism, which contextualizes the therapeutic moment, is peculiarly political. Fanon's counsel to those clients suffering from racial degradation was for them to become politically active. This was because their suffering was actually a mark of them being psychologically healthy enough to realize, at a subconscious level, that something was wrong. An unhealth client could appear "happy" or, in some instances, not angry at a vicious system but only discontented at it having an impact of any kind on her, him, or them. Again, it's not that there aren't ethical dimensions and implications of oppression, but ethics – or, for that matter, normative life – requires important restructuring, in fact also decolonizing, of its normative framework for the Other as human being to appear. Since psychoanalysis doesn't exist in a vacuum but through institutions that set the conditions of possibility for practitioners to do their work, that means there is already a political dimension to be addressed, even if reluctantly or, worse, defensively so.

On this matter of defensiveness, a thought comes to mind on Dorothy Holmes's (2021) description of racism in her abstract as "a disavowed marauding presence in the white psyche, a pathological formation that weakens psychic structures and creates a vulnerability to acting out that is hateful, discombobulated, and destructive." It captures wonderfully the pathology of what is at work with living under supported and entitled notions of "superiority." But we should bear in mind that the impetus, here primarily about how white supremacy affects blacks and whites, suggests that a transformed white psyche doesn't get rid of antiblack racism. The society in which this reflection is taking place is one marked by both. As it is possible to dissolve white supremacy but maintain antiblack racism, the result would at its best be an increase in the number of allies against antiblack racism. Here there is opportunity for profound psychoanalytical in addition to political work or, perhaps, a fusion of the two. After all, as antiblack racism is not peculiar to any group but can be actions of all, including black people, then the affective elements of a shifted social structure would need serious therapeutic intervention. This was an insight from Fanon's final work *Les Damnés de la terre* (1961), where he offered clinical studies of the damage done to people through national liberation struggles. Building a better society includes not only material conditions of living better lives but also effective practices of overcoming the consequences of its members taking themselves too seriously. Getting over oneself is an ongoing, therapeutic practice.

It is striking how affected some (perhaps many?) white critics are to Donald Moss's "On Having Whiteness," especially his descriptions of white expectations of affirmed entitlements, at the expense of his ultimate point, which is that:

Epistemologies of identificatory obligation aim to reverse Freud's famous axiom and to arrive, finally, at this: Where ego alone once was, there id too must also be.

Psychoanalytic work, then, need not properly target Whiteness itself here. Instead, it can effectively target the psychic receptor sites that provide Whiteness the interior vertical mapping on which it depends. The vertical map disrupts the identificatory bond that might once have bound subject to object. The bond persists, though, reshaped and hardened now into a vertical format. Identification morphs into disidentification, similarity into difference, affectionate care into sadistic cruelty. Diminish the spread and influence of these interior vertical receptor sites and, indirectly, the parasite of Whiteness is dislodged, loosed, itself becoming susceptible to exposure, as a differentiated and alien presence. Psychoanalytic work, in its most radical, fundamental, and, finally neutral forms, targets any and all of the effects of vertical mapping. Where verticality was, there horizontality will be.

(Moss, 2021: 365)

Many black people would consider Moss's descriptions of whiteness and his concluding point not only correct but also actually mild. There are many ways to talk about whiteness and notions of white supremacy. That such a piece occasioned outrage is revealing of (a dreaded word these days) fragility. I should like to illustrate an additional consideration succinctly here through an example that has occasioned similar responses to my book *Fear of Black Consciousness* (Gordon, 2022). I was an external examiner of a thesis in which there was a chapter entitled, "What Do Whites Want?" Now, the author was not referring to every individualized or embodied individual designated "white," but, instead, the structural one about whom we may have this classic rephrasing of a well-known gendered theme of psychoanalysis. The student had elaborate illustrations from literature, but he did not get to the actual point. So, I simply asked him if he were aware that the answer is well-known among most people of color and among many whites deep down. What do the people we have come to know as white people want? *Everything.* Add to this the presupposition of limited resources, and everything boils down to haves who want more, which includes not only what is materially at the table but also its symbolic offerings. The parasitism of which Moss wrote pertains also to the labors and creativity of others. Recent history has grown tired of white claims of building houses that were in fact built by enslaved, colored, and female labor. The white-washing – and I would add masculinizing – of history is, after all, well known, with similar defensive responses when challenged.

Holmes reflects on some of these defensive responses to deflated whiteness as follows:

> To mourn certain aspects of whiteness is a huge undertaking. Specifically, it is a painful undertaking to no longer have license to hate on the basis of one's unexamined whiteness as an entitlement. After all, that entitlement arrogates undue power to oneself while denying power, rank, and dignity to nonwhites.
>
> (Holmes, 2021: 242)

She is spot on in identifying "license" as a crucial expected entitlement of whiteness. Although it is fashionable to speak of "white privilege," a problem with it is that privileges have limits and can be goods, at times rights. License, however, pertains to exceptions, to being beyond reproach; to be licensed is to lack constraints over one's liberties; to be able to do, like spoiled children, whatever one wants. I should add that this insight is one of the reasons I have argued against the notion of white privilege and have argued for, instead, the characterization of white license as the perverse offering of white supremacy. From posing for photographs in publicly advertised lynchings to countless examples of volatile actions marked by a lack of accountability, the promise of white supremacy is an absence of limits – except, of course, against fellow whites when determined as white, in a word, enough.

Holmes's use of mourning is linked to her use of the word "ghost." In her words:

> When elements of one's personal psychology of whiteness are split off and disavowed, they constitute a ghost that interferes with psychotherapy, particularly with the process of grieving. In general, as psychoanalytic psychotherapists, we know that our job includes an essential aspect of mourning in which, as Loewald formulated many years ago, we transform ghosts into ancestors.
>
> (Holmes, 2021: 237)

Many whites are not transforming their ghosts into ancestors. By extension, a white supremacist society is haunted by its racism. I have argued elsewhere that ghost metaphors pertain more to indigenous displacement and settler colonial logic, but there are also temporal elements in which truth could be structured as past or hidden, where the displeasing truths could be "buried" in pleasing falsehoods. I take Holmes's point to be such. This form of bad faith, although I'm aware psychoanalysts prefer the terms "dissociation" and "unconscious," is well characterized as, as Holmes formulated it, "white-out." Here we find an analysis of a form of covering over instead of the usual presuppositions of opacity or darkness. For some psychoanalysts, this threatens the unconscious as a bedrock of psychoanalysis. Yet, harkening back to the call against orthodoxy, why not consider the possibility of some appeals to *the unconscious* also meeting a need for escaped responsibility. It's one of the reasons terms such as "unconscious bias" and "epistemic ignorance" hold sway in contemporary discussions of race and racism. They are preferred to a deeper, displeasing truth experienced by many black and brown people each day, which is that these tropes are at times more opportune than causal. I've rarely encountered antiblack racism from whites that was not conscious but then became "unconscious" when challenged. But this is part of the game of narcissistic devolution. It is accompanied by shame when identified, which requires, strangely, a conscious effort of unconscious designation, which requires a double move of burying the initial conscious act. In short, white supremacy and antiblack racism often place black people into witnessing dissociation and degeneration in real time.

We should bear in mind that the unconscious is not a discovery of psychoanalysis. The idea is as ancient as the theory of emanation in East African thought in the times of Akhenaten and Nefertiti, and more ancient as even writers in their time referred to tapping into dreamlife and concealed forces among their ancients. As Barnaby Barratt concludes on this matter in his trilogy, a major innovation in what is formally known as psychoanalysis is the methodological approach of free association through which to access unconscious life.

Returning, then, to narcissism, there is something that whites who personalize critiques of white supremacy also fear, and it strikes me that Corpt, Fanon, Holmes, and Moss have identified it—namely, ultimate white irrelevance. Perhaps the most famous metaphor on this matter is Audre Lorde's (1984) dictum that the master's tools cannot dismantle his house. On this matter, I should like to add Haki Madhubuti's (2021) reformulation from "master" to "enslaver." This brings to the fore a response from Jane Anna Gordon and me in our introduction to our anthology *Not Only the Master's Tools* (2006). We should remember that enslavers – and all exploiters taking on the moniker of "masters" – don't actually build houses; indeed, they rarely build anything. Regarding the enslaved, history actually reveals that most were skilled labor whose tools brought prosperity to the lands in which their enslavement continued. Jane Anna Gordon and I have argued over the years about the importance of building other houses (institutions and conceptual frameworks). Building other, better homes would render the "master's house" isolated and eventually obsolete in its delusions of mastery. Having healthier homes elsewhere disarms the centrality of domination or supremacy.

If the work is done well to undermine white supremacy, that achievement would mean, for white supremacists, the end of the world. But for the rest of humanity, including those designated whites who have let go of that perverse attachment to their inhumanity, what a wonderfully relevant irrelevance that would be.

References

Barratt, Barnaby (2012) *What is Psychoanalysis? 100 Years after the "Secret Committee".* "Rediscovering Psychoanalysis" Trilogy. Routledge.

Barratt, Barnaby (2016) *Radical Psychoanalysis: An Essay on Free-associative Praxis.* "Rediscovering Psychoanalysis" Trilogy. Routledge.

Barratt, Barnaby (2019) *Beyond Psychotherapy: On Becoming a (Radical) Psychoanalyst.* "Rediscovering Psychoanalysis" Trilogy. Routledge.

Biko, Steve Bantu (2002) *I Write What I Like: Selected Writings,* edited with a personal memoir by Aeired Stubbs, preface by Desmond Tutu, an introduction by Malusi and Thoko Mpumlwana, with a new foreword by Lewis R. Gordon. University of Chicago Press.

Bulhan, Hussein Abdilahi (1985) *Frantz Fanon and the Psychology of Oppression.* Plenum.

Du Bois, W.E.B. (1903) *The Souls of Black Folk: Essays and Sketches.* A.C. McClurg & Co.

Corpt, Elizabeth (2021) *Ethical Labor: A Step Toward Reparations Within Psychoanalysis.* Presented at the Online Psychology and the Other Conference.

Fanon, Frantz (1952) *Peau noire, masques blancs.* Éditions du Seuil.

Fanon, Frantz (1961) *Les Damnés de la terre.* Preface by Jean-Paul Sartre. François Maspero ed.. S.A.R.L.

Fanon, Joby (2014) *Frantz Fanon, My Brother: Doctor, Playwright, Revolutionary.* Translated by Daniel Nethery. Lexington Books.

Firmin, Anténor (1885) *De l'égalité des races humaines (Anthropologie positive).* F. Pichon.

Gordon, Jane Anna and Lewis R. Gordon (2006) Introduction: Not Only the Master's Tools. In Jane Anna Gordon and Lewis R. Gordon (Eds.) *Not Only the Master's Tools: African-American Studies in Theory and Practice.* Routledge, pp. ix–xi.

Gordon, Lewis R. (2006) *Disciplinary Decadence: Living Thought in Trying Times.* Routledge.

Gordon, Lewis R. (2008). *An Introduction to Africana Philosophy.* Cambridge University Press.

Gordon, Lewis R. (2015) *What Fanon Said: A Philosophical Introduction to His Life and Thought.* Fordham University Press.

Gordon, Lewis R. (2021) *Freedom, Justice, and Decolonization.* Routledge.

Gordon, Lewis R. (2022) *Fear of Black Consciousness.* Farrar, Straus, and Giroux.

Greenberg, Gary (2013) *The Book of Woe: The DSM and the Unmaking of Psychiatry.* Plume.

Holmes, Dorothy Evans (2021) "I Do Not Have a Racist Bone in My Body": Psychoanalytic Perspectives on What is Lost and Not Mourned in Our Culture's Persistent Racism. *Journal of the American Psychoanalytical Association,* 69(2), pp. 237–258.

Madhubuti, Haki (2021). Acceptance Speech, Frantz Fanon Lifetime Achievement Award Ceremony, Caribbean Philosophical Association. https://www.facebook.com/watch/?v=315301673413520.

Morrison, Toni (1995) Racism and Fascism. *The Journal of Negro Education,* 64(3), pp. 384–385.

Moss, Donald (2021) On Having Whiteness. *Journal of the American Psychoanalytical Association*, 69(2), pp. 355–371.

Pizan, Christine de (1405) *Le Livre de la Cité des Dames.* Possibly originally published in Burgundy, France.

Pizan, Christine de (1405) *Le tresor de la cité des dames de degré en degré.* Possibly originally published in Burgundy, France.

Robcis, Camille (2021) *Disalienation: Politics, Philosophy, and Radical Psychiatry in Postwar France.* University of Chicago Press.

Chapter 6

Unthought, Concealment, and the Problem of the Lacanian Unconscious

John L. Roberts

Modern subjectivities have been increasingly linked to diverse historical expressions of psyche and struggle, such as in narcissism, trauma, and madness. In this essay, my efforts follow this trajectory, in situating the modern subject of the dynamic unconscious within its historical light, while avoiding essentialism. The influence of Foucault (1966/1973) cannot be overlooked, with two points of emphasis. First, Foucault's late avowal of Heideggerian thought finds hermeneutic ground for his earlier Nietzschean proclivities (Raynor, 2007). Second, both positive knowledge and aporia warrant address. In *The Order of Things,* the early Foucault (1966/1973) discerns a vortex of non-knowledge threatening the human sciences through what he refers to as the "analytic of finitude," including a problematic doubling of the subject and its temporal fragmentation, but also what he nominates as the "*cogito* and unthought." Regarding the unthought, Foucault (1966/1973) suggests it is precisely psychoanalysis that pursues its excavation. In avoiding the dangers of lapsing into a naively empirical rendering, Foucault obliquely points to Lacanian psychoanalysis as a potential "counter-science," which might remain at a similar level to his own historical analysis, to take such lacunae of finitude into account rather than descend into impossible sedimentations. Thus, Lacan and his heirs retain the possibility of avoiding conflation of the unconscious as an ontic matter with that of its historically ontological structure. Still, in the main, the philosophical supports for Lacanian analysis have mostly originated in forms of German Idealism, and while these perspectives avoid reductive operationalism of unconscious life, they also fall prey to forms of metaphysics that obscure the historical emergence of the unthought as the dynamic unconscious. Returning the Lacanian project to its grounding through historical ontology will require a joining of Foucauldian insight into discursive problematization and subjectification with Heidegger's hermeneutic understanding of the clearing, and the withdrawal of being, or concealment. In other words, the problem of how the Lacanian unconscious itself arises as a problem implicating knowledge and its disappearance for the subject must be approached by reference to the appearance and disappearance of, and phenomena within, historical worlds

DOI: 10.4324/9781003394327-7

themselves. In what follows, I will first examine Foucauldian perspectives on unthought as the unconscious within the modern period before locating these problems within Heidegger's analysis of concealment and unconcealment. Second, I will position the Lacanian subject of the unconscious, where repression operates via the signifier to produce lack – as a particular form of un/concealment arising from strife between earth and world. Finally, I will offer insight into Lacanian subjectification as a historically emergent form of ethics.

The Unthought as the Dynamic Unconscious and as Concealment

Foucault (1966/1973) argues that the classical episteme of the Enlightenment – as unproblematic, transparent representation – falls into crisis at the beginning of the nineteenth century. The masterful *cogito* cannot account for its foundation as an ideal gaze presiding over synchronically arranged taxonomic grids of knowledge. Consequently, in so many philosophical forms – in rationalist and empiricist inquiries – epistemic limit finds a vanishing point. For Descartes (1641/2008), an external guarantor in the presence of God is summoned to ground the rational intelligibility of world that precedes us. The logical necessity of prior events and involvements portending gaps in remembering or access require an ontotheological warrant providing a correspondence of *thinking* and *being*, one that Lacan will reverse. Similarly for Leibniz (1686/1991), *petites perceptions* which are confused and clouded with appetition or sentiment must be clarified through an apperceptive peak of logically necessary analyses, culminating in the discernment of God's teleological cause. For Spinoza (1687/1992), an epistemic point of disappearance involves that of the necessarily inadequate basis for rational intuition, always already mired in conative direction and striving, and the immanent deconstruction of will and causality. The various empiricist rejoinders continue to work themselves out in the shadow of representation, culminating in conundrums of primary against secondary qualities and the point of access for such distinctions (i.e., Locke), further theological justifications (i.e., Berkeley) or abject skepticism (i.e., Hume). In these philosophical forms, variously reliant on ideal representation or rational intuition, the location of entry invariably recedes into logically aporetic, or impossibly and theologically distant, positions. The philosophical solution to this conundrum, as chronicled by Foucault (1966/1973), manifests in Kant (1781/2007), where the limits of knowledge as a matter of the subject's own transcendental capacities become structural for a finite subject. Foucault (1966/1973) continues his scrutiny of the modern episteme through an examination of the modern empirical sciences wherein foundations of knowledge increasingly find themselves emanating from historico-temporality – i.e., grounding in the unfolding of events within the world. As related herein, what engages

Foucault's interest is the emergence of the human sciences (e.g., psychology) and their relation to epistemic incongruities in validating their claims. That is, to found such claims to knowledge in a historically grounded subject would problematize concomitant claims to universality. For example, psychological research is never able to provide a full account of its object – i.e., the sedimented qualities and attributes of human beings. The inquiring subject's own transcendental conditions withdraw in response to the shifting *techne* and pragmatic ends bringing them to light. This doubling of subject and empirical object always involves a referential overflow into worlded background, with its darkened periphery. As Foucault (1966/1973) argues, an analytic of finitude – expressing an empirico-transcendental doublet, conjoined with a return and retreat of the origin (which touches the problem of time), as well the *cogito* and the unthought – plague efforts to establish the security of enduring knowledge.

Pursuant to the analytic of finitude, non-knowledge that under the classical Enlightenment episteme eluded the transcendental subject as an ideal gaze, that became evacuated into a void of reference, arrives within shifting and worlded engagements touching the subject as object to itself. In other words, this properly modern subject becomes alienated or *other to itself*, not as an indication to exterior being-in-itself but as exterior to its *own being*. In previous writings, I have suggested that this impasse – involving the return and retreat of the origin – relates to the genesis of traumatic temporality (Roberts, 2018). Thus, also on the plane of temporality, traumatic suffering links to the enigma of the *cogito* and unthought, where alterity hidden in the subject's own being upsets the psy-disciplines' efforts to close the circuit of human being. As such, the rotation of thinking and being – the dream of the Enlightenment thought from Descartes through its destruction in Hume – spawns an alienation in the subject as the unthought, "not lodged in man like a shriveled-up nature or a stratified history; it is, in relation to man, the Other" (Foucault, 1966/1973, 326). As Foucault argues, at the beginning of the nineteenth century, after Kant – the final arbiter of how the experience of nature might offer necessary judgments about the world – the question becomes "How can man think what does not think, inhabit as though by a mute occupation something that eludes him, animate with a kind of frozen movement that figure of himself that takes the form of stubborn exteriority?" (Foucault, 1966/1973, 323). The historical answers to this question span a continuum from the sedimentations of economic thought to philosophies of negation, or the underside of phenomenology. Still, any attempt bringing the unthought closer into illumination also push it farther beyond the horizon of thought, which Boothby (2001) notes in situating Foucault's unthought as an ineffaceable other of cogent representation. As mentioned, for the human sciences, the exteriority of knowledge maintains a fissure in being that is captured in biopolitical administrations of the psy-disciplines, which both bring the unthought closer and simultaneously obscure other possibilities.

Regarding unthought as the dynamic unconscious, representationalist psy-discourses reifying the nature of the suffering subject have contributed most notably to the pernicious problem that Foucault describes as falling into an "anthropological sleep." By way of positive knowledge, unthought itself becomes seduced into distorting illuminations. The historical origin of these efforts extends from Mesmerism through Puységur's modification opening into a theory and practice of hypnosis (Ellenberger, 1970). As is well known, Freudian constructions follow in the wake of hypnosis as formulated in the Nancy School (e.g., Hippolyte Bernheim) and especially the Salpêtrière school that locates Charcot's (1889) contributions to theory of "second mental states." French psychiatric contexts of double consciousness, related to trauma and multiple personality – including the work of Janet (1925) and Ribot (1882) – are well historicized by Hacking (1995), and the legacy of German Romantic medicine is sketched by Ellenberger (1970). Early psychoanalytic thinking and practice, thus, constellate in the effort to give a natural science footing to the speculative enterprises of the Romantic age, an early expression of which is evident in Freud's (1895/1950) "Project for a Scientific Psychology." Other psychological-scientific sources for Freud's formulations include Brentano, Meynert, and Herbart. Though complicated with sociological (Freud, 1930/1961) and hermeneutic leanings (Ricoeur, 1977), Freud (1923/1961, 1905/2000) never abandoned an ever-changing scientific model of the subject framed through structural divisions and bent towards a hydraulic conception of psychic energy finding its epiphenomenal form in embodied sexuality. Freudian psychoanalysis, as the twentieth century unfolded, would produce several iterations. In the main, these generational changes privilege the subject's early relationships at the expense of drive theory, and often presume a theoretical/empirical foundation in the analyst's own experiential reporting through case studies. From the object relations theories of Klein, Fairbairn Winnicott, and Kohut (Greenberg and Mitchell, 1983), through the interpersonal school of Sullivan and his successors (e.g., Stern, 2003), we find the psychoanalytic subject as developmentally etched with unconscious dynamics that are predominantly relational, and often painful and self-defeating. Janetian understandings continue to compete with classical Freudian practice, and the relational tradition – borrowing from neuro-cognitivist perspectives on trauma (e.g., Putnam, 1997) – conjoins Freud's repressive hypothesis with discourse on dissociation. In the light of relational and Bionian approaches (e.g., Ogden, 2016) that follow Klein, the analyst's position as a container for unformulated experience, and the symbolic appearance of truth in a dyadic in-between, also mirror a rhetorical style of scientific justification. As such, the analyst's own theoretical ruminations, and countertransferential self-reflection on the unconscious as emergent in process, merge with the client's report. Post-Freudian variations so described exhibit a continuum between strongly representationalist depictions of unconscious life (as repressed sexuality, for instance) to weakly representationalist ones foregrounding in-process symbolic utterance (e.g., Ogden, 2016). Nonetheless, a commitment to Freud's original aim of producing a natural science justification for psychoanalysis continues in forms of neuropsychoanalysis and others (Brakel, 2009), seeking to bring the Freudian project back within the orbit of general psychology.

The German Idealist philosophical tradition expresses, perhaps, the most archaic lineage pertaining to the historical emergence of the dynamic unconscious, installing Foucault's doubling of the subject as unthought into the very fabric of being. Ffytche (2011) and McGrath (2011) have recently explored the legacy of Schelling for psychoanalysis, and others such as Mills (2012) illuminate the Hegelian position. Žižek (1989) and his supporters (e.g., Johnston, 2008) advocate for a convergence of Freudo-Lacanian psychoanalysis with its putative origin running from Kant to Fichte, Schelling, Hegel, and Schopenhauer, and their heirs. In a broad view, the thread running throughout this tradition is that of a divided human subject expressing contradictory and opposing impulses *within the natural order itself.* As observed by Altman and Coe (2013), and as signaled in Foucault (1966/1973), Kant (1781/2007) anticipates Freudian thinking through extending the possibility of deterministic knowledge of ourselves, yet – through its phenomenal, not noumenal, character – only by degree. The post-Kantian, Fichtean (1796–99/1992) effort is to challenge Kant's dogmatic epistemological empiricism through discerning the "unknown root" that would mediate between a direct realism and the positing activity of the "I" or self. Such selfhood is an act, a doing intertwined with knowing, always finite and embodied. Through its encounter with the resistance of the "not-I," the *Anstoss*, the self comes to find in its being concrete manifestations of finitude. Schelling, however, attempts to find a deeper ground for the subject-object divide, which is framed as a non-ground of being, containing a "preponderant mass of unreason," that may be apprehended in a potentially revelatory "self-appropriation" of the striving/desiring underlying worldly phenomena. McGrath (2011) contends that the middle Schelling (1815/2000) foresees contemporary psychoanalysis, where a dark ground of being (*das Seyn*), retreating and without otherness, stands out of itself in existing (*das Seyende*), generating rupture capable of affective unification. This may be overcome in a Jungian gesture of integrative return, yet the Žižekian and materialist reading of middle Schelling expresses the subject's alienation as emergent from a constitutive lack in its being eliciting desire for exteriority emanating out of the dark ground, and its retrospective fantasy of being fulfilled. Within this logic of an oscillation of mind passing through contingent forms of life, Hegel's (1807/1977) gambit is the most far-reaching in positioning the splitting of being as a dialectical overcoming, originating in a metaphysical idealism touching the subjective, objective, and absolute. Consequently, within the unfolding of the mind in the world, Hegel pins fate onto perpetual negation, having both subjective and objective trajectories. As is well known, in the master-servant dialectic, recalling Kojève's (1947/1980) influence on Lacan, consciousness itself is projected outside of itself and mirrored back as exteriority. As Johnston (2008) notes for Žižek, the unconscious as unthought in the Hegelian understanding surpasses a merely epistemically ungraspable reality, and subject and substance are outside themselves in perpetual negation. Significantly, this bifurcation of the subject continues throughout the nineteenth century in Schopenhauer, where will and representation form a fundamental antagonism, which become explicit sources for Freud's early formulations (Gödde, 2010), and in the neo-Romantic and synthetic accounts of the unconscious of C. G. Carus, writing in shadow of Schelling, and von Hartmann's appropriation of Hegel and Schopenhauer (Gardner, 2010).

It is difficult to overestimate the influence of German Idealist philosophy on conceptions of the unconscious taken up in the Freudian legacy, in its natural science forms, more experience-near guises (e.g., Kohut), its heresies (e.g., Jung), or its structuralist revisions in Lacanian theory. For our purposes, what links this philosophical ancestry, especially, to the attempts of the psy-disciplines to fashion discourses around a psychodynamic conception of the unconscious is a bent toward essentializing a dynamic unconscious life in ways that obscure or distort its historical appearance. Representationalist depictions drawn on through the psy-disciplines posit underlying neo-evolutionary, developmental, interpersonal bases resting on conflict between affective and symbolic forms of life, though more phenomenologically and narratively inflected approaches somewhat escape this tendency. In parallel, overtly metaphysical accounts drawn from the philosophical tradition of German Idealism – informing the entire trajectory of the psychoanalytic endeavor – locate a tension between a non-rational Real and its symbolic mediation as exteriority in the *things-in-themselves*. As Foucault writes:

> The whole of modern thought is imbued with the necessity of thinking the unthought – of reflecting the contents of the *In-itself* in the form of the *For-itself*, of ending man's alienation by reconciling him with his own essence.
>
> (Foucault, 1966/1973, 327)

To apprehend the dynamic unconscious as a historical emergence, it would be necessary to bracket such metaphysically laden understandings and, instead, treat the appearance of the unthought as related to the gaps and lacunae that appear in our worlded relation to ourselves. Without fictionalizing, or exposing its nature as "constructed," the dynamic unconscious may be approached through the conditions of its appearance and disappearance. As such, the unthought discloses simultaneous and related forms of concealment and unconcealment. Something withdraws from illumination, as something is brought into view. Thus, it would seem a wider process is at work, one involving the historically ontological character of the unthought, and those at work within any epoch. Foucault's reliance on Heidegger signals a historical analysis that would pay due attention to movements of unthought, as a matter of hiddenness and disclosure, which would avoid unnecessary rationalist intuition as to an underlying metaphysics, or scientistic and positivistic reductions. Moreover, to examine this process *in vivo* it may be beneficial to attend to forms of psychoanalysis positioning themselves within present and absent manifestations of life occurring within the structure of the unthought. Consequently, alongside Foucault's Heideggerian leaning is his oblique nomination of Freudo-Lacanian psychoanalysis – its concern with Death, Desire, and Law – as that which "leaps over representation, overflows it on the side of finitude" (Foucault, 1966/1973, 374) traversing the epistemological space that would suture the analytic of finitude rather than necessarily dwell within its vortex.

Withdrawal and Concealment

In its hermeneutic approach to ontology – i.e., in overcoming the onto-theological tendencies of representationalism, idealism, or naïve realism – Heideggerian understanding of the historical clearing of being may avoid the trap of substantializing the unconscious. Heidegger (1989/2012) finds in the history of Dasein's relation to being a pernicious tendency, stretching from the pre-Socratics to the advent of modern *techne*, to obscure being as *phusis* – as presencing, coming into the open, coming forth into light, gathering, or "eventing." In this continuance, Western philosophical and scientific traditions have translated the flux of appearance and disappearance into a nihilistic elsewhere, namely the interplay between substance and *logos*, entity and idea. Positioning an historical ontology of the dynamic unconscious back within Heideggerian origins, as worlded occurrence, confronts us with Dasein's own involvement in 1) concealment and unconcealment, and 2) the epochal withdrawal of being. Heidegger's enigmatic phrase, "Language is the house of being" pertains to the originary way that language binds itself to truth as *Aletheia*, or unconcealment: "Language is the law-giving gathering and therefore the openness of the structure of beings ... Something previously inaccessible and veiled is torn from its concealment and set into un-concealment, ἀλήθεια, that is, truth" (Heidegger, 2001/2010, 91). This hermeneutic outlook gives language a world-forming power, gathering phenomena together through Dasein, and setting out the visible contours of what is brought into unconcealedness against what withdraws or is concealed. More pointedly here, Heidegger (1987/2001) warns against blindly accepting Freudian repression, and the unconscious, as a retreat into the methods of the natural sciences. As Heidegger illuminates, "Concealment belongs to the clearing ... In the proper sense the clearing of *concealment* [*Lichtung des Sich-Verbergen*] means that the inaccessible shows and manifests itself as such – as the inaccessible" (Heidegger and Boss, 1987/2001, 183). According to Sheehan (2015), Heidegger's lecture "On the Essence of Truth" constitutes a profound shift in his thinking, wherein he articulates that it is the undisclosed facing of the clearing, its inherent hiddenness in its appropriation, that is its essence: "The concealment of beings as a whole, un-truth proper, is older than every openedness of this or that being. It is older even than letting-be itself" (Heidegger, 1967/1998, 148).

Wrathall (2010) outlines several aspects of Heidegger's view of truth, differentiating forms of concealment that may guide an understanding of the unthought as unconscious. First, unconcealment involves uncovering entities or phenomena that may be potentially disclosed – i.e., *there is a place for them in the world* – but are concealed because we lack the skill or attention to do, *or* because we have fallen into commonplace coping or constriction. In other words, we must engage in an artful and courageous discernment of entities and phenomena to bring them into any possible illuminated comportment. Heidegger writes, "Truth originally means what has been wrested from hiddenness ... The hiddenness can be of various kinds: closing off, hiding away, disguising, covering over, masking, dissembling" (Heidegger and Boss, 1987/2001, 171). Many received psychoanalytic renderings of the unconscious reside within possibilities that already flesh out a *world* – whether we are talking in the usual way about repressed or dissociated affect, relationality, or disavowed elements of selfhood. Even those analytic approaches drawn from phenomenology or hermeneutics continue a neo-Freudian tendency to draw out reified "expectations, interpretive patterns, and meanings, especially those formed in the contexts of psychological trauma – losses, deprivations, shocks, injuries, violations, and the like ... as prereflectively unconscious" (Stolorow, Orange, and Atwood, 2002, 45) or theorize an "unformulated experience" (Stern, 2003). Second, as Wrathall suggests, unconcealment and concealment touch the epochal presencing and withdrawing of worlds. As Dreyfus (2003) remarks, worlds open and close – and Dasein flashes up in Homeric Greece as hero or slave, in the Middle Ages as saint or sinner, or more recently as someone struggling with neurosis and unbearable affect, and its expression. Early on, Breuer and Freud (1895/2000) find the root of hysterical symptoms in trauma, and the "strangulated affect" given effect in this wounding, which Freud (1915/1957) would later intimately connect with repression of the representative of the instincts, and its trace in memory. Beyond Freud, Cushman (1995) notes in his historical study of psychodynamic psychotherapy that in the case of object-relations and Kohutian theory, troublesome affects are seen as fallout empathic failures in parenting, which specifically arise in a neo-Romantic, modern world where affect is the mainspring of authentic relational life. And, is it not precisely these tensions that psychoanalytic *techne* shares with its philosophical forebears in forms of German Idealism? Does psychoanalysis not recapitulate at the level human science the worlded emergence of the self and Not-I, the non-rational ground over against otherness or representation, or the negation of the thing by the word? Because being withdraws, and forms of worldedness are eclipsed by other possible worlds, psychoanalytic formulations or their metaphysical formulations also belong to this passing away. In a Foucauldian turn, the withdrawal of certain forms of self-understanding, such as those that place the subject within a great chain of being or ideal point of reflection, have given way in the modern period to a different configuration. Importantly for the human sciences, especially, is the emergent episteme of historicality – replacing representation or resemblance – not necessarily characterized by negation but by nihilation.

Historicality brings to light a third dimension of concealment/unconcealment – *a concealing or unconcealing where worlding itself is at stake*. Wrathall emphasizes how the ready apprehension and availability of beings in a world depends on the invisibility of things showing themselves *as* showing, well described by Withy's (2017, 2022) distinction of *kruptesthai*, or self-concealing where worlding itself is concealed, from *lethe* (prior concealment) or *kruptein* (other concealment). Withy writes that self-concealing requires that "the worlding of the world can happen if, when it does, that the very worlding is hidden from us" (Withy, 2017, 1510). Heidegger (1989/2012) writes of the withdrawal or withholding of being as the abyssal ground (*Ab-grund*), the essence of truth, which is that of "staying away." This is not a pure nothingness as a lack in being itself – as it might be argued in Hegelian renderings of Lacanian psychoanalysis – but a holding back, related to a dislodgement of a particular historically worlded clearing made possible by self-concealing. The untruth that must accompany truth – as withholding or withdrawal – of the event of appropriation (*Ereignis*) rests on the abyssal ground, the oscillation of clearing and concealment that protrudes in a time and place as a gathering embrace. The self-concealing of the clearing affords a "sheltering" to what is unconcealed in worldedness. Moreover, Heidegger (1956/1971) also speaks of the intersection of world, withdrawal, and earth, the last term elaborated in his later work in the fourfold (earth, sky, gods, mortals). In an earlier formulation, the worlding of the world takes on the position of the self-disclosing openness, where historical worlds occur and are displaced, and the earth occupies the role as the groundless ground of the world, a self-secluding withdrawing that draws the world back into it. For Heidegger at this stage, the earth expresses a materiality that – in conjunction and disjunction with worldedness – allows for oscillation of *beyng*. The relation of world and earth is one of strife: "The earth is not simply the Closed but rather that which rises up as a self-closing. World and earth are always intrinsically and essentially in conflict" (Heidegger, 1956/1971, 53). As Mitchell (2015) notes, Heidegger's discussion of earth includes stones, water, plants, but also animals, and such an account often veers toward anthropocentrism; however, another view is also supported. Heidegger (1959/1971) who, in a treatment of the poetry of George Trakl, speaks of the "blue deer" who enters the twilight of mortality, of the excentric reaching out to the beyond as being-toward-death, allows a blurring of the mortal and animal (Mitchel, 2015). Furthermore, what also is implied here is how *beyng* self-conceals through earth's withdrawal, and how Dasein's animality is related to world. In other words, Dasein, given over to the clearing by the later Heidegger as "Da-sein," becomes the very location of historical selfhood in "the 'there': the open, clearing-concealing 'between' in relation to earth and world, the center of their strife" (Heidegger, 1989/2012, 255). For the truth of the clearing, then, what is engaged in our inquiry is the sheltering of being through its withholding, canceling, or the pound of flesh extracted in the withdrawal of being through Da-sein's own earthly abyssal grounding.

The Problem of the Lacanian Unconscious as Repression

The confluence of Heideggerian perspectives with that of Foucault will, perhaps, allow a discernment of how the unthought as unconscious in its Lacanian form – as un/concealment – would find its way into the modern epoch, and how specifically it would insinuate itself into the being of the subject as problem. In this pursuit, it may serve to place Heidegger's notion of *Ereignis* in dialogue with Foucault's concept of "problematization." Often translated as "enowning," "the event" or "the event of appropriation," *Ereignis* allows a distinctly different vantage point on Dasein's relation to its worldedness, existence, and concealment. Heidegger writes that "in the essence of truth of the event, everything true is simultaneously decided and grounded, beings come to be, and nonbeings slip into the semblance of beyng" (Heidegger, 1989/2012, 21). *Ereignis*, thus, pertains to the thrown-openness of ex-sistence (appearance) and appropriating as belonging (occurring) to the clearing in its thrownness (*Geworfenheit*). Foucault, writing under Heidegger's influence, reflects on the history of truth as it touches the subject through the "*problematizations* through which being offers itself to be, necessarily, thought" (Foucault, 1984/1990, 11) and practiced. Raynor (2007) observes that Foucault's (1984/1990) problematization parallels *Ereignis* as "eventalization" (*événementialisation*). Critically, what is problematized, or gathered in the historical event of the modern period concerns the unthought as a form of withdrawal that in epistemic terms results in aporetic impossibility, though in Heideggerian ontology pertaining to a sheltering for what arises as truth. As de Boer (2000) argues, in dialogue with Hegel, Heidegger refigures negation from privation as an essential absence (*steresis*) to withdrawal in which absencing occurs as a positive condition. As with so much German Idealist philosophy, Hegel's perpetual negation lies beyond the ken of human understanding, a perpetual and naturalistically endowed overcoming that may actualize its full potentiality. As de Boer goes on to suggest, Heidegger radicalizes Hegel's negativity in locating it fully within the historical light from which it appears and by understanding the "not" as nihilation, as always denying us the possibility of turning to the thingliness of beings as entity or substance for grounded security:

> This "not" must be distinguished from the negativity that is rendered harmless by reducing it to the force which derives the absolute toward its own completion. We may now infer that the "strife within being itself" pertains to the strife between a mode of being that is pervaded by the "not" and a mode of being that expels this "not" from itself to become constant presence.
>
> (de Boer, 2000, 299–301)

In other words, Heidegger takes up a Hegelian trajectory, submitting it to temporality of the historical worlding of the world, and the self-concealing or nihilation that would only be apprehended phenomenally from within the clearing and not from a metaphysical access point of nowhere. The self-concealing (*kruptesthai*) occurring as the sheltering of being in the clearing would manifest in those forms of subjectification in the human sciences that – as counter-sciences – might preserve the vortex of unthought of withdrawal as the death that makes a world possible. The self-concealing of unthought at this stage may be more centrally figured within Lacan's own formulations, which – compared with other psychoanalytic discourses – move most proximately to the Real and its confrontation with the signifiers that open and close world horizons, and away from the psy-disciplines. In theorizing the Real – which may be profitably connected with Heidegger's understanding of earth in some respects – Lacan (1966/2006a) arguably places the furthest distance between conscious life and the unconscious.

In mediating the conflict or strife between drives and the civilizing matrix, Freud's (1915/1957) repression pertains not only to ideational representatives of instincts inadmissible to consciousness but also to their derivatives, including future associations. As related thereto, the problem of the Lacanian unconscious concerns the strife within the flashing up of the subject's world, and what must stay behind or remain inaccessible. As such, the self-concealing of unthought may, thus, be centrally figured within Lacan's work. In theorizing the Real effects of the unconscious – connective to Heidegger's understanding of earth – Lacan places utmost distance between the unthought and worlded life, as unified in psychological appropriations of psychoanalysis, or in metaphysical absolutisms. Markedly, for Lacan (1973/1981, 1986/1992), the unconscious is structured like language, though not identical with its processes. In a reversed parallel with Heidegger, one might say that language is the house of non-being. As such, through deferring actions of metaphor and metonymy signifiers in the unconscious work differentially, spacing out Real remainders, to disrupt any harmony of *thinking* and *being* at the level of an inversely Cartesian subject. Lacan (1973/1981), thus, writes of non-meaning occurring at the intersection of thought and being which is realized in the subject as the unconscious. This first etching of unthought, as non-sense and non-being, produces an alienation, where signifiers cross the subject's being – as a translation of demand into misrecognition. The elemental lack is, thus, inaugurated, opening a gap or void, giving rise to Lacan's understanding of the subject as a "want-to-be" (*manque-à-être*), where names bear with them unnamaeble embodiments. Relating the worlded incursions of what is *said* – with residues of nonknowledge, the leftovers of being – and the visible other, Lacan writes "the unconscious is the Other's discourse ... the beyond in which the recognition of desire is tied to desire for recognition" (Lacan, 1966/2006b, 436). In a Levinasian vein, the symbolic Other's *said* silently underwrites any answer to the imaginary other's *saying*. The receding of being from the symbolic universe finds its way into the Oedipal knot of desire, the swearing in of the typically neurotic subject's symptomatic suffering. The separation of the subject and its earthly, maternal embrace – falling out from the impossible Cartesian link, no longer guaranteed by God – retains its repressed placeholder as a primordial signifier. Thus, the paternal metaphor, as what stands in the world of thought as signified return to wholeness with the m/other's being, bars the way in its vanishing from the open clearing of possibility. The impossibility of the subject's return to the m/other and aligning its being with their being precipitates the circuits of desire emanating from the otherness of the unconscious. This second engraving, as the Name-of-the-Father, is given to the subject in the world of its origin where its repression presents a positive void, carved out of flesh by the signifier of maternal desire. In Lacan's refiguration of Cartesian unity, the paternal metaphor governing through separation is routed through metonymic search for signified derivatives. The lost unity of subject and maternal being – falling out as *objets a,* or fragments of the Real – return to cause the subject's desire. In these pathways alongside visible others circulates a promise, the fantasy that some signified happening in the subject's existence will finally authorize an intelligible answer to the other's desire. Yet, as the subjects' desire is that of the Other, Lacan writes, "A lack is encountered by the subject in the Other, in the very intimation that the Other makes to him by his discourse" (Lacan, 1973/1981, 214). Issuing from the other scene, repression becomes that absence, that shadow – cast by the forever lost object – finding its position only within memory offered through signifiers snaking their way through the future and then back toward to those historical events that will have been. From its expulsion from the open expanse in lit surroundings that might be spoken, expressed, or represented, the lost Thing – as pulled forcibly into materiality through its obverse opening in a name – may only be accounted for *après-coup* (*Nachträglichkeit*), pursuant to later events, deferred to other signifiers, and caused by yet other things. For that reason, the origin of trauma appears retroactively, arriving from the future. Traumatic temporality – the effect heralding its cause via "afterwardness" – constellates the Name-of-the-Father, in the Lacanian drama, as the blurred stain of the "I am" that illegibly persists, if not in its signified arrivals, in further failed authorizations for, and dissolutions of, life. This feverish non-arrival is none other than the death drive, which bestows upon the subject (*es gibt*) its cherished projects, its animation in meeting the world, even as the dead hand of the symbolic Other exacts the discontent of mourning, of cadaverization. The later Lacan, raising the stakes, abandons positioning the Name-of-the-Father as a metaguarantor of the symbolic order itself and, rather, radicalizes the signifier of lack in the Other as identifiable with the phallus, which carries with it desire to realize the fantasy of return. Where to return? That there is "no Other of the Other" means that the point of disappearance in the subject's being will allow for no final accounting in the symbolic order for its incursions into the subject's real history. Still, those psychoanalytic practices marching under the banner of understanding – those fixated on ego identification, early relations with relational objects, or strangulated affect – continue to find within tacit experience realities ready to be unconcealed as patterns of meaningful suffering. Such psychodynamic conveyances point outward toward an Other of the Other, offering epistemic settlements imagined from an ideal, generalized gaze that fill in and suture the unthought as it withdraws from empirical knowledge, and assign a universalist conception of the unconscious as touching both the subject, and the subject as object. The problematization of the Lacanian unconscious, thus, occurs historically in the modern period as a negation through nihilation, taken together in shearing updrafts and downdrafts of subjectivity, expressive yet materialized. The sheltering of fantasy and identification – the innumerably lived existential projects taken up – simultaneously bestows truth for the subject that recedes mercifully away and withdraws from any deterministic capturing through the dyad of the Ego Ideal and the symbolic identifications in an Ideal Ego.

The modern epoch, in its event of appropriation, gathering its world and horizons into being, provides a historical clearing for the Lacanian subject's life, disclosing the scars of its temporal disunion, its own fantasies of fulfillment according to the logic of its desire, and the Real remainders that drive it. The various horizons that signified realities obtain – as fantasies would give them imagined or realistic contours, authentic beginnings, or potentials for actualization – are emasculated by the arbitrary cuts of signifiers. If Lacanian analysis were to remain at the level of signified desire, and its explanations, concealment of the *worlding of world* would remain, as above; however, *Ereignis* as process is unconcealed, in part, because worlding through self-concealing (*kruptesthai*) is exposed in its lacunae. Lacanian perspectives allow an incomplete, yet resonant, grasp of the receding of a material earth from world, in the Heideggerian idiom, through the impossible relation of signifier to the subject's Real being, and through the subject's subsumption within its own symptom, which is meaninglessly, if stubbornly, knotted together. Lacan (2005/2016) goes on to gesture toward the gravitation of the subject's suffering and vitality around particular unconscious formations, as given through primordial signifiers and the worlded realities that be might unfeasibly assembled as fallout. The *sinthome*, as Lacan elaborates, is well depicted in James Joyce's relation to his own enjoyment in creation:

> It is so far as the unconscious is knotted to the sinthome, which is what is singular to each individual, that we may say that Joyce ... has earned the privilege of having reached the extreme point of embodying the symptom in himself.
>
> (Lacan, 2005/2016, 147)

The *sinthome* may be designated as the manner by which the unconscious, enjoyment, and the death drive find themselves coiled in a manner that may not be fully translated. Verhaeghe and Declercq (2002) distinguish the subject's relation to the jouissance and the death drive according to which one believes in their symptom – as it may stand apart from their own conception of ego or selfhood – and where one embraces embodiment with their *sinthome*, wherein it incorporates and stands before any emanation therefrom. Believing in one's symptom encircles a fantasy of a completed signification, where a complete Other will guarantee the meaning of the symptom that might be translated into the Heideggerian "as structure" of imagined possibility. Under the biopolitical and epistemic strategies of the psy-disciplines this may be revealed through certain cognitive or behavioral patterns, or in received forms of psychoanalysis undertaking detective work in uncovering fundamental conflicts, or in the here-and-now junctions of relational disturbance. These projects undercut the historical unfolding of worlds, and the process of concealment itself because there would be an Other of the Other who might guarantee the arrest of interpretation. To embody one's *sinthome*, in distinction, entangles one in the destitution arriving when one has given up answering the Oedipal question in a way that would solve the subject's uncanny relation to the world. Thus, no response completing any plausible narrative would eradicate the unthought at the heart of subjective being, the recession of being in the Nothing (*Das Nichts*). As such, Verhaeghe and Declercq suggest a different positioning, one portending the incorporation of the impossible Real, and the maelstrom of unthought, within the subject's being: "Before, the subject situated all jouissance on the side of the Other ... after this change, the subject situates jouissance in the body, in the Real of the body" (Verhaeghe and Declercq, 2002, 10). Significantly, to embody the *sinthome* is move into a different subjective structure in relation to one's ownmost history as related to historicality. The primordial signifier, as a vanishing point leaving a wound, takes up its position as unbelievable even in its all too evident effects: "This is what the subjects is missing in thinking he is exhaustively accounted for by his cogito – he is missing what is unthinkable about him" (Lacan, 1966/2006a, 694). Desire becomes possible as related to what is missing, what gives its Real effects the silhouette of loss – flesh finds its unknowable glimmering in the interstices between worlded symbolic articulation and the withdrawal of material being. In other words, Lacanian perspectives allow an incomplete sense of the receding of a material earth in the Heideggerian idiom – through the impossible relation of the signifier to the subject's Real being. In this, Lacan comes closest to Heidegger's admonition that the concealment belongs to the historical clearing as inaccessible.

Ethics and the Lacanian Unconscious

In returning to the later Foucault's (1983) work on ethics, it is possible to frame the form of subjectification inhabiting the unthought as a counter-science, in not turning away from the difficulties, the aporias occasioning the modern epoch. Put differently, how might an ethical self-relation finds its space within the problematic of the unthought as unconscious, rather than as a premature closing, a suturing of the structural dimension of historicality itself? Very schematically, Foucault (1983) sketches ethical subjectification across several dimensions, which takes ancient Greek models to heart, such as that of Aristotle – meaning ethics involves a self-cultivation that would precede any moral or normative way to live one's life. These elements encompass the ethical substance (*substance éthique*), mode of subjection (*mode d'assujettissement*), means of subjection (*practique de soi*), and aspirations of the subject (*teleologie*). The question of ethical substance pertains to those aspects of oneself concerned with moral conduct. For Greek antiquity, the ethical substance unites the unity of pleasure and desire with mastery in will and action. For older forms of Christianity, ethical substance touches the question of flesh and desire, later altered in the Cartesian moment as passions that might be rationally tracked and regulated. Candidates for a modern ethical substance would consist of, as in Kant, rational intention, or one's repressed psychosexual impasse for classical psychoanalytic thought. The mode of subjection probes *the manner* subjects are impelled to realize their moral commitments, whether that is divine command, procedural rationality, or for Kantian ethics forms of law arrived at through reason alone. Further, as regards the form of address, the means of subjection concerns the multiple forms of *techne*, the pragmatic skills or *savoir faire* facilitating the actualization of ideals – practices and techniques such as forms of confession, modern therapeutic dialogue, or the many thought and behavioral modifications currently offered in psychological self-administration. The final element in Foucault's ethical analysis relates to what is aspired to, the ends or *telos* of the subject's practices. As a historical matter, this involved self-mastery in service of the *polis*, spiritual purification, or rational freedom.

Though a more complete analysis under Foucault's ethical schema is beyond the current scope, it is possible to touch on the second (mode of subjection) and last of these elements (aspirations of the subject). Inasmuch, the Lacanian subject's mode of subjection relates most deeply to the problem facing the subject in the modern epoch – that is, the historical relation of a knowledge not mired in a totalizing intelligibility of its embodied being. The unconscious as repression for Lacan expresses an ethics emanating from the strife at the heart of the worlding of the world. Lacanian ethics does not remain at the level of a mentalized ego, in which its failures up against the analytic of finitude would amount to an epistemic collapse. In aligning the subject *within* the analytic of finitude, inside its rotations of impossibility separating thinking and being, Lacan traces the subject to its original traumatic dissolution, hollowed out as symbolic wound to earthly materiality. In examining the repressed unconscious – as ethical substance, having great similarities in Freud and Lacan – Foucault's mode of subjection, *specifically for Lacan*, involves the subject's *alienation through the signifier*. This means that the otherness that confronts the subject concerns the ways that language as the symbolic order, as not merely embracing the meaning of words, divides the subject from its Real being. For Lacan, the castration threat as imaginary, is relocated in the symbolic register as the mark, Name-of-the-Father, that will stand in for the m/other's desire forever out of reach, the symbolic phallus being what arises as worlded value and as desire (Fink, 2004). Importantly, the phallus, being the signifier of the m/other's desire, is installed in its absence. Because the phallus is missing, it is often conceived of as a positive lack yet inside the universal set of signifiers, thus amounting to an impassible contradiction (i.e., the empty set) (Muller and Richardson, 1982). Such a lack – obeying the greater logic of nihilation as negation – vibrates positively in its Real effects. So, rather than signifying sheer absence, the signifier of the lack of the Other indicates a murder of the Real that occurs only in a pure past, which nonetheless retains its problematization within the historical world. The disquieting epiphany is that there is no purely Real otherness, any potentially represented form of unthought. The Real simultaneously trespasses the boundaries of the symbolic and is fastened to it. The Thing (*das Ding*) as a fictional primordial object, as withheld through the conflict of earth and world, was always already lost, continually concealed within a world where desire might be realistically signified, and the unconscious forming the unspeakable delineations around such loss. What was forever lost has its Real effects that are both within the unconscious and without it, as an *extimacy*. The *objets petit a* (causes of desire) that arise and occupy the void as fragments of non-knowledge will become the recessions of earth which fantasies pursue. In our epoch, these often assume the moral and psychologized forms of life offered through biopolitical apparatuses that enjoin us to understand our dysfunctions and affective suffering in the realistic idioms of human science. In other words, the alienating effects of the signifier will register themselves within the modern world as desire, though their object causes might only be supposed as fragments of earth unknown to any named history but needed through the subject's life within the symbolic and imaginary. For subjects uncovering their own origins in their own time, the ethical injunction is to discern how such fundamental fantasies of fulfillment might be structured, what signifiers they may enfold, and what signified realities imaginary life may promise. Significantly, as the Name-of-the-Father amounts to an impossible simultaneous outside and inside of the symbolic order – as a positive lack – the signifiers that retroactively attempt to complete the desire inevitably run into the limit of castration. In the main, this pertains to the subject's inability to find the historical origin of its suffering, the ineradicable place of fantasy in discerning what the other wants, or what the subject takes itself to be. Because the originary signifiers that cross our existence relate to a nihilating negation that creates a Real wound or lack in being, signaling the withdrawing of being through the subject's own being, those efforts to positively signify this reality inevitably exhaust themselves in the fury, or slow burn, of everyday miseries. The task at hand bears some similarity to the familiar existentialist edict – that our experiences and histories are always subject to revision in light of the opening of future possibilities as they are understood (Heidegger, 1927/1962); however, for Lacanian ethics, the not-all of the subject's being lies not in its intact if outward facing toward an ineffable beyond. The inevitable and continual undoing from the future pertains not to an undivided subject, but to inevitable lapses of the signifier to reify the subject's being, or to find its way home to a true origin. Žižek writes of the Kantian impossibility (aligned with the First Antimony of Pure Reason) at the heart of the subject's historical encounter with unthought as signified, as a return and retreat of the origin: "The basic paradox of the psychoanalytic notion of fantasy consists in a kind of time loop ... for the subject to be present as a pure gaze before its own conception" (Žižek, 2002, 197). The modern subject's mode of subjection, therefore, relates specifically to its alienation by the signifier and through fantasied and impossible return to a completion, or signified origin of suffering in a world where the effects of marking the body are spelled out in bio-temporal tracings of desire, the lifting of the veil of concealment of one's being-in-time.

The *telos* of the Lacanian subject's accounting to itself as failure orients toward its symptomatic suturing, to the logic of the symbolic debt owed to its worldly project, errands, and relations. Following Foucault's ethical analysis, the subject's fragmented temporal being as alienation – refracting Heidegger's (1927/1962) argument in Division Two of *Being and Time* – and spawning desire, proposes another kind of revelation. Instead of authentically seizing one's pre-existent possibilities as interpreted via Heidegger, Lacan contends that "from an analytical point of view, the only thing which one can be guilty is of having given ground relative to one's desire" (Lacan 1986/1992, 319). Neill (2011) notes that Lacanian ethics is not a decree to

straightforwardly express desire or an aspect of the Real but is an acknowledgement of desire for what it is, as given over to primordial fantasies of
presence, of consolidated origins. Further, confronting desire as such
becomes nothing less than "assumption of responsibility for and as the
cause of desire that is in one" (Neill, 2011, 241). In Foucault's outlook, as
inflected through Heidegger, the subject finds its self-relation through a
legacy of worlded desire, and apart from the inheritance of possibility as
what it might find alongside itself as tool-use, or idioms of understanding, it
finds its desire emerging from the etchings, the markings this machinery
leaves on its flesh. Within the scarifications of factical origins – as Descartes'
doubt began in the embodied search for the warmth of a stove – fantasies of
desire, and who one will have been, meet the subject from the future. Retroactively enacted in a world governed by historicality, the arrival of any
fantasy of finalized identification becomes indefinitely postponed. In
addressing the release from suffering as traversal of fantasy, Lacan asks:
"What, then, does he who has passed through the experience of this opaque
relation to the origin, to the drive, become? How can a subject who has
traversed radical fantasy experience the drive?" (Lacan, 1973/1981, 273).
Traversals of fantasy engage the adoption of a different orientation to alienation in the symbolic order, that of assuming the cause of one's being –
occasioned by the downdraft of material suffering – and through desire and
its futural updraft as being-in-the-world, in a drive to death. In a sense, this
assumption amounts to the subject taking responsibility for its being-in-the-
world as correlated with the *worlding of the world*. Dasein must subjectify
those signifiers associated to the repressed and disappearing paternal metaphor the barring m/other's desire, and how the earthly splinters of its being
were withdrawn or concealed under duress having no counterfactual. Signified realities barred by the unconscious as unthought would include not
only the gentle and intimate hope of identity or generativity falling out of
Eriksonian developmental trajectories, but also the numerous ways that the
subject would find its being directed according to biopolitically framed understandings of health and disease. Consider, for instance, how interpersonal relationships might be managed through more skillful communication, or how
family systems may be arranged as to achieve boundaries with others, or that
the meaning of individuation would surround fixed coordinates of realistic ful-
filments in love and work. In the main, such projects for concluding significa-
tions assemble the appearance of that which might be archived in biopolitical
institutions. Following Foucault, Esposito (2011) suggests that subjectification as a
biopolitical matter increasingly comes under the protection of an immunizing
function. That is, to augment the vitality of the governed, immunization extends
beyond its juridico-political limits to colonize the lifeworld and its embodiment. In
its psychologized forms, the biographical dissolution of the subject, as well as its
relationships and functionality, would be sheltered through the implementa-
tions of the psy-disciplines, at the cost of asserting the adequation of knowledge

and being. Yet, such constriction brings paralysis, and concealment of world-ing itself (*kruptesthai*). In contradistinction, the Lacanian subject unearths within its own being the point of *withdrawal* for the Name-the-Father – the hollow of a chasm whose cavity in flesh arrests the signified, and whose void returns the emblems of the Real. This indispensably failed search deprives the signifier of its signified endings and fulfillments, given over to fate, and stain-ing the subject's historically material being with the imprints of trauma. Lacanian ethics, then, extends to the subject the task – worlded through his-torical temporality – of fathoming the effects that unintelligible messages have for its unfolding. And, as well, a glimpse of the path of those fantasies that have guided desire, and the subject's own truth, under an unnameable burden. This nominates the crossing of the unthought, as symbolic and worlded exteriority, into the modern subject's material being as the event of the unconscious.

References

Altman, M. C. and Coe, C. D. (2013) *The fractured self in Freud and German philo-sophy*. Palgrave.

Boothby, R. (2001) *Freud as philosopher: Metapsychology after Lacan*. Routledge.

Brakel, L. (2009) *Philosophy, psychoanalysis, and the a-rational mind*. Oxford Uni-versity Press.

Breuer, J., and Freud, S. (2000) *Studies on hysteria* (trans. J. Strachey). Basic Books. (Original work published 1895.)

Charcot, J. (1889) *Clinical lectures on diseases of the nervous system delivered at the infirmary of la Salpêtrière* (trans. G. Sigerson). New Syndenham Society.

Chiesa, L. (2007) *Subjectivity and otherness: A philosophical reading of Lacan*. MIT Press.

Cushman, P. (1995) *Constructing the self, constructing America: A cultural history of psychotherapy*. Da Capo Press.

de Boer, K. (2000) *Thinking in the light of time: Heidegger's encounter with Hegel*. SUNY Press.

Descartes, R. (2008) *Meditations on first philosophy, with selections from the objections and replies* (trans. M. Moriarty). Oxford University Press. (Original work published 1641.)

Dreyfus, H. (2003) "Being and power" revisited. In A. Milchman and A. Rosenberg (Eds.), *Foucault and Heidegger: Critical encounters*. University of Minnesota Press, pp. 30–54.

Ellenberger, H. (1970) *The discovery of the unconscious: The history and evolution of dynamic psychiatry*. Basic Books.

Esposito, R. (2011). *Immunitas: The protection and negation of life*. Polity.

Ffytche, M. (2011) *The foundation of the unconscious: Schelling, Freud, and the Birth of the Modern Psyche*. Cambridge University Press.

Fichte, J. G. (1992) *The Foundation of Transcendental Philosophy* (trans. D. Breazeale). Cornell University Press. (Original work published 1796/99.)

Fink, B. (2004) *Lacan to the letter: Reading Écrits closely.* University of Minnesota Press.

Foucault, M. (1973) *The order of things: An archaeology of the human sciences* (trans. A. Sheridan). Vintage. (Original work published 1966.)

Foucault, M. (1983) The subject and power. In H. Dreyfus and P. Rabinow (Eds.), *Michel Foucault: Beyond structuralism and hermeneutics.* University of Chicago Press, pp. 208–226.

Foucault, M. (1990) *The history of sexuality, volume 2: The use of pleasure* (trans. R. Hurley). Vintage. (Original work published 1984.)

Freud, S. (1950) Project for a scientific psychology. In J. Strachey (Ed. and Trans.), *The standard edition of the complete psychological works of Sigmund Freud.* Vol. 1. Hogarth Press., pp. 281–391. (Original work published 1895.)

Freud, S. (1957) Repression. In J. Strachey (Ed. and Trans.), *The standard edition of the complete psychological works of Sigmund Freud.* Vol. 14. Hogarth Press., pp. 141–158. (Original work published 195.)

Freud, S. (1961) The ego and the id. In J. Strachey (Ed. and Trans.), *The standard edition of the complete psychological works of Sigmund Freud.* Vol. 19. Hogarth Press., pp. 1–59. (Original work published 1923.)

Freud, S. (2000) *Three essays on sexuality* (trans. J. Strachey). Basic. (Original work published 1905.)

Gardner, S. (2010) Eduard von Hartmann's Philosophy of the Unconscious. In A. Nicholls and M. Liebscher (Eds.), *Thinking the Unconscious: Nineteenth-century German thought.* Cambridge University Press, pp. 173–199.

Gödde, G. (2010) Freud and nineteenth-century philosophical sources on the unconscious. In A. Nicholls and M. Liebscher (Eds.), *Thinking the Unconscious: Nineteenth-century German thought.* Cambridge University Press, pp. 261–286.

Greenberg, J. R.., and Mitchel, S. A. (1983) *Object relations in psychoanalytic theory.* Harvard University Press.

Hacking, I. (1995) *Rewriting the soul: Multiple personality and the sciences of memory.* Princeton University Press.

Heidegger, M. (1962) *Being and time* (trans. J. Macquarrie and E. Robinson). Harper. (Original work published 1927.)

Heidegger, M. (1971) The origin of the work of art (A. Hofstadter, Trans.). In M. Heidegger, *Poetry, language, thought.* Harper, pp. 17–86. (Original work published 1956.)

Heidegger, M. (1971) Language in the poem: Discussion on Georg Trakl's poetic work (P. Hertz, Trans.). In M. Heidegger, *On the way to language.* Harper, pp. 159–198. (Original work published 1959.)

Heidegger, M. (1998) On the essence of truth (trans. J. Sallis). In W. McNeill, *Pathmarks.* Cambridge University Press. (Original work published 1967.)

Heidegger, M. (2010) *Being and truth* (trans. G. Fried and R. Polt). Indiana University Press. (Original work published 2001.)

Heidegger, M. (2012) *Contributions to philosophy (from enowning)* (trans. R. Rojcewicz and D. Vallega-Neu). Indiana University Press. (Original work published 1989.).

Heidegger, M., and Boss, M. (Eds.) (2001) *Zollikon seminars: Protocols-conversations-letters* (trans. F. May and R. Askay). (Original work published 1987.)

Hegel, G. W. F. (1977) *The Phenomenology of Spirit* (trans. A. V. Miller). Oxford University Press. (Original work published 1807.)

Janet, P. (1925) *Psychological healing. Vol.* 1. Macmillan.

Johnston, A. (2008) *Žižek's ontology: A transcendental materialist theory of subjectivity.* Northwestern University Press.

Kant, I. (2007) *Critique of pure reason* (trans. M. Weigelt). Penguin. (Original work published 1781.)

Kojève, A. (1980) *Introduction to the reading of Hegel: Lectures on The Phenomenology of Spirit.* Ithaca, NY: Cornell University Press. (Original work published 1947)

Lacan, J. (1981) *The four fundamental concepts of psycho-analysis* (trans. A. Sheridan). Norton. (Original work published 1973.)

Lacan, J. (2006a) The subversion of the subject and the dialectic of desire (trans. B. Fink). In *Écrits: The first complete edition in English.* Norton, pp. 671–702. (Original work published 1966.)

Lacan, J. (2006b) The instance of the letter in the unconscious (trans. B. Fink). In *Écrits: The first complete edition in English.* Norton, pp. 412–441. (Original work published 1966.)

Lacan, J. (2006c) Science and truth (trans. B. Fink). In *Écrits: The first complete edition in English.* Norton, pp. 726–745. (Original work published 1966.)

Lacan, J., and Miller, J.-A. (Ed.) (1992). *The seminar of Jacques Lacan: Book VII, the ethics of psychoanalysis, 1959–1960* (trans. D. Porter). Norton. (Original work published 1986.)

Lacan, J., and Miller, J-A (Ed.) (2016). *The seminar of Jacques Lacan: Book XXIII, the sinthome, 1959–1960* (trans. A. R. Price). Polity Press. (Original work published 2005.)

Leibniz, G. W. (1991) Discourse on metaphysics. In *Discourse on metaphysics and other essays* (ed. and trans. D. Garber and R. Ariew). Hackett. (Original work published 1686.)

McGrath, S. J. (2011) *The dark ground of spirit: Schelling and the unconscious.* Routledge.

Mills, J. (2012) *The unconscious abyss: Hegel's anticipation of psychoanalysis.* SUNY Press.

Mitchel, A. (2015) *The fourfold: Reading the late Heidegger.* Northwestern University Press.

Muller, J. P. and Richardson, W. J. (1982) *Lacan and language: A reader's guide to Écrits.* International Universities Press.

Neill, C. (2011) *Lacanian ethics and the assumption of subjectivity.* Palgrave Macmillan.

Ogden, T. H. (2016) *Reclaiming unlived life: Experiences in psychoanalysis.* Routledge.

Putnam, F. W. (1997) *Dissociation in children and adolescents.* Guilford.

Raynor, T. (2007) *Foucault's Heidegger: Philosophy and transformative experience.* Continuum.

Ribot, T. A. (1882) *Diseases of the memory: An essay in the positive psychology.* Kegan Paul, Trench.

Ricoeur, P. (1977) *Freud and philosophy: An essay on interpretation* (trans. D. Savage). New Yale University Press.

Roberts, J. L. (2018) *Trauma and the ontology of the modern subject: Historical studies in philosophy, psychology, and psychoanalysis.* Routledge.

Schelling, F. W. J. (2000) *The ages of the world* (trans. J. M. Wirth). State University of New York. (Original work published 1815.)

Sheehan, T. (2015) *Making sense of Heidegger: A paradigm shift.* Rowman and Littlefield.

Spinoza, B. (1992) *Ethics: Treatise on the emendation of the intellect, and selected letters* (trans. S. Shirley). Hackett. (Original work published 1687.)

Soler, C. (2014) *Lacan – The unconscious reinvented* (trans. E. Faye and S. Schwartz). Routledge.

Stern, D. B. (2003) *Unformulated experience: From dissociation to imagination in psychoanalysis.* The Analytic Press.

Stolorow, R., Atwood, G., and Orange, D. (2002) *Worlds of experience: Interweaving philosophical and clinical dimensions in psychoanalysis.* Basic Books.

Verhaeghe, P., and Declerq, F. (2002) Lacan's analytical goal: "Le sinthome" or the feminine way. In L. Thurston (Ed.), *Essays on the final Lacan: Re-inventing the symptom.* The Other Press, pp. 59–83.

Withy, K. (2017) Concealing and concealment in Heidegger. *European Journal of Philosophy,* 25(4), pp. 1496–1513.

Withy, K. (2022) *Heidegger on being self-concealing.* Oxford University Press.

Wrathall, M. (2010) Unconcealment. In M. A. Wrathall (Ed.), *Heidegger and unconcealment: Truth, Language, and History.* Cambridge University Press, pp. 11–39.

Žižek, S. (1989) *The sublime object of ideology.* Verso.

Žižek, S. (2002) *For they know not what they do: Enjoyment as a political factor.* Verso.

Chapter 7

Confessions and Quantum Uncertainties

The Violence of Language, Organismic Cells, and the Incarnation of Words

Nahanni Freeman

Politically-motivated rhetoric marginalizes the pursuit of the impeccability of language, forging an invalidating cultural war against "political correctness." Consumed like miasma, this rhetoric legitimizes hegemony, justifies systems of oppression, and minimizes awareness of the transformative and violent power of language. Resurfacing, recycling, there remain the mutations, the resistant viral forms, of cultural narratives that perseverate, for humans have "image-making habits" (Watson, 1982). The projected image emerges in racial stereotypes, undergirding a symbiotic word-image connectivity, which is also mapped onto neural networks. The attempt to reduce, classify, and essentialize is endemic to political and journalistic discourse, accentuating the divide the divide between self and Other. The relationship between images and words is conjoined, clarifying meaning while also preparing the possibility of stereotypic representations and motivated persuasive campaigns. While flaws are "inherent to images," the ability to critique images is essential to their responsible usage, and may awaken reason and awareness of higher forms beyond the world of imitation and appearance (Smith, 2007, 12).

This chapter will seek to examine language in its many permutations, including its inculcation from sociocultural, religious and historical forces, and its emergence within a developmental context that includes interiorization into private speech. The limitations of language for simulating the mind of the Other, the distance between minds, and the constant dynamism of words will be evaluated in light of the theme of the value of recognizing subjectivity and acknowledging layers of meaning in the quest for truth and legitimacy. Metaphors of the body are used to represent ecological and systemic forces in language, also emphasizing the potency of mind-word-body interactions for immune functions. Reconciliation with the Other will be reviewed within the context of transcendent self-examination and dawning consciousness. Ultimately the power of the word, and the quest for confessional atonement, are prospected here.

As invented signification, naming attempts to create boundaries around what is known; this mutates into marginalization in political polarities and

DOI: 10.4324/9781003394327-8

cultural hegemonies. Lacan speaks to the web-like, symbolic construction of the sentence, adding that a principal task "is to not become poisoned by this sentence that always continues circulating and seeks only to re-emerge in a thousand more or less camouflaged and disturbing forms" (Lacan, 1955/1993, 113). Recounting the work of Thomas Szlezák, Bowery points out that narrative frames and precautions may function as "hermeneutic keys" (Bowery, 2007, 83). Language can alter consciousness, symbolize violence and annihilation of the Other, and yet in more adaptive contexts may transform, heal, and help to solidify a self, as observed in the case of atoning confession. Ultimately, language has the power to transfigure matter, as observed in the epigenetic changes within the human body that arise in response to trauma. Attacks on "political correctness" are observed as non-compassionate forms of denial of personal responsibility for the ethical usage of this powerful medium; by de-emphasizing the significance of language, permission for violent linguistic replication and egocentrism is offered. The notion that meaning and transcendent self-examination emerge within the space between the listener and the narrator is expanded from Bowery (2007, 90).

Interiorization, Transformation and Emergentism

An epigenetic change alters what is manifest, yielding material plasticity in response to environmental stimulation, trauma, and internalizing of the exterior world. Introjection of prejudicial and sexist language into the self-system may prompt epigenetic changes in egocentric inner speech and embodied matter. Internalized prejudice risks opaque effects for individuation, orientation toward the world, coping, and may stunt linguistic development by truncating the transition from interpsychic to intrapsychic function (Vygotsky, 1934/1986). The interiorization of language and cultural patterns into the unconscious is described by Sapir as a "condensation of energy" (Sapir, 1949, 556, 564).

One form of interiorization is inherently social. While both Vygotsky (1934/1986) and Wittgenstein (1945/2009) examine the social functions of language, the latter's skepticism about private language suggests a mechanism and pragmatism that limits the creative and transcendent functions. Nevertheless, Wittgenstein's focus on the invented aspects of signification may imply the emotional and spiritual damage of arbitrary classifications, and he refers to naming as an "occult" process, "like the baptism of an object" (Wittgenstein, 1945/2009, 23).

The current project will seek to examine co-existing notions of language and transformation, considering confession, essentialism, hidden structure, and ambiguity in the works of Wittgenstein, Augustine, Lacan, and Vygotsky within a model that reflects upon the effects of language on emerging consciousness, introspection and physical dimensions of personhood. Authentic self-examination and access to intuition are offered as one route towards greater racial justice and gender equality. This process emerges with rising emotional awareness, aporia, reassessment of knowledge and beliefs, and the epistemic motivation that develops within an interpersonal context (Bowery, 2007). Self-examination in the Platonic sense may advance with incremental, longitudinal, and "thoughtful reflection on experience" (Bowery, 2007, 96).

Confessional Modes and the Unknown

The encounter with the indeterminate is the place where justice originates. This region, beyond egocentric overgeneralizations, is infinite, personal, and relational, yet may be bordered by an unknown organizational structure (Milbank, Ward and Pickstock, 1999). Confession moves one beyond the self, towards racial and gendered reconciliation. The myopia of self-examination is acknowledged. Peters (2000) discusses the possibility of Wittgenstein's confessional mode as a genre examined through philosophy, taking the writing of the self beyond the deception of autobiography, and outside of the Cartesian notion of privileged access to the mind. It is also interesting to consider Boulding's (2002) contention that Augustine's confessions are not truly autobiographical, but rather reveal multiple facets of confession as: re-enactment of fall, praise, prayer to enable contrition, transcendent word, and co-creation.[1] Within Augustine's account, confession is a statement of what is – a truth – and constitutes a self. Wittgenstein's (1945/2009) opening reflections on Augustine's theory of language lack acknowledgement of the transformative and incarnational elements essential to Christian thought. However, Porter argues that Wittgenstein's work can expand upon and correct Augustine's view, prompting greater cohesion with "the grammar of Christian theology," warning against the "fantasy of sublime or absolute meaning" (Porter, 2019, 452–453).

Lacking universal clarity, language can isolate, move us past the literal, illuminate, and distance us from action and the Other. Language is a mixed bag. The ambiguity of language has the potential to limit human evolution and the construction of the heavenly city of humankind, derailing progress towards superordinate goals. Webs of linguistic meaning, this cultural scattering by region, may also curtail narcissism and reveal an underlying potency of diversity and uncertainty. Nevertheless, linguistic scattering also sequesters individuals into the isolation of individual consciousness in ways that inhibit mutuality and intimacy. In response to the people settling in the land of Shinar, who desire unlimited power, the prohibition arrives, for "come, let us go down and confuse their language so they will not understand each other" (Genesis 11: 7, NIV).

Literalism concretizes the self and the Other. The dream-like quality of language and image can provoke the sensory elements of knowledge – the hyperactive detection systems – which represent a cognitive power distinctive from belief, for "not all dreams are mere phantasms" (Smith, 2007, 4). Lacan cautions against the tendency to only extract that which is clear from a delusion, pointing out that intuition lies beyond appearances (Lacan, 1955/1993, 122). Incoherence in being, alienation, contributes to the empty speech referenced in Lacan, a culmination of narcissistic mirage fused with thoughts of possibility (Lacan, 1953/2002, 43).

The inaccessibility of communication is implied with Lacan's discussion of analytic inadequacy, for there are no other "ears" that could allow a "trans-audition of the unconscious by the unconscious" (Lacan 1953/2002, 46). The misleading assumption of truly contacting another's reality is exposed (Lacan 1953/2002, 45). Naming is shown as an oversimplified linkage in de Saussure (1916/1960), who reveals through his treatment of speaking circuits how the process of verbal classifications assumes that ideas exist before the words. Naming converts the listener, for a concept "unlocks a sound image" (De Saussure, 1916/1960, 65). The ineffable features of language leave humankind in an isolated space, but also with the possibility of illumination. By recognizing one's inability to truly access the Other, prejudicial labeling may collapse.

Uncertainty, Violent Language, and Organismic Cells

The uncertainty and persistence of language, and its imagistic qualities, may be inferred from Wittgenstein's claim that "where our language suggests a body and there is none: there, we should like to say, is a spirit" (Wittgenstein, 1945/2009, 22, 36). Heisenberg's uncertainty may yield a metaphor for contemplating language and its non-deterministic effects, where at the subatomic level, the foundation, only probabilities of movement, rather than pragmatic utility, can be ascertained (Humphrey, Pancella, and Berrah, 2015). The subatomic capacity of language to transform and destroy is implied.

The Spell

It is noted that the spell, the incantation, the curse, the prayer, and the liturgy are all bound by the medium of language. The notion that language alters physical realities is an ancient one, demonstrated in the Christian narrative with the wedding at Cana, the command to Lazarus to arise, and through ex nihilo creation. If observation by a conscious and self-aware mind may alter the properties of matter, this may govern the introjection of reflected appraisals into the self-system, which in postmodern spiritual contexts of Ruiz (1997), built from Castañeda (1969) emerge as a spell that alters the consciousness of the hearer. While the mystical origins of Ruiz, and the anthropological claims of Castaneda, arrive with considerable controversy (Braga, 2010; Kostićová, 2019; Krantz, 2006; Shelburne, 1987; Trichter et al., 2009), the underlying principle of the social responsibility attached to language, and the potency of its impact on the Other, are taken up here. The spell is also considered in Whorf (1941/2012) with his discussion of man-tram, incantation, and magic. Sapir, in reflections on tribal societies, con-siders the notion of intimacy between words and objects, the saturation that occurs with labels (Sapir, 1949, 11). Sapir identifies the genetic and struc-tural forms of language, its planned and unintentional symbolism, the way that it conserves authority structures and uniformity, and its capacity to substitute for actions and transmit culture (Sapir, 1949, 16–18). Language as substitution may reveal the latent aggressive impulses in utterances that seek to disintegrate "political correctness".

Subjectivity is the ground of justice, made manifest in the physical reduc-tions of language. The physicality of language connects the material to con-sciousness – that realm of ontology and experience that cannot be fully contained by, or reduced to, matter. Mind-body relationships yield evidence of the destructive and restorative power of words for the body. Linguistic forms unite (apparent) objective and subjective qualities in ways that sustain and invigorate scientific creativity, while also illuminating word-body rela-tionships. However, the subjectivity of science is often underemphasized. The invalidation of linguistic potency in political rhetoric surfaces as disembodiment.[2]

Language unifies the body and the immaterial. Connections between the muscular features of speech and the representation of sound are examined by Ferdinand de Saussure (1916/1960, 65–67), who presents the linguistic sign as a two-sided entity of concept (signified) and sound image (signifier). The sound image is only a "potential language" (de Saussure, 1916/1960, 66), for the motor is subordinate and implied. De Saussure reveals that the bond between the signifier and the signified is arbitrary, protecting immutable aspects of language as a law of the signifier, tolerated by a community and prevented from revolution by the collective. Yet rapid change can occur with a shift in relation. Whorf also discusses the plane of sound waves, muscles, and speech organs, but argues that language fosters a premonition of a realm more cast, an order "stolen from the universe" (Whorf, 1941/2012, 319).

Language, both physical and nonphysical, remains as a chemical conduit for hidden structures that connect to racial and gendered justice and its absence; however, the compound can only be viable within a medium of sub-jectivity and aporia, and is subject to constant change. The subjectivity of language is seen in the notion that it is never entirely translated from one conscious mind to another. Quine points out that a community standard, plausible but wrong, may exact a boundary that creates an epigenetic change in linguistic usage (Quine, 1960/2013, 26). An epigenetic process transforms an outer manifestation, leading to structural changes, while retaining an interior genetic map or intention. Like a virus, transmutations of language convert and recombine, interacting with cultural substrates in ways that can lead to entropy or evolution towards humanistic ideals. Translation, inde-terminate and non-equivalent, arises from linguistic viral mutations, Delta variants and copying errors that seed in response to nonverbal stimulation and simulations of the Other that traverse across persons.

The centrality of language for consciousness, forms of existence and sentience strengthens the argument that the impeccability of speech may be an ethical ideal worth pursuing, even if the goal is unattainable. The significance of word for consciousness and self-examination may be extended from Williams' statement that

> language, for Heidegger, is the "house of Being", which is to say that language is the primary way we dwell in Being. Or put another way, Heidegger says: "In language there occurs the revelation of beings …. In the power of language man becomes the witness of Being".
>
> (Williams, 2017, 11)

Language may not only impact being, but also constrain the nature of thought. In a chartered journey through linguistic relativity in French, English and German philosophy, Harvey begins his discourse with reference to Quine's untranslatability, Derrida's universal ambiguity, Ricoeur's metaphor as understanding, and Heidegger's concept of language as the "house of being" (Harvey, 1996, 273). By extension, the eminence of language for culture and politics is endorsed, devaluing the idea that "political correctness" is unnecessary and extreme.

Essentialism, the Unrevealed, and Signification

The weightiness of uncertainty may redirect attention towards intuitive forms of knowledge, yielding esteem for transcendence. According to Milbank et al. (1999), the value of self-expression, aesthetics, sexuality, embodied life, and political community is sustained and nourished through exploration of the transcendent. Transcéndere connotes ascent as climbing over and above. Thompson (2002), introduces his consideration of ascent in both Wittgenstein and Augustine with a quote derived from Drury's notes from conversations with Wittgenstein, where the latter is purported to have said that "he could not help seeing every problem from a religious point of view" (Drury, 1984, 153). This religious viewpoint may refer to the introspective enterprise, self-transformation, and dynamic processes in thought (Thompson, 2002). Although Augustine is not typically found in discussions of linguistic theory (Watson, 1982), it is not surprising to consider parallels between his work and Wittgenstein, and Thompson reports that Wittgenstein often carried the *Confessions* with him later in his life, referring to the work as "the most serious book ever written" (Thompson, 2002, 153).

The precariousness of delving into subjective religious phenomenology in the current discussion includes the risk of concretizing the infinite. With references to *King Lear* and *Measure for Measure*, Ward et al. warn that the worst forms of Puritanism confined and banned groups of people, hiding tyrannical politics behind external piety (Ward et al., 1999, 3). As an early developmental form, a referential-style approach to language will elevate the labeling and classification process. Essentializing references to religious thought can reflect a cursory review of theological literature.

In Wittgenstein's *Philosophical Investigations,* he begins with Augustine's notion of language as label, referencing the signification of nouns, as might be observed with essentializing references to the Other (Wittgenstein, 1945/2009, 5–7: 1–4). Wittgenstein critiques what he perceives as Augustine's over-simplification and reliance on language as instrument and script, yet the former seems to omit much of the deeper linguistic work that is revealed in *The Confessions.* The argument to counter Wittgenstein's critique of Augustine is well-presented in the work of Watson (1982). The Stoic theory of language presented by Watson is shown to undergird Augustine's understanding, and includes the assertion by Sextus Empiricus that "a thing is 'whatever is sensed or understood or which lies hidden.' A sign 'is something which shows itself to the sense, and besides itself, shows something to the mind'" (Watson, 1982, 12).[3]

Religious interactions with language and philosophy need not be confined to objectivism, certitude, and a referential-style approach that labels and delimits. Indeed, faith is sometimes construed as a will to believe in the midst of uncertainty and inexhaustibility. Building from this model, Augustine's views were likely less concretized than they have often been presented. Watson posits that Augustine's theory of language included the notion that mere sound, the ephemeral vibrations the travel through the air, is not equated with dialectic, nor is truth engaged by reason. Watson states in his analysis, based on Augustine's work *On the Greatness of Soul,* "so in a word, just as in some living being, the sound is the body and the meaning is, as it were, the soul. The meaning…animates and integrates all the letters of the word" (Watson, 1982, 13). The ambiguity of language is treated in Augustine's De Magistro when he references the "if," which

is an indication of doubt…something in the mind, not a concrete object in the world. Or again, nihil (nothing)…it signifies some state of the mind when it sees no reality, yet finds, or thinks that it finds, that the reality does not exist.

(Watson, 1982, 14)

In Augustine's conversation with Adeodatus, the question of whether humankind can make anything known without signs remains unanswered. Like the Stoics, who focused largely on the incomplete in the lekta (the meaning attached to a proposition), Augustine sought to "emphasize the *limits* of signs and particularly the most important class of these, words" (Watson, 1982, 16). The juxtaposition of the pointlessness of signs with illumined reality is a theme in Augustine's De Magistro, yet he argues that they should still be used, despite their inadequacy. While natural signs reveal something without intention, in book II of De Magistro, conventional signs are purposive and convey "motions of their spirit of something which they have sensed or understood" (Watson, 1982, 17).

The power of language is exposed by its versatility; it has both boundaries and an absence of boundaries, containing tradition, convention, revolution, crisis, and assumption. Wittgenstein queries about words as tools of modification with the potential to mutate reality, yet he also implies the arbitrariness of language rules and the notion of words as samples of meaning (Wittgenstein, 1945/2009, 10–11, 14, 16). The epigenetic impact of essentializing claims about the racial, political and religious Other would seem to be implied with Wittgenstein's statement that "a name signifies a thing, and is given to a thing" (Wittgenstein, 1945/2009, 10, 15). The inaccessibility of the mind of the Other is hinted with Wittgenstein's contention that "to imagine a language means to imagine a form of life" (Wittgenstein, 1945/2009, 11, 18). The language games are prismatic, for words are simultaneously or chronologically: preparations, defined by contrasts, limited by mutual understanding, goal-directed and confined by rules, contextualized, learned, representational, associationistic, incomplete and synthetic, approximations, obsolete, existing beyond the object, and deriving meaning from secondary qualities (Wittgenstein, 1945/2009, 11–44). When considering his argument of language as both an activity and form of life, the reader may question whether the superfluous, arbitrary, and invented linguistic forms may also be transformed to vivify the inanimate – word speaking into existence ex nihilo.

A discussion of language is a treatise on meaning. Signification is audited in the context of Lacanian anthropology by Kodre, who identifies language as gap and tyranny, highlighting the tendency to "suppose the existence of a guarantor of meaning...the Lacanian...big Other" (Kodre, 2011, 54). Discussions of racial reconciliation unfold in the context of cultural symbols and system-justifying hierarchies. Kodre argues that Lacan's contention that social realities may be supervised by a general unconscious structure was constructed from the latter's reading of Lévi-Strauss (Kodre, 2011, 56). Kodre contrasts de Saussure's algorithm of the signified with Lacan's revision, with its added sense of instability of the relation between signified as meaning (a mental event) and signifier as behavior (a material event).

To understand something merely due to its edges and contrasts is distinctive from deeper forms of knowledge. Like Wittgenstein, de Saussure's (1916/1960; Kodre, 2011) appeal to meaning as emergent from contrast, may hold explanatory power for the tendency to look for edges between white and black, self and other, male and female, living and invisible, literal and subjective, ontological and metaphysical. Meaning and signification will develop within the context of internalized representations, lodged in culture. In a visual representation of Lacan's "Name-of-the-Father," Kodre juxtaposes Sapir's cultural pattern with Lacan's sentiment of paternal function as introduction to a culture's symbolic architecture and codes (Kodre, 2011, 59). Symbolic architecture defines the power distance between the governors and the subjugated. The inability to authentically apprehend another's cultural identity, and the pliancy within a quantum world, suggest the inadequacy of fear-infused, power-distant language to capture. Yet, words also convince the adjudicator of the Other's lack, building the narcissistic edifice of prejudice and sexism. The confining parameters of judgment are thus retained.

Biological and quantum metaphors enhance an understanding of hegemonic systems. From this analysis that includes Lacan, Hegel, and Sapir, one may envision the unseeing linguistic warden as a cellular nucleus, self-contained by a semi-permeable boundary and influenced by the intentions of a sociopolitical construction of a genetic map. Yet, the adjudicator of culture and gender comes with projections, with axons of transference that seek to communicate with a vast neuro-cultural network. The failure to see oneself within a projective sociopolitical context evokes reference to subject-object fusion.

What is the identification of another's lack without desire? How might one gain sufficient perspective to reflect about the singularity and aporia within one's own linguistic paradigms? The absence of metalanguage outside of desire shows human egocentrism and the fusion between the mind and the word. Painful pleasure and desire modify observation. A folk psychology assumes a reality script as if it were quantifiable; movements and actions in the social world project this reality as an externalized object. The metaphor of the quantum world is greater than the sum of word picture elements – it contains a boundaryless vantage point for conceiving of physical and supra-physical subjective realities. This would imply that projections of the Other have quantum principles, taking on a life course that is dynamic, affected by observation, and unpredictable. Žižek also speaks to the quantum as a recollective failure to apprehend the real (Žižek, 2006, 75), and when symbols are removed, a void remains. Projective processes answer the terror of the void.

Mystery, Confession, and Racial Reconciliation

Desire and a vision of the *hoped-for* must intersect with the aggressive impulse in language. In the midst of uncertainty, change, racial trauma, and quantum principles, one form of cultural healing comes in the combined practice of atonement and confession, exercised within probing self-examination. In Book II of *The Confessions, Adolescence*, Augustine explores the disintegration of self, the great omission of cultivation, and the silence of God in the context of sexual awakening and pillage. At great length, Augustine discusses the stolen pears, the social elements of violation, the virginal state of the uncorrupted orchard, and the gravity of waste, for this consumption was unnecessary and outside of desire. The restorative power of confession and noncontingent forgiveness is expressed, for Augustine incorporates into his narrative the language of Psalms 130:1–2, *The Song of Ascents,* where Solomon commends the internal to the evoked companion with the words, "out of the depths I cry to you, O Lord...hear my voice. Let your ears be attentive to my cry for mercy" (NSVB, 1973/2021; Augustine, ca. 397/2019, 35: 3:5).

Augustine confers the restorative power of the language of God through song in vessels of humankind (Augustine, ca. 397/2019, 36), yielding to an admission of the dark fog that impeded the light of consciousness (Augustine, ca. 397/2019, 37), as might be observed in the implicit darkness of prejudicial depravity. Contrasted with the divine, from whom nothing can be taken away, and who is the source of the vestiges of beauty of the pears, Augustine illumines the sadness at the pleasure of greed for another person's loss, concluding with the omnipresence of the observing Other, for "where can I flee from your presence?" (Psalm 139:7; NSVB, 1960/2021; Augustine, ca. 397/2019, 40–42).[4]

Racial reconciliation and a return to reason in political discourse may be enhanced through greater veneration of mystery, including the unknowable in the Other. In Book III of *The Confessions,* in his discussion of his student years at Carthage, Augustine (ca. 397/ 1997) describes the movement from distaste to passion with his burgeoning ability to approach the language of the biblical text as "something veiled in mystery" (Augustine, ca. 397/2019, 48; 4:9). This appreciation for uncertainty is also seen in the transition described in Book Six from his Manichean views of the divine to his assertion of God as spirit, unconfining, life-giving (Augustine, ca. 397/2019, 98; 4:5). The movement from materialism was influenced by his relationship with Bishop Ambrose, and he writes that the mentor, when teaching his students "drew aside the veil of mystery and opened to them the spiritual meaning of the passages which, taken literally, would seem to mislead" (Augustine, ca. 397/2019, 99; 6).[5] At the same time, he acknowledges his desire for certitude in the unseen, a fear of entertaining false beliefs, and the juxtaposition of the seeming absurd with "holy and profound mysteries" which also "guard a mysterious dignity" for their inaccessibility (Augustine, ca. 397/2019, 100; 8).

Consciousness and Language

The intersection of language with religious practice, cultural and historical influences, group dynamics, and thought can be grounded in a developmental and social context, informing an understanding of the identity consolidation process in ways that can illuminate discussions of racial reconciliation. Lev Vygotsky begins his discussion of the relationship between thought and word with a quote from Osip Mandelstam, which suggests that the connection between cognition and language is "a product of...[the] development of human consciousness" (Vygotsky, 1934/1986, 210). Strikingly, Vygotsky then goes on to claim that there is no specific form of interdependence between the lineage of thought and word. Word meaning is conveyed as amalgamation, which cannot be considered as elemental. Vygotsky denotes that preverbal, unconscious associations (similar to Augustine's gestures and tones), stamped in through reinforcement, are insufficient explanations for word meanings (Vygotsky, 1934/1986, 213).

After exploring the limits of associationism in the Wurzburg and Gestalt schools, Vygotsky fixates on the psychological nature of inner speech, with endophasy conceived as silent recitation, memory, imagination, and governed by its own operational principles (Vygotsky, 1934/1986, 224–225). The inner speech is the seed of egocentric thinking, which Vygotsky observes to derive from insufficient differentiation of one's own speech from that of others, with collective monologue being a prime example (Vygotsky, 1934/1986, 231). Egocentric speech is conjoined with "the illusion of being understood" (Vygotsky, 1934/1986, 233), and only provides an appearance of social speech (Vygotsky, 1934/1986, 234). The great distance between dyadic minds is hinted when Vygotsky credits Jakubinsky and Polivanov with the observation that, "shared apperception...is a necessary precondition of normal dialogue" (Vygotsky, 1934/1986, 238). This sharing of a perceptual world may be unattainable in the complete or authentic sense, but can represent an ideal of racial reconciliation to aspire towards.

Biological metaphors help to reveal the dynamic sense of potential that is found in language and consciousness, which provides an optimistic scrim for discussions surrounding diversity, identity and justice. In Lacan's (1955/1993) work *The Psychoses*, Book III within the Seminar, language manifests as an organism that contains the "all" of consciousness, implying word-as-possibility. Five principle domains of linguistic consciousness may be intuited, including paradox, social construction, the language of the unconscious, superficial structure, and language as generative. Lacan explores a range of paradoxical possibilities within language, such as meaning and nonsense, mechanism vs organism, the motivated and the symbolic, classification and superstition, reality and unreality, experienced and vicarious, and the exercise of opposite words. The reader might infer that these paradoxes cohere in ways that extend existence, for the organism contains both mechanistic and indeterminate processes and systems. The simultaneous existence of meaning and nonsense, like the possibility of becoming either particle or wave, reveals the generative qualities of language as epiphenomenon, with the potential to become teratological or restorative.

Social Constructions and Expectancies

Knowledge of the Other is socially-constructed and also wrought in the unconscious projections that are guided by desire and awareness of lack. Language-as-social-construction reveals its symbiotic qualities, for "the unconscious is the also the discourse of the Other" (Lacan, 1955/1993, 128). Internalizations of the words of others became calcified in self-narratives. Continuously evolving in ways not entirely random, the social elements of internalized language develop from prepared hearing, representing a pre-potent or canalized response – a need to distinguish between self and other, ingroup and outgroup. Prepared hearing is rooted in neural expectation, which guides what is observed, attended to, and recalled. That which is canalized will emerge as native unless strong countervailing forces prevent it. Language-as-social-construction is an edifice upon precedent, history, human ecology, and cultural analysis, elevated in societal manifestations of the good, and darkened in the penumbra of the materialization of the culture of death.[6] Prepared hearing serves implicit and explicit prejudice, with motivated processing that creates a new retrospective account, based in a sense of lack and emptied of meaning.[7] One may encounter the prepared hearing – the anticipation of language – as a recipient of the narrative, as vicarious participant, or as the prodigal; priming renders it difficult to bracket imported assumptions. In the presence of system justifying myths, cultural voices convey enslavement, denial, yet there remains the hope of eventual emancipation.[8] Lacan writes that voices become "part of the very text of lived experiences" (Lacan, 1955/1993, 113). The real may reside somewhere outside of the mutually co-created, symbolic world – the world as perceived by others – the homonyms where meaning is doubled, the both, the capturing, the classifications.

The language of healing speaks to power and limitation. Words escape, as Lacan describes in the French phrase by Saint-Amant regarding absence (Lacan, 1955/1993, 115), for the implicit meaning is "lacking now is the leading thought" (Lacan, 1955/1993, 114). Culturally-transcribed metaphors convey meaning as anticipated and repeated, with impressionistic narratives rife with fear, vicarious experience, assertions, and pattern-search. Cultural images reveal blurry truth-boundaries – a sense of something – rather than the precision of pointillism. The ego protective function circulates in collective language while also obfuscating truth, as Lacan enlists with his biblical reference, "they have ears so as not to hear" (Lacan 1955/1993, 113), a notion cross-referenced throughout the Bible and also described in the Gospels with the words, "and in their case the prophecy of Isaiah is being fulfilled, which says, 'You shall keep on listening, but shall not understand; and you shall keep on looking, but shall not perceive...'" (NSVB, 1960/2021, Mt 13:14). Also conveyed in Psalms 115: 5–7 is the notion of a lifeless effigy contrasted with living spirit, for the uninhabited "have mouths, but cannot speak; they have eyes, but cannot see; they have ears, but they cannot hear…they have hands, but they cannot feel."[9] Such is the reduction of a human life to a caricature, or the materialization of that which is ineffable and irreplaceable.

An Internal Saboteur – Language, Structures, and the Unconscious

Recognition of the relativity of language, the influence of the unconscious, and the developmental impact of private speech on identity formation may evoke a form of self-examination that can be employed for fruitful dialogue on matters of diversity. Lacan (1955/1993) probes the interaction between the unconscious and private speech, and without dismembering the notion of imageless thought, he circles around the propositions of linguistic relativity. Language as unconscious thought admits omission. The internal interlocutor may serve as saboteur, critic, or elucidator, arresting motivated thoughts with both fictional and evidentiary truths in the midst of lack. The interlocutor is a behavioral guide, recounting, reciting memoirs, and recycling. Ego protective, the interlocutor compounds associations until a superstructure emerges, with the misconstrued as an essential fixture in that which is both mechanical and epigenetic. The words of the unconscious are as superstitions, compartmentalized and displaced to support symbolic immortality and continuity of the self. When engaged in an attempt to understand or unearth the meaning of the internal interlocutor, an appreciation of paradox may be enlisted, for Lacan writes that, "in order to understand what one is saying it's important to see its lining, its other side, its resonances, its significant superimpositions" (Lacan, 1955/1993, 131).

An analysis of linguistic structure may advance the understanding of narratives within interpersonal encounters with the Other. The superficial structure of language reflects movement, change and rhythm, synthesis and decomposition, a chemical reaction between thought, motivation and experience. Spherical movement, continuous development, and multi-directional influence guide the relation between consciousness and word. Conscious life is a *moving-away-from*, while still persisting and re-emerging, as shown also by the metaphor of multidirectional motion in Wittgenstein (1945/2009; Thompson, 2002, 155). Lacan (1955/1993) circumnavigates linguistic structure with consideration of: suspension / slowing, continuous modulation, scansion / metric, the rote and the scripted, the interrupted thoughts, refrains, calculation, intervals, resolution and adjournment, all of which is encased in the non-confined, the symbolic laws that follow inertia as both continuous and non-continuous. By averting preoccupation with linguistic structure, a pointillist image emerges as the vast – the void – in the categories of thought. Pointillism, sometimes referred to as divisionism or chromoluminarism, applies dots of paints to a surface in ways that can only reveal meaningful structure from a distance, Within its structure is the impossibility of language to capture, and "may there be forgiveness for the word," a pause, "sit venia verbo."[10] There is a sentence that persists within this structure, this internal monologue that overlaps with the discourse of the Other as in a Venn Diagram. The persistence is an apology.

The endophasic qualities of language, as introjections of reflected appraisals, remain in an unconscious sarcophagus, resurrecting and changing forms to camouflage and protect the fragile, skeletal ego. Yet the worthlessness of "things which are easily worked out" was shown in Augustine, who "saw all the world as a sacrament or sign of a hidden reality, and among the signs the most striking were words" (Watson, 1982, 5). The fragmentary, ineffable qualities of word processes were expressed in emergent sentences in Augustine's writings. Beneath the surface structure is the metaphor – the implicit. Lacan (1955/1993, 114) points to Molière, where words express beyond intention. Double negatives – mind-benders – convey the inverse and Lacan asserts that "the state of language can be characterized as much by what is absent as by what is present" (Lacan, 1955/1993, 115). This is an irony that is also observed in Plato.

Dawning Consciousness

The excavation of the unconscious is the starting point for racial reconciliation, social justice, and the transcendence of sexism and other forms of alterity. In his analysis of Lacan, Žižek states that the unconscious, using idiosyncratic grammatical forms, is a locus where "traumatic truth speaks," adding that the ego's function is to "dare to approach the site of my truth" (Žižek, 2006, 3). In a place where every truth is sectarian, there is a mythic creature, a lamella, an embodied alien and nightmarish in its ignorance of human limitations (Žižek, 2006, 62–63). The lamella, unrepresentable, enters as violent language, a transubstantiation of the material where a tiny, imperceptible object of implicit prejudice transforms an organism at the cellular level. The horrifying, with bi-directional influence and an internalized violence, may hide behind a "wall of language" in a collective monologue, an egocentric illusion, ordained by the "big Other," which Žižek calls the "symbolic order" (Žižek, 2006, 4).

Self-examination within a transcendent consciousness assists with the analysis of linguistic structures and their impact on self and Other. In Book I of the *Confessions, Infancy and Boyhood*, Augustine examines the sense of dawning consciousness and awareness, miraculous paradox, divine indwelling, and the nature and emergence of language. His narrative of existence applied to speech and development, intimates the role of memory in light of preconsciousness and the remnants of Neoplatonic ideas in the Intellect, which may be communicated with the higher soul.[11] Augustine explores language in many forms, such as: invocation, praise as the initiation of joy, call for rescue as the source of knowledge of the Other, argument, addressing self to mercy, controlling changes and activating renewal, and attempting to contain that which is beyond containment (Augustine, ca. 397/2019, 14–17; 1:1 to 5:5). Augustine reveals language as that which fills, enters into, while remaining elusive, hidden and present (Augustine, ca. 397/2019, 15). Language conveys debts, losses, praise for what cannot be recalled, and confession of the diminutive knowledge that follows infantile amnesia – the existence before memory (Augustine, ca. 397/2019, 17–18). Augustine regards the possibility of language to mine and extract deeply hidden riches of creation, flow from divine spirit, animate the material, and expand the capacity for restraint from craving. Augustine describes language as prayers for deliverance from suffering, confession of God's nature as a baptism, requests for elucidation, and pursuit of cleansing from guilt (Augustine, ca. 397/2019, 17–18). The structures of linguistic forms embody the conception of consciousness. The birth of dawning consciousness illuminates awareness beyond the self. Language welcomes the newborn.

Dawning consciousness may be considered as a collective movement towards reconciliation with the marginalized, oppressed, and enslaved Other. This reconciliation requires a confession. In Book I, Augustine refers to seeking a divine audience regarding the sins of humankind, considering the urge for individual and collective confession and the agony that precedes freedom, sought by a call (Augustine, ca. 397/2019, 19, 23; 7:11). He describes the disentanglement from error, the efforts of language to hide what is shameful, poetic fantasies, the embrace of the prodigal, and the silence of the encounter with the divine (Augustine, ca. 397/2019, 27–30). Humankind might collude with violence towards the Other through silence, anticipation, passivity. Augustine sees divine silence not as apathy, constructing a theodicy and a hope for human restoration, and states, "will you always remain silent? From this vast, deep sea you are even now drawing out to safety a soul that seeks you..." (Augustine, ca. 397/2019,; 17:27).[12]

One feature of dawning consciousness is awareness of conscience and deeper commitment to ethics. Language as social, spiritual, original and potential unfolds in Book I, as Augustine speaks to the conscience that lies deeper than education. The communicant may dominate, praise, offer gratitude, self-promote, lie, provoke pleasure or cope with great anxiety (Augustine, ca. 397/2019, 30–31; 19:30). The preservation of origins, an integrated self through the Word, is invoked when Augustine speaks of his desire to remain whole, to "preserve the trace in me of your profoundly mysterious unity, from which I came" (Augustine, ca. 397/2019, 32). In Augustine, the incorruptible is contained within the perishable, longing for an unknowable unity, in the presence of silence, in the pursuit of ongoing existence. Augustine anticipates a form of self-actualization as intimacy, and mutuality as existence, stating, "will you preserve me too, and what you have given me will grow and reach perfection, and I will be with you; because this too is your gift to me – that I exist" (Augustine, ca. 397/2019, 32). Preservation serves as a harbinger of announcement of light, annunciation, and conversion to a new mode of being. Confession, with its restorative power for the relation to the marginalized Other, may seek to unify material and immaterial dimensions. Perhaps confession, in order to be properly restorative, must be anchored in some form of radical apology (Katz, Grand, and Sugarman, 2021).

Ascent, Descent, Purity, and Atonement

While the pursuit of impeccability of language is advocated in this chapter, there is also acknowledgement of the dangers of moral perfectionism and self-aggrandizement. The impulse to ascend out of confusion, which Wittgenstein comes to view as unachievable, is demonstrated by his conclusion that language does not have the formal unity once envisioned, for "the preconception of crystalline purity can only be removed by turning our whole inquiry around" (Wittgenstein, 1934/ 2009, 51e, 108:47). This rejection of the fantasy of perfection is also seen in Augustine's *Confessions*, which may have influenced changes in Wittgenstein's work from his early to later writings (Thompson, 2002). The desire for ascent is noted in Book IX of the Confessions, representing remaining influences from Neoplatonic and Platonic thought of perfection and perfectibility, respectively. In Augustine, ascent finds its reversal, for "incarnation inverts...ascent as participation in Christ's descent" (Ables, 2015, 286). The inauthentic quest for impeccability and purity, and yet the hypocritical descent into the depths of human cruelty, is revealed by the history of the Magdalen Laundries, which call for papal atonement (Katz, Grand and Sugarman, 2021).

Puritanical eradication of the Other is one form of captivity that abuses language in the service of grandiosity. While this chapter does not seek to explore sexuality in light of Augustine's perspective, his venture into the unconscious dimension of motivation, sensation and sexuality is relevant for psychological inquiry, as well as his contention of the enigmatic hiddenness of the self, for "no one knows what he himself is made of, except his own spirit within him" (Augustine, ca. 397/2019, 184, 5:7).[13] Likewise, religious and secular institutions that have failed to explore their harmful impact on human flourishing should make atonement through a process of bringing that which is hidden into the light. Augustine's process of atonement involves admission of his inability to reach perfection, pursuit of honest introspection, and the assumption of personal responsibility (Thompson, 2002), a process that should be reflected as the church approaches the victims of travesties like the Magdalen Laundries. Like Augustine, who must "grieve at his 'imperfect state'" (Thompson, 2002, 160; Augustine, ca. 397/2019, X: 4,5:19,20), the church must express the lamentation of the distance between her ideals and her history. This confession is also called for by the hypocrisy observed in secular institutions of politics and journalism, which relentlessly employ the language of dehumanization and essentialism towards the racial, gendered, political, socioeconomic, and religious Other. Modern American journalism, the symbiotic appendage of political and financial agendas, will naturally incline towards *I-it* language, or the language of the naïve object, as a form of life. Politics, guided by artificial intelligence that serves as a mechanism of unconscious control and monetary exploitation, retains an elusiveness that resembles the depth of human depravity. Indeed, politics is not the answer.

Incarnation of Word and the Hiddenness of Language

Augustine's chief argument is that "we must rise to the level of knowledge purified by love" (Watson, 1982, 18). When language becomes rooted in love, there is the fruition of Augustine's psychological analogy, whereby participation in the divine mind reforms the faculties and knowledge, unfolding in the pursuit of introspective illumination and the restoration of the Imago (Ables, 2015). In a reflection on Augustine's De Trinitate, Ables shows the paradox of Word as incarnation, which "enflames us for the love of the Spirit," yet the participation in the divine is also presented as the source of the existence of knowledge, for "divine ideas are in the Word...the eternal Verbum is in some form the expression of divine light" (Ables, 2015, 287).

Reconciliation with the other relies upon enlightened self-awareness and may be enhanced through a process of theosis, a transformative deification discussed in Orthodox Christianity. Self-alienation thwarts the process of illumination, for reflection on the good reflects the mind of the summum bonum (Ables, 2015). Language that is grounded in love will yield transformative power for the body, resembling the "biological love energy" discussed by Sorokin and Hanson in their cellular analysis of the creative act (Sorokin and Hanson, 1953, 133). The movement from the literal analysis of language structure, and the failure to derive the "completely unambiguous statements" (Thompson, 2002, 163) that derive from scientism, corresponds with Wittgenstein's contention that it is impossible to find perfect clarity of expression. Creating a transformational grammar in the humanistic sense must acknowledge the fact that meaning is not reliant on syntax; there is inexact correspondence (Chomsky, 1957). The difficulty of using language to construct a linguistic theory, the tautology, is reflected in Wittgenstein's analogy of using the clumsiness of fingers to restore a torn spider's web (Watson, 1982, 15). The conclusion that it may be impossible to attain impeccability of speech is derived, but in no way does this negate the significance of our absolute linguistic responsibility to the Other.

The dynamic and evanescent qualities of language influence its impact, yet the words may also retain profound lodging in recollection. In Book IV of *The Confessions*, Augustine comes to consider language as a series of extinctions, signifying the transience of created things and restoration by Word, with a new fixed place for dwelling after the individual is summoned as thunder for unity with the Other, and relinquished to transcendence over disintegration (Augustine, ca. 397/2019, 66–67; 10:15; 70–71, 73). The part and whole of language, considered together, create a new life of transmission and liberation from grief, as if "one lover can be set on fire by another" (Augustine, ca. 397/2019, 70). The dwelling place is a womb, a returning to "him in his hidden place" (Augustine, ca. 397/2019, 68), a calling. Radiance, the origination of beauty, and anchorage is provided as the home that language finds in Truth, spoken with the "fire of charity" by Spirit. Mystery in Augustine's work also conveys intimacy and being fully known, for the human is an "immense abyss" restored "from the valley of weeping" (Augustine, ca. 397/2019, 69). Movement from the dead letters of literalism, towards the elucidation gained from uncertainty, is implied in our refrain – the chorus. This is recycled in Augustine's recounting of the teachings of one with a name signifying immortal, for we repeat our chorus refrain in the music of words, "he drew aside the veil of mystery and opened to them the spiritual meaning of passages, which taken literally, would seem to mislead" (Augustine, ca. 397/2019, Book VI, 4:6). By venturing beyond a mechanistic and material understanding of communication, Augustine came to regard the incarnational element of language as that which is beyond mere pragmatism and use, where layers of meaning conceal and guard a "mysterious dignity" to be encountered only through "narrow openings" (VI, 5:8) when the beginning was the Word.[14]

Notes

1 See Boulding (2002), pp. 12–13.
2 The violence and intentionality of language, its interplay between the internal and the external of consciousness, and its social effects are likewise examined in Matthew 15:11 when Jesus confronts the Pharisees and responds to questions of what is consumed, saying "It is not what enters the mouth that defiles the person, but what comes out of the mouth; this defiles the person" (NASB, 2021).
3 Watson references Sextus Empiricus Adv. Math, 8,80.
4 The discussion of light and dark in Psalms 139 may have relevance for Augustine's discussion of evil as the absence of good, also being significant for his theodicy. For reference, "Where can I go from Your Spirit?
   Or where can I flee from Your presence? 8 If I ascend to heaven, You are there; If I make my bed in Sheol, behold, You are there. 9 If I take up the wings of the dawn, If I dwell in the remotest part of the sea, 10 Even there Your hand will lead me, And Your right hand will take hold of me. 11 If I say, 'Surely the darkness will overwhelm me, And the light around me will be night," 12 Even darkness is not dark to You, And the night is as bright as the day. Darkness and light are alike to You.'"
5 See 2 Corinthians 3:14–16.
6 In the Evangelium Vitae, Pope John Paul II refers to the culture of death in contrast to the "incomparable worth of the human person." It is in the context of Christian humanism and its connection to racial and gender equality and social

justice that this term is invoked. The reference to ecology imparts the notion of contextualization as seen in Bronfenbrenner (1979).

7 For more on implicit prejudice, see Karpinski and Hilton (2001).
8 System justification theory is empirically examined in Jost and Banaji (1994).
9 The idea is cross-referenced throughout the biblical text, as seen in Ezekial 12:2 (NASB) "Son of man, you live in the midst of the rebellious house, who have eyes to see but do not see, ears to hear but do not hear; for they are a rebellious house," and also in Psalms 135:17 "They have ears, but they do not hear, Nor is there any breath at all in their mouths."
10 Lacan (1955) references Freud's Traumdeutung, *The Interpretation of Dreams*, but Miller points to *Sexuality and the Aetiology of Neuroses* and *The History of Neurosis* (Lacan and Miller, 1993).
11 The background of Neoplatonism, which influenced Augustine prior to conversion, is summarized by Maria Boulding (2002), pp. 9–10.
12 Ps 85:13; Is 33:5.
13 Also see I Corinthians 2:11, NIV, "For who knows a person's thoughts except their own spirit within them? In the same way no one knows the thoughts of God except the Spirit of God."
14 Matthew 19:24; Mt 7:13.

References

Ables, T.E. (2015) The word in which all things are spoken: Augustine, Anselm, and Bonaventure on Christology and the metaphysics of exemplarity. *Theological Studies*, 76(2), pp. 280–297.

Augustine (2019) *The confessions* (trans. M. Boulding). New City Press. (Original work published ca. 397.)

Boulding, M. (2002) Introduction. In J. E. Rotelle (Ed.) and M. Boulding (Trans.) *The works of Saint Augustine: A translation for the 21st century, part I, books, vol. 1: The confessions*. New City Press, pp. 9–36.

Bowery, A.M. (2007) chapter-title>Know thyself: Socrates as story teller. In G. A. Scott (Ed.) *Philosophy in dialogue: Plato's many devices*. Northwestern University Press, pp. 82–110.

Braga, C. (2010) Carlos Castañeda: The uses and abuses of ethnomethodology and emic studies. *Journal for the Study of Religions and Ideologies*, 9(27), pp. 71–106. http://ezproxy.ccu.edu/login?url=https://www-proquest-com.ezproxy.ccu.edu/scholarly-journals/carlos-castaneda-uses-abuses-ethnomethodology/docview/816629189/se-2?accountid=10200.

Bronfenbrenner, U. (1979) *The ecology of human development: Experiments by nature and design*. Harvard University Press.

Castañeda, C. (1969) *The teachings of Don Juan: A Yaqui way of knowledge*. University of California Press.

Chomsky, N. (1957). *Syntactic structures*. Mouton & Company.

Drury, M.O'C. (1984) Some notes on conversations with Wittgenstein. In R. Rhees (Ed.) *Recollections of Wittgenstein*. Oxford University Press, p. 79.

Garcia-Linares, M. I., Sanchez-Lorente, S., Coe, C. L., & Martinez, M. (2004) Intimate male partner violence impairs immune control over herpes simplex virus type 1 in physically and psychologically abused women. *Psychosomatic Medicine*, 66(6), pp. 965–972. https://doi.org/10.1097/01.psy.0000145820.90041.c0.

Harvey, W. (1996) Linguistic relativity in French, English, and German Philosophy. *Philosophy Today*, 40(2), pp. 273–288.

Humphrey, M., Pancella, P. V., and Berrah, N. (2015). *Quantum physics*. Dorling Kindersley Limited (DK).

Jost, J. T. and Banaji, M. R. (1994) The role of stereotyping in system-justification and the production of false consciousness. *British Journal of Social Psychology*, 33(1), pp. 1–27. https://doi.org/10.1111/j.2044-8309.1994.tb01008.x.

Karpinski, A. and Hilton, J. L. (2001) Attitudes and the Implicit Association Test. *Journal of Personality and Social Psychology, 81*(5), pp. 774–788. https://doi.org/10.1037/0022-3514.81.5.774.

Katz, C., Grand, S., and Sugarman, J. (2021, September 17–19) From Magdalens to dress codes: Embodied shame, radical apology and the promise of justice. [Paper presentation]. Psychology and the Other, virtual.

Kodre, L. (2011) Psychoanalysis for anthropology: An introduction to Lacanian anthropology, *Anthropological Notebooks*, 17(1), pp. 53–72.

Kostićová, Z. M. (2019) Castaneda's Mesoamerican inspiration: The Tonal/Nagual, the cardinal points and the birth of contemporary Toltec spirituality. *Religio*, 27(2), pp. 247–268.

Krantz, D.L. (2006) Carlos Cataneda and his followers: Finding life's meaning in your local bookstore. *The Journal of Popular Culture*, 39(4), pp. 576–598.

Lacan, J. (1993) *The seminar of Jacques Lacan, Book 3: The psychoses 1955–1956* (ed. J.-A. Miller, trans. R. Grigg). W. W. Norton & Company. (Originally published 1955.)

Lacan, J. (2002) The function of speech and language. In *Écrits: A Selection* (trans. B. Fink). W. W. Norton & Company. (Original work published 1953.)

Lacan, J. and Miller, J.-A. (Eds.). (1993) *The seminar of Jacques Lacan, Book 3: The psychoses 1955–1956* (trans. R. Grigg). W. W. Norton & Company.

Milbank, J., Ward, G., and Pickstock, C. (1999) Suspending the material: The turn of radical orthodoxy. In J. Milbank, C. Pickstock and G. Ward (Eds.) *Radical orthodoxy: A new theology*. Routledge.

NASB (New American Standard Version Bible) (2021) NASB online. https://www.biblegateway.com. (Original work published 1960.)

New International Version Bible (2021) NIV online. https://www.biblegateway.com (Original work published 1973.)

Peters, M. (2000) Writing the self: Wittgenstein, confession and pedagogy. *Journal of Philosophy of Education*, 34(2), pp. 353–368.

Porter, P.G. (2019) Inheriting Wittgenstein's Augustine: A grammatical investigation of the incarnation. *New Blackfriars*, 100(1088), pp. 452–473. https://doi-org.ezproxy.ccu.edu/10.1111/nbfr.12358.

Quine, W. van O. (2013) *Word and object: New edition*. The MIT Press. (Originally published 1960.)

Ruiz, D. M. (1997) *The four agreements*. Amber-Allen Publishing.

Sapir, E. (1949) *Selected writings in culture and personality* (ed. D. G. Mandelbaum). University of California Press.

Saussure, F. de. (1960) *Course in general linguistics* (eds. C. Bally, A. Sechehaye, & A. Redlinger, trans. W. Baskin). Peter Owen. (Original work published 1916.)

Shelburne, W. A. (1987) Carlos Castañeda: If it didn't happen, what does it matter? *Journal of Humanistic Psychology*, 27(2), pp. 217–227.

Smith, N. D. (2007) Plato's book of images. In G. A. Scott (Ed.) *Philosophy in dialogue: Plato's many devices*. Northwestern University Press, pp. 82–110.

Smith, A. K., Conneely, K. N., Kilaru, V., Mercer, K. B., Weiss, T. E., Bradley, B., Tang, Y., Gillespie, C. F., Cubells, J. F., and Ressler, K. J. (2011) Differential immune system DNA methylation and cytokine regulation in post-traumatic stress disorder. *American Journal of Medical Genetics Part B: Neuropsychiatric Genetics*, 156(6), pp. 700–708. https://doi.org/10.1002/ajmg.b.31212.

Sorokin, P. A. and Hanson, R. C. (1953) The power of creative love. In A. Montagu (Ed.), *The meaning of love*. Julian Press Inc., pp. 97–167.

Trichter, S., Klimo, J., and Krippner, S. (2009) Changes in spirituality among ayahuasca ceremony novice participants. *Journal of Psychoactive Drugs*, 41(2), pp. 121–134.

Vygotsky, L. (1986) *Thought and Language* (trans. and ed. A. Kozulin). The MIT Press. (Original work published 1934.).

Thompson, C. (2002) Wittgenstein, Augustine and the fantasy of ascent. *Philosophical Investigations*, 25(2), pp. 153–171.

Watson, G. (1982) St. Augustine's theory of language. *The Maynooth Review*, 6(2), pp. 4–20.

Whorf, B. (2012) Language, mind and reality. In J. B. Carroll, S. C. Levinson, and P. Lee (Eds.) *Language, thought and reality: Selected writings of Benjamin Lee Whorf*, 2nd ed. The MIT Press. (Originally published 1941.)

Williams, D. (2017) Introduction. In *Language and being: Heidegger's linguistics*. Bloomsbury Academic, pp. 1–12. http://dx.doi.org/10.5040/9781472594433.0007.

Wittgenstein, L. (2009) *Philosophical investigations* (trans. G. E. M. Anscombe, P. M. S. Hacker, and J. Schulte). Wiley Blackwell. (Original work published 1945.)

Žižek, S. (2006) *How to read Lacan*. W.W. Norton & Company.

Chapter 8

Anti-Black Racism in the Anthropocene

A Lacanian Reading of a Birder and a Dog-lover in Central Park

Sheila L. Cavanagh

On the morning of May 25, 2020, Christian Cooper, a gay, black, male, birder asked Amy Cooper (no relation) to put a leash on her cocker spaniel. The spaniel was running free in the Ramble (a semi-wild area) where the Central Park Conservancy requires dogs to be leashed. Amy Cooper refused to leash her dog. Christian Cooper said, "Look, if you're going to do what you want, I'm going to do what I want, but you're not going to like it." Christian Cooper, apparently accustomed to intransigent dog owners in the park, had dog-treats on hand and coaxed the spaniel toward him. The gesture alarms Amy Cooper who yells, "Don't you touch my dog!" Christian Cooper starts to video-record Amy Cooper with his cell phone. The video begins with Amy Cooper asking Christian Cooper to stop recording her, which he does not do. Amy Cooper, in N-95 mask and yoga tights, clutching the dog standing in as a transitional object-like blanket (soon to be suspended in mid-air), walks over to Christian Cooper. She points at him and grips the dog's collar tightly, effectively hoisting the dog up off the ground.

Christian Cooper (who we do not see in the video) says repeatedly: "Please do not come close to me." She continues to march toward Christian Cooper and says: "I am taking a picture and calling the cops." Christian Cooper responds calmly, "Please call the cops." Amy Cooper says: "I'm going to tell them there's an African-American man threatening my life." Knowing full well that Amy Cooper is operationalizing anti-black racism in the dispute, he responds: "Please tell them whatever you like." She calls the police and while she waits on hold (and the video recording is still in progress), puts the cocker spaniel in a choke hold. Amy Cooper not only endangers the life of Christian Cooper by calling the police and making a false allegation, but has a strangle hold on her dog, whom she claims to love on her Instagram account.

Amy Cooper moves back and away from Christian Cooper as she makes the police call. Her voice is breathless, mimicking grave danger and distress, as she tells the operator:

> "I am in a Ramble and there is a man, [an] African American man, he has a bicycle helmet. He is recording and threatening me and my dog.

DOI: 10.4324/9781003394327-9

[Pause.] There is an African- American man, I am in Central Park, he is recording me and threatening myself and my dog. [Pause.] I am sorry I cannot hear you either, I am being threatened by [voice amplifies] a MAN in the Ramble. Please send the cops immediately. [Pause.] I am in Central Park in the Ramble".

By the time police arrived, both Coopers were nowhere to be found. But the scene in Central Park reappears, albeit in a different spectral form, on social media. Christian Cooper posted his video-recording on Facebook and his sister, Melody Cooper, posted the same video on Twitter. Christian Cooper's video, of Amy Cooper calling the police and reporting that "*an African American man is threatening myself and my dog*" went viral. Like all traumatic repetitions it does not stop. The confrontation in Central Park was viewed over 45 million times. By early afternoon, the entire nation, and many around the globe, knew about the non-existent threat upon Amy Cooper's life, the fraudulent police call, and she was dubbed the "Central Park Karen."

Amy Cooper later told CNN that her actions (in calling the police) were inexcusable, but she was scared and alone in the park. She explains, "When you're alone in the Ramble, you don't know what's happening" (Vera and Ly, 2020, para. 33). Christian Cooper seemed to just appear, as she says, "out of the bush", taking her by surprise. In the metonymic slide from Ramble to bush (the latter term more easily racialized through its association with savagery and primitivity), Amy Cooper depicts a scene in which Christian Cooper is a likely predator. She describes Christian Cooper as a "birdwatcher with a history of aggressively confronting dog owners in Central Park who walked their dogs without a leash. It was [Christian] Cooper's practice and intent to cause dog owners to be fearful for their safety and the safety of their dogs." On the podcast, *Honestly with Bari Weiss*, Amy Cooper says "I don't know that as a woman alone in a park that I had another option [but to call 9–1-1]."

In this chapter, I offer a Lacanian reading of the case to illustrate how desire and *jouissance* (a painful pleasure) operate in what I would like to call the racist beating fantasy in the Anthropocene. The Anthropocene is a period in human history when we have altered the environment to such an extent that the continuation of the human species is at risk (or, at least, difficult to imagine). I suggest that these risks engender symptoms expressed through animals that are not neutral with respect to race. Both Coopers use animals to inscribe something relevant to being at risk in the natural environment. My argument is that the anti-black racism central to the Cooper case involves unconscious sexuality, desire, and *jouissance* but also animals. What Sigmund Freud originally called the beating fantasy is racialized in the contemporary case and mediated by dogs and birds. In what follows, I trace the "Central Park Karen" (meme) back to the hysteric who, in psychoanalytic terms, enacts things that cannot be remembered or enunciated as such. I take my interpretive cues from Christian Cooper who knows that the Real (unrepresentable) solution to the problem of anti-black racism is to be found in the signifier (the metaphorical leash) and in World Building (alternative fictions), as opposed to the Law (of the Father).

The Beating Fantasy and Memorial Day

In "A Child is Being Beaten" Sigmund Freud (1955) argues that there is masturbatory pleasure in the beating fantasy. Moreover, he notices that there is a transitive quality to the fantasy that obscures the subject (agent) and object (recipient) of the beating, generational, and natal sex differences. Freud associates the beating fantasy with sex-indeterminacy and pre-Oedipal (incestuous) longings for whom he believes to be an opposite sex parent. Important segments of the beating fantasy are unremembered but persist into adult life. Notably, they involve an excess of excitation that obscures the reality of the situation for the one having the fantasy, thereby diffusing responsibility for the imagined beating. This diffusion of responsibility helps us to understand the contemporary case in which Amy Cooper declares that an African American man is threatening her life when he is not.

While Amy Cooper is most certainly aware of the fact that she is lying, the hysterical call about an African American man threatening her life bears an uncanny resemblance to the beating fantasy theorized by Freud. I do not believe Freud intended to discount real experiences of physical and sexual assault, but neither did he take his patient's word at face value. His primary interest was in how what is said operates at the level of fantasy but does not square with reality. There is, as Lacan notes in his return to Freud, something more real than reality that occurs, something beyond signification involving not only a traumatism but a phantasy, an unconscious desire mediated by *jouissance* and the Other (as legal agent).

Not only does Amy Cooper enact a racist fantasy by making a false allegation, but in so doing she demonstrates an understanding of how anti-black racism works. Moreover, she can weaponize it and does so with an assumed impunity that involves something more than white privilege and entitlement. Although Christian Cooper is video-recording her, Amy Cooper does not seem to think she will be seen and held liable. This is because the beating fantasy is, like the Lacanian mirror stage, predicated upon an oscillation between seeing and being seen that is not only alienating (in Lacanian terms), but delimited by the gaze. In Jacques Lacan's interpretation of the beating fantasy, he focuses on the structure of the gaze in the fantasm. In his account, the fantasizer is reduced to an eye, a "mere unconcerned spectator, no longer symbolic mediator between the punishing figure and the victim" (Viñar, 1997, 183). In other words, the one having the beating fantasy or, in the case of Amy Cooper, the one reporting upon the threat of a non-existent beating to come, feels as though they are anonymous (unseen) and will not be held accountable. Much like the subject's being is alienated by the gaze of the other in the mirror, the one imagining a beating is, similarly, not-there fully, that is subjectively.

The jubilance Lacan notices in the child who recognizes themselves in the gaze of the Other (as parent) is, like the one having a beating fantasy, dependent upon a finding (recognition) of oneself elsewhere (in the gaze of the Other). But while the mirror stage is subjectifying, the beating fantasy involves a "breakdown of symbolization (diluting and blurring of the subject and of the characters on [the imagined beating] stage…)" (Viñar, 1997, 183). Lacan calls this desubjectification and links it to the perverse structure. The important point being that the beating fantasy involves not only forgetting (and subject-object confusion), but a proportionate evasion of responsibility for the prohibited content of the fantasy (or false report). If we think about beating fantasies as universal, as opposed to features of the perverse structure only, we may better understand the lack of personal responsibility white Americans take for anti-black racism.

Given that Freud refers to Harriet Beecher Stowe's *Uncle Tom's Cabin*, an anti-slavery novel that paved the way for the American Civil War in his chapter "A Child is Being Beaten", it is unfortunate, though perhaps not surprising, that he ignores the centrality of race to the beating fantasy. As Freud explains, the structure of the beating fantasy is delimited not only by aggression turned inward, but by what is desired but forbidden and thus forgotten. To the extent that the fantasy goes unremembered, it is subject to repetition.

Let us remember that the confrontation between the Coopers occurs on Memorial Day, a day to remember and mourn those who lost their lives in international combat who are, disproportionately, African American. In retrospect, we know that Christian Cooper's life was put at risk the same day George Floyd was murdered by Derek Chauvin in Minnesota. Just before Black Lives Matter (BLM) protesters took to the streets of Minneapolis the video of Amy Cooper calling the police on Christian Cooper was being shared on multiple social media and news platforms.[1] Although the day is about remembrance Amy Cooper, like many whites living in the US, choose not to remember or, in fact, understand the legacy of American slavery, the realities of police violence, and anti-black racism more generally. But as Freud suggests, what goes unremembered cannot be forgotten (at the level of the unconscious) and is destined to repeat itself through an enactment. It may be that Amy Cooper was acting out, through a false allegation, something relating not only to anti-black racism, and its traumatic legacy dating back to the trans-Atlantic slave trade but negating her own positioning in relation to it through a phantasmatic substitution: *it is not Christian Cooper, but I, Amy Cooper who is about to be beaten*. While I do not believe that Amy Cooper believed that her life was in danger, she was strangely at ease with the substitution. She informs Christian Cooper that she is going to tell the police that an African American man is threatening her life as if the reversal is not a falsehood but somehow plausible or, perhaps, logical. The ease through which she tells the lie is not only shocking, but eerily familiar. As Trevor Noah, television host of *The Daily Show*, who never fails to enunciate the cultural complexities of racism in the US says (on a YouTube video):

> It was like a "got ya" [moment]…the curtain had been pulled back. Ah ha! So you do this [white women]. Because it has always been spoken about [falsifying reports to police implicating black men] but it is powerful to see it being used. And I think a lot of people were triggered by that…damn, we knew it was real but this is like real, real…
>
> (Comedy Central, 2020)

As Noah says, there is something going on that is more real than real. In Lacanian terms, the falsified police call is irreal (or Real). There is, in other words, something more real than reality motivating the call to 9-1-1. Whatever is going on in Amy Cooper's imagination at the time of the racially motivated call, it cannot be video-recorded. My suggestion is that Amy Cooper acts out an internal drama through a racist beating fantasy and uses the (false) allegation of endangerment to her person (and to her dog) to justify it. It is also worth noting that the fantasy is enacted in a cultural moment when white Americans are being asked to account for anti-black racism and women are coming out with their experiences of sexual assault (#MeToo). It is also interesting that the false report is made in a nature preserve where ideas about the end of life as we know it set the phantasmatic stage.

Let us also remember that the beating fantasy is not only about a refusal of what Lacan would later call the law of the father, but about an overarching fear of mortality (the ultimate law). The beating fantasy is, according to Marcio Giovannetti and Philip Slotkin a "confession of rejection of the oedipal law, at least in part, insofar as that law places the individual within the chain of the species and of genealogies" (Giovannetti and Slotkin, 1997, 105). Not only is there a refusal to acknowledge sexual difference (which Lacan equates with the hysterical structure), mortality, and the Oedipal law of the father, but there is an enactment of desire that, in the Cooper case, concerns not only sexuality and survival, but gender and race in the nature preserve. As such, beating fantasies are defenses against castration (lack), but also death. Beatings, real and imagined, are about life and death which feel like the end of the world. But time does not really stop in the beating fantasy. It is, perhaps, more accurate to say that the difference between the past and the present is elided in a figurative loop, much like the difference between subjects, Amy Cooper and Christian Cooper, is elided in an alarming reversal as evident in the 9-1-1 call.

Like the phantasmatic beating scene described in Freud's account, the Ramble is saturated by sexual taboo, prohibition, and fantasies about nature. It is a thirty-eight-acre protected nature preserve with forested area, diverse vegetation, rough topography (including rocky outcrops), a lake and labyrinth-like paths. It is listed on Centralpark.com as an ideal location for weddings, bride and groom photography following the ceremony. But despite the heterosexual and pastoral depictions of the Ramble it is a notorious venue for gay male cruising. The two most popular activities in the Ramble, excluding walking, may, in fact, be birding and cruising. Dense thickets and statues of dead poets throughout the park, including a bronze of Hans Christian Anderson (posthumously remembered as a homosexual), make it ideal for public gay sex. Although there is nothing to suggest that Christian Cooper uses the park for cruising, he is metonymically associated with illicit sex as a gay man. Let us remember that he leaves his boyfriend in bed at what some reporters have called an obscenely early hour, jumps on his bike, and peddles to Central Park not for unlimited sexual encounters but to view any one of the 230 species of birds in the trees and vegetation. But his interest in the birds, as a black gay man, does not offset the danger he encounters in the Ramble. The intricate network of paths in the Ramble designed to encourage wondering, intimacy, and surprise also enable anti-black racism, anti-gay and gender-based violence.[2]

Christian Cooper, a gay African American birder, along with the birds in flight, are not threats to Amy Cooper's physical being (despite the fraudulent police call), but threats to her sense of entitlement to be in the Ramble without limit. Her dog's right to run-free parallels her own desire to be free in the Ramble, that is without regard for other humans and animals (including birds). In effect, she transfers her desire to be free onto her dog (whom she refuses to leash) and accuses Christian Cooper of threatening her life. While the libelous report does not square with the reality of the situation it may be read as a hysterical (albeit racist) response to an existential threat to being in the Anthropocene that must be read through what cannot as of yet be said about race and gender.

While much has been written about Freud's hysterical patients, gender and the Lacanian formalization of the hysterical structure, less has been written about how racism, and the use of animals to enable racism, figure in fantasies about the end of the world. This is unfortunate because, as Giovannetti and Slotkin explain, the beating fantasy dissolves the "symbolic dialectic of differences...between I and other, between animate and inanimate, and between life and death – that is, ultimately, the human dialectic" (Giovannetti and Slotkin, 1997, 107). But differences between the human and the non-human animal are also obscured. The denial of difference linked as it is, in Freud's analysis of the beating fantasy, to a denial of mortality is, for Lacan, about the problem of being which, in this paper, I elucidate in terms of the feminine not-all which the hysteric, perhaps better than anyone, is not only attuned to, but animated by. While I use the term hysteric in a more generic (non-diagnostic) way, I suggest that hysterics suffer because part of their being-experience is not inscribed in the socio-Symbolic. My suggestion is not that Amy Cooper is a hysteric but that the discourse of the hysteric animates something that has not yet been enunciated or symbolized in the cultural milieu.

Although the discourse of the hysteric, in Lacanian terms, poses a challenge to the discourse of the master (the university and to what is now called the discourse of capitalism), it can also be regressive (conservative and racist). What defines the hysteric is not a politic but an acute sensitivity to what does not exist as such or is, relatedly, unspeakable. Racism, like sexism, involves trauma that cannot be fully represented. Both Coopers suffer from a degree of erasure in the social field that is Real. This is not only due to sexism and racism respectively, but to the way both demographics lack and are vulnerable to (often white) hetero-masculine aggression in the Anthropocene.

The Woman and the African American man do not exist in Central Park

It is an open secret that woman, along with Black, Indigenous, and People of Color (BIPOC) communities are not well represented in Central Park. Consider, for instance, the bronze statues and memorials erected in the park. There are fifty-one statues, most of which are of (white) men. The remaining sculptures, less than ten, are, with one exception, not exactly (white) women. Prior to 2020, there were no statues of actual historical women. Those walking through Central Park can see imaginary (white) girls and women like Alice in Wonderland and Mother Goose. Juliet, of the Shakespearean tragedy, appears in the park alongside Romeo. There is even a statue of Balta, a husky sled dog, a dancing bear, and a dancing goat, but no actual women, or African Americans, were, until 2020, memorialized.

Monumental Women, a non-profit committed to the construction of statues of women adopt a masculine solution to the problem of the Woman's non-existence in the park. They want to "break the bronze ceiling" by erecting statues. The lack of real historical women in Central Park received nationwide publicity in the same year the video of Amy Cooper calling the 9–1-1 went viral. In an article on the website, *Quartz*, Mya B. Dosch, an American art professor, is quoted as saying that the "erection" of statues [in Central Park] is phallocentric: "Heroic statues are very phallic; it's a very masculine way to take up space." Women, Dosch continues, are metaphors, "fictional ideals, allegories, or mythic creations, such as Liberty, Justice, Beauty, half naked nymphs, angels of water" (Quaglia, 2019, para. 11). Dosch is not wrong. Women do have an absent (or allegorical) presence in the park. But the problem cannot be rectified by constructing female-statues in the park because the problem of representing the feminine not-all is Real. What Monumental Women call a lack of real historical women is a Real problem that cannot be symbolized. There is, in Lacanian terms, no way to represent the Other (feminine) *jouissance*. We can erect phallic-women but insofar as they are phallic-monuments the feminine continues to be eclipsed. In other words, the feminine not-all persists. The problem of being that was, perhaps, felt by Amy Cooper to be an actual risk in need of police-intervention is more closely associated with the problem of representation as opposed to the problem of her actual physical being.

While almost a hundred confederate statues were torn down across the US in 2020, following the killing of George Floyd, Monumental Women were unveiling a bronze statue of Susan B. Anthony (organizing), Elizabeth Cady Stanton (writing), and Sojourner Truth (speaking) around a table, 100 years after the passing of the Ninth Amendment giving women the right to vote. In an interview in the *New York Times,* the president of Monumental Women, Pam Elam, said "nobody, for a long time, even noticed that women were missing in Central Park" (as cited in Gupta, 2020, para. 6). While it is unlikely that nobody noticed the missing women of Central Park, African Americans did notice the non-existence of black suffragettes in the original plans for the feminist commemorative statue. While the originally planned sculpture by Meredith Bergmann included only Anthony and Stanton, Monumental Women decided to include Truth after criticisms were launched by members of the Washington Street Advocacy Group, the Harlem Historical Society and The Sojourner Truth Project about the erasure of African American women in the memorial-like sculpture (Small, 2021). But criticisms were not allayed by the late addition of Sojourner Truth to the sculpture-table. It is an unfortunate truth that Anthony and Stanton did not support the 15th Amendment because they believed their suffrage, as white women, should take precedent over African American voting rights and, also, that Truth did not do feminist organizing work with Anthony and Stanton. The sculpture is also misleading because it obfuscates anti-black racism in white female suffragette work.[3]

The Central Park Karen and the Beating Fantasy

While Amy Cooper, Anthony, and Stanton are not the same people and divided by multiple generations, they share a white presumption that their lives, as white women, matter more than Black lives. The genesis of the "Karen" meme is contested but it dates back (at least) to the white suffragettes, who, according to Aja Romano in an article on *Vox,* are "officious white women ruining the party for everyone else" (Romano, 2020, para. 5) The epithet captures the dual positioning of white women as not having an actual agentic voice due to sexism – a legal agent (coded as masculine) must be called in to the scene, and to the way white women are now being asked to address anti-black racism and to give cultural and symbolic space over to non-white folks.

In psychoanalytic terms, "Karens" are contemporary instantiations of the Freudian hysteric (who cannot speak) and are, until they can speak (authentically, as distinguished from false speech), committed to the re-enactment of a beating fantasy (dating back to a real or imagined sexual encroachment). The fabricated story Amy Cooper tells the operator fits this strange (inner) inditement on speech that Freud noted in his case studies of hysteria. It stands to reason that the Central Park Karen is not a person like Amy Cooper (although she wears the name like the scarlet letter) but a signifier of a symptom in Lacanian terms. The epithet is a popular cultural name (a meme) for what happens to a subject when unconscious desire is compromised, thus posing a threat to being in imaginary, not physical terms. It is not only that Amy Cooper lies to the police and endangers Christian Cooper, but that she enacts a beating fantasy to convey something of consequence to herself and, potentially, of relevance to Christian Cooper (as an African American).

Amy Cooper seems to be narrating something Real through a lie, a false report implicating Christian Cooper, that is not only symptomatic, but tied to what cannot be remembered (memorialized). The real-life example of Trisha Meili, the Central Park jogger who was raped, gagged, tied, viciously beaten, and left to die in a park ravine on April 19, 1989 comes to my mind. Five African-American and Latinx men were wrongly charged with the attack.[4] Like Amy Cooper, Meili, prior to the attack, worked in finance for an investment bank, the Salomon Brothers. She, like Cooper, excels in economics. Meili has a degree in economics from Wellesley College and an Masters in Business Management from the Yale School of Management. She was, compared to the racialized youth wrongfully accused of the crime, educationally privileged, affluent and had the sympathy of New Yorkers.[5]

Although Meili did not make false allegations like Amy Cooper, there are wrongful allegations made against racialized men and actual instances of violence against white women that coincide. The Karen meme is a way to characterize the wrongful accusations white women make against black men, but it gains cultural currency by tapping into the sexist ways women's real experiences of physical violence and sexual assault are often disregarded. As people of color can attest, the police are more likely to investigate assaults against (white, cis) women and, also, relatively minor (or non-existent) misdemeanors, when a racialized man is accused of having committed the crime. White women, like Amy Cooper, seem to understand this. There is, in the contemporary moment, a growing awareness of both police violence against African Americans enabled by the organizing efforts of the BLM movement, and sexual violence against women enabled by the organizing efforts of the #MeToo movement (which was, not coincidentally, coined by Tarana Burke, an African American woman, on Myspace. But it gained traction when white women used it to draw attention to their own experiences of sexual assault). Instead of understanding how racism and sexism are intersectional there is, as evident in the Cooper case, a way in which the threat of sexual violence is used to enable anti-black racism. But more than this, there is a resemblance and substitution. While Amy Cooper imagines (and reports upon) a threat to her life she puts Christian Cooper at actual physical risk by calling the cops.

But the substitution (Christian for Amy) is accompanied by an all too real linguistic resemblance. Consider, for instance, the coincidence of the common surname: Cooper. The shared surname suggests that Amy and Christian have a common familial or genetic heritage. Although genealogists know that the surname is, like all signifiers, unreliable it prompts those following the case to imagine a likeness, a shared familial ancestry that confounds racial difference and is an affront to those opposed to "inter-racial" sex. The imagining is amplified by the number of times those reporting on the case insert the "no relation" clause in their descriptions of the Coopers. As Lacan notes, two (or more) nots (as in "not" related), posits a relation (that does not exist as such). But this non-existent familial relation harkens back, if only unconsciously (or, perhaps, metonymically), to a common heritage relating to slavery whereby those enslaved along with the slave owner's wife, take on the white man's name. This is not to say that the position of the white woman (who may be married to a white man) and the Black man (who may be a descendant of slaves) are the same (certainly they are not), but it is to say that there are analogies at play relating to their subordination to white paternal law. These analogies, however imperfect and misleading, are animated, in part, through animals. To put this in psychoanalytic terms, the beating fantasy analyzed by Freud and the threat articulated by Amy Cooper – *there is an African American man threatening myself and my dog*, involves not only subject-object confusion at the level of race and gender but human subject-animal confusion in need of interpretation and clarification.

Animals and Anthropocentrism in the Anthropocene

While Freud attends to the way beating fantasies obscure the subject and object of the beating (at the level of the Imaginary) along with the sexual, temporal, and generational differences pertinent to the imaginary scene, the contemporary instantiation of the beating fantasy reported by Amy Cooper involves race and animals in ways that appear to be sexuated in the Anthropocene. There is something in the panic-stricken (though performative) allegation (of a beating to come) that is not only the voice of white entitlement, racism, and privilege, but of a subject who hears the signifier-leash (which she is supposed to put on her dog) as an obstacle to her desire. The dog is like a little phallus which will, in Amy Cooper's fantasy, be castrated should he be leashed. The dog-phallus belongs to her, and Christian Cooper's enjoyment of the birds requiring that she abide by the sign is felt, by Amy Cooper, to be arresting which is why she turns-the-tables and calls the police. Amy Cooper's dog is a phallic object that should not be leashed whereas the birds are for Christian Cooper to be seen (through binoculars), heard, enjoyed, but not owned (like pets). Like the Other *jouissance*, birds are not fully subject to the phallic (dog) premise and while birds can be pets it is the undomesticated birds that interest Christian Cooper.

In Lacanian terms, the animals are *jouissant* (objects) and sexuated accordingly. Amy Cooper owns a cocker spaniel and Christian Cooper is a birdwatcher. But, like the sexual non-rapport of concern to Lacan, the fantasies each Cooper has about their respective animals, including the *jouissant* ways they enjoy their animals, is subject to a structural impasse. Christian Cooper's sensitivity to the (uncaged) birds is at odds with Amy Cooper's investment in her domesticated cocker spaniel.[6] She owns her dog much like she acts as though she owns or has unlimited access to the park. The dog is felt to be an extension of her rights and entitlement. Henry's right to run through a bird sanctuary without a leash is an expression of Amy Cooper's desire to be without limits. The spaniel is like the Lacanian phallus (imaginary object and symbol of lack) while the birds are, for Christian Cooper, non-phallic. The dog-animal that Amy Cooper refuses to leash interferes with the birds in flight, signifiers of the Other (supplementary) *jouissance*. The unleashed (phallic) dog also interferes with Christian Cooper's right to enjoy the park and watch the birds. This puts the Cooper's at socio-political-environmental loggerheads. The impasse can also be seen in the stories they tell, and are told about, their lives through their respective animals.

According to an article in the *New York Times*, as a young boy Christian Cooper was given a book titled *The Birds of North America* while on a road trip with his family (Nir, 2020). During the trip in the family Volkswagen, Cooper memorized the book and could identify the birds flying by. Now, as an adult, the article continues, he compares the bird songs he strains to hear to the uniqueness of his mother's voice and they figure in his science fiction (to be discussed in a later section). Amy Cooper, by contrast, does not listen to Henry (the dog), but talks through him to convey something about life, death, and risk management. Notably, she is an actuary and works in finance. Only days before the confrontation with Christian Cooper in Central Park, Amy Cooper posted a story about the near-death experience of her dog. She writes the post in Henry's voice:

> Today my Mommy wants to tell the world how thankful she is to have me. Last night I gobbled something and choked. I was unable to breath. I laid on my side and my tongue turned blue. My Mom was fast to act and used infant CPR to remove the object and save my life. We have since learned that a pupper can choke in 20 seconds or less. If you are not familiar with the techniques my Mommy is asking while we all have a little more time [given

COVID] to please learn. She prays you will never need it like we did last night.

(as cited in Cleary, 2021, para. 35)

Reading this post (which has since been taken down) after the killing of George Floyd by Derek Chauvin who knelt on Floyd's neck for nine minutes and twenty-nine seconds, effectively suffocating him, is truly uncanny. While Amy Cooper could not have known about Floyd's death at the time of the post and people are free to anthropomorphize their pets at will there is a conspicuous way in which the animal (as pet) is used as a medium for the expression of injuries (real and imagined) of the (often white) dog-owner in the present-day. In Lacanian terms, Amy Cooper acts out by speaking on behalf of her dog.

Prior to the fictitious threat to her life, Amy Cooper had an Instagram account where she posted photos of Henry's romps in Manhattan. He appeared to be a happy dog. The day after Christian Cooper and his sister posted videos of Amy Cooper calling the police online, the images of Henry posted on her Instagram account took a sinister turn by documenting injuries to the dog. There is a disconnect between Amy Cooper's manifest concern about her dog's welfare, including Henry's near-death experience, and the way she is seen choking her dog in Central Park without seeming to notice or care. Amy Cooper ventriloquizes her own anxiety about risk through her dog and in so doing dissolves a difference between herself as adult-subject and the dog-animal (anthropomorphized as Henry). The defensive and projective tactic must be unnerving and upsetting to African Americans who have been dehumanized by racist comparisons made between themselves and animals, including dogs, and having those racist comparisons used to deny their access to civil rights and personhood. It should also be remembered that dogs have been violently used by police against African Americans to obstruct civil rights marches and "race riots." Amy Cooper's identification with her dog does not dehumanize her in a negative way or curtail her civil liberties as it likely would for African Americans. In fact, her over-identification with Henry-the-dog expands her sense of entitlement to public space. But more than this, her claim to love Henry and to act on his behalf makes her appear selfless and above reproach until, of course, the charade is shown by Christian Cooper and his sister on social media to be a ruse and cover for anti-black racism.

The adage…*my dog*, as in *an African American man is threatening myself and my dog* seems to add an extra layer of urgency to the police call and positions the cry for help as innocent and above reproach. While it is usually white children who are to be vigilantly protected against improbable threats, it is, in Central Park, the domesticated animal who occupies the position of (fantasized) endangerment. The blond cocker spaniel is metonymically associated with a (white) child-at-risk (about to be beaten) while BIPOC children are more likely to be at actual risk due to the deleterious effects of racism. But the domesticated cocker spaniel, like the white child (and, in fact, all human animals) are not extensions of nature but ruptures in nature. As Alenka Zupančič (2017) explains, we are the lack or gap in the Anthropocene, the exception to the structure of nature. This natural impasse mirrors what Lacan calls the non-existent sexual relation and animals cannot ameliorate the schism.

While BIPOC communities were enraged about the police call on May 25, animal rights advocates were irate about Cooper's treatment of the cocker spaniel (although many of these animal rights advocates acknowledged the anti-black racism central to the fraudulent police-call). The trouble is that animal rights activists are often uncritical of the anthropomorphic tactics they use to protect animals, and of the way these tactics can be racializing. Animal protectionists, like Amy Cooper, anthropomorphize Henry. Animal protectionists complain about the lack of psychological assessments done on prospective dog-owners like, presumably, Amy Cooper. They also lament how dogs cannot hire attorneys while dog-owners can, conveniently forgetting that proportionately few BIPOC dog-owners, compared to white dog-owners, have the financial resources to access legal assistance for themselves when they are criminalized by police, let alone for their pets. One animal protectionist raises Henry, quite literally, to the dignity of an abandoned angel. Addressing his comment to the Abandoned Angels Cocker Spaniel Rescue Facebook group, the poster says: "When you say 'abandoned' angels you really mean it, huh?" (as cited in Cacich, 2020, para. 7). While anti-racist groups do not oppose animal welfare, they are legitimately critical of how white animal protectionists seem to care more about the well-being of abandoned dogs than BIPOC children.

Responding to dog-rights advocates, Amy Cooper returned Henry to the non-profit Rescue. Following a veterinarian inspection establishing that the dog was in good health, the non-profit returned Henry to Amy Cooper ten days later. The dog's return to Amy Cooper caused widespread anger and backlash from both animal protectionists and BIPOC communities, but for different reasons. Animal protectionists worried about Henry-the-dog while BIPOC communities noted how white privilege operates. If Amy Cooper were not white she would not have gotten her dog back so quickly or, in fact, at all. In the same video referenced above, Trevor Noah explains:

> ...a lot of people felt like it would have been great if the dog shelters had the same power...or if the police department were run by the people who run dog shelters because they seemed to act like this [snaps]. They didn't waste time. They were like nope, we'd like our dog back lady. That was a hell of a punishment [said sarcastically]. Her job is one thing, taking a white lady's dog, [that is another thing].
>
> (Comedy Central, 2020)

After the incident went viral, Amy Cooper was cyber-bullied and doxed online but less for her racism than for animal cruelty. The blond cocker spaniel received nation-wide sympathy while BIPOC children subject to racism in American institutions, including the criminal justice system and state-parks, not only fail to garner comparable sympathy but are largely ignored. Animal rights activists online accuse Amy Cooper of abusing her dog and wonder how many times this has happened but not been caught on video. BIPOC communities ask the same question about how often racism occurs but goes unrecorded.

Although Amy Cooper evades political responsibility by fabricating a story about her life, her dog, and endangerment in Central Park, Christian Cooper's investment in nature and the birds is not at odds with his commitment to anti-racist politics.[7] He is not only concerned with African American civil rights but is, if his media interviews, fiction, and YouTube videos are any indication, equally concerned about nature and bird-preservation. In an interview with the *Los Angeles Times* about what transpired before he turned the video-recording device on, Christian Cooper explains: "My approach is always to first be polite, tell the rules and ask for a leash". When dog owners, like Amy Cooper, fail to comply, he coaxes the dogs with treats to protect the birds along with the planting. While not all birders in the park agree with Christian Cooper's tactics, using food to curb unleashed dogs (thereby upsetting, predominantly white, law un-abiding dog owners), he is well respected in the bird and environmental conservation community. Cooper is one of few black birders in the park and is a mentor to BIPOC interested not only in birding but in accessing city park lands and green spaces. He is a powerful force curtailing what the The Center for American Progress calls a racialized "nature gap" relating to the larger problem of "environmental racism."[8] There is a growing recognition that green spaces are racialized as white and anti-racist advocates and birders, like Christian Cooper, help to make nature more inclusive.

Christian Cooper could hear Amy Cooper calling Henry as the dog ran freely through the Ramble on Memorial Day. He was, by contrast, quiet: listening and watching for the birds. The dog running rough shod on protected grounds endangers the birds. Christian Cooper explains to Whoopi Goldberg on *The View* (an ABC production) that the Ramble is a protected area because there is a "lot of wildlife there and a lot of delicate planting" which is why the signage prohibits un-leashed dogs. He explains that people are not obeying the signage and "we" (who I assume to be likeminded birders) have been trying to get better enforcement which is why he, and others, have been video-recording those, like Amy Cooper, who disobey the signs. Christian Cooper suggested that Amy Cooper take her dog to an off-leash area outside the Ramble, but she refused stating that the off-leash area is too dangerous.

In the Anthropocene the problem of desire and risk is articulated through animals. As suggested above, Amy Cooper's desire seems to take refuge in her dog (Henry). As written in *The New York Times*, Amy Cooper was regularly seen in the company of her dog, taking the spaniel on morning walks, and making appearances at dog-birthdays. She was, also, said to engage in "combative behavior with other dog walkers and the building staff" (Nir, 2020, para. 4). A resident living in a building not far from Cooper's building was quoted as saying that she is "devoted to her animals" but "never spoke directly to a person. She always spoke through her dog, and in a baby voice. It was really bizarre" (Nir, 2020, para. 5). Speaking through one's dog may be bizarre, but it is common in (white) pet cultures prone to anthropomorphizing their dogs and not without psychoanalytic precedent. Freud was, like Amy Cooper, a dog-lover (who kept Chow Chows), and his daughter, Anna, had a German Shepherd (named Wolf). As a blog post on the Freud Museum London website reports, each year Freud's dogs delivered a poem on his birthday. While Anna or Martin wrote the poems, the dogs would deliver the scripted rhymes, affixed to their collars with a ribbon (as if they were the authors), to the father of psychoanalysis (Davies, 2020). While Freud's children spoke through their dogs to commemorate their father's birthday, Amy Cooper's spoke through her dog in a way that put Christian Cooper's life at risk.

X-Men in Science Fiction and Fantasy

Beating fantasies are not only about sexual indeterminacy but ways to process and manage perceived threats to life. While Freud understood the beating fantasy in terms of the masculine protest (in girls), Lacanian theory suggests that there is a search for a phallic signifier to bar the unmitigated tyranny of the Other. The masculine (in Freud) and the phallic (in Lacan) are not bound to males and masculinity but are, nevertheless, paired with gender and sex in the social field. What I find interesting is the way both Coopers, despite their gender and differences in sexual orientation, are looking for alternative men or phallic signifiers other than the ones on offer in the Symbolic field. Both want to mitigate a lack in or threat to being that has something to do with men and hetero-masculinity (or, in Lacanian terms, the phallic function). Amy Cooper works in finance capitalism (a masculine enterprise), pursues and sues men who lie to, fire, endanger, or disappoint her, while Christian Cooper invents X-Men (comic superheroes) who are not like other men. He is not only a social justice advocate, but an animator, author, and World Builder. Amy Cooper's corporate world is, by contrast, defined by her job at Lehman Brothers, the now infamous investment bank that filed for bankruptcy in 2008 (following the subprime mortgage lending crisis) and Citigroup, a US investment bank that was, like Lehman Brothers, branded "too big to fail."

Like the masculine protest Freud observes in his female patients (which he, unfortunately, analyzes in sexist and bi-gender terms), Amy Cooper is described in the news-media as having more than her fair share of troubles with men. According to *The New York Times*, Amy Cooper's friends say "she can be sensitive and caring…but also seems to have a more contentious side. Neighbors said she had a tendency to get into personal disputes" with people, like the doorman who she said she wanted to get fired because he cursed her. According to a neighbor, Alison Faircloth, Cooper cursed at the doorman (not the reverse), "barged into a security booth and had to be removed by a guard." The incident seems to have been precipitated by a broken elevator. According to Ms. Faircloth, "There's always a narrative from her about someone who has done her wrong" (Nir, 2020, para. 8).

In the media-generated accounts, Amy Cooper is described as having been wronged whether it be by her lover (Martin Priest), the doorman (unnamed), Franklin Templeton (for wrongful dismissal), or Christian Cooper. She is also always in danger (in the Ramble, on the streets of Manhattan, and in her residence). To protect herself in fantasy, or to receive recompense, she hires lawyers and calls police. Agents of the law (phallic supports) are called in to act and to arbitrate on her behalf. Prior to suing Franklin Templeton for wrongful dismissal,[9] she filed suit against Priest in 2015 to regain $65,000 she lent him on the assumption that he would leave his wife. According to *The New York Times*, the money was to "help speed his divorce and pay another woman he was involved with to abort her pregnancy" (Nir, 2020, para. 12). The results of the settlement are confidential, but Martin Priest denies having had a romantic relationship with Amy Cooper and referred to her as a stalker.

While Amy Cooper's relationship with Martin Priest did not work out, she did build a friendship with his ex-wife. The friendship was consummated when Amy Cooper told Tianna Priest about her husband's infidelity (Nir, 2020). Apparently, Amy Cooper and Tianna Priest "now spend holidays together." As reported in *The New York Times*, Amy Cooper is a hero who, according to Tom Selby (Tianna Priest's father), saved his daughter from a toxic marriage. Selby sees Martin Priest as a toxic person and refers to Amy Cooper as "just another one of his victims."[10]

Tianna Priest is quoted as saying that Amy Cooper is all about "Work, work, work, work, work – she's a workaholic…She loves numbers, so she gets it and she's good at it" (Nir, 2020, para. 20). Christian Cooper, by contrast, makes fiction and animation his life work. He wrote for the anthology *Marvel Comics Presents*, edited *X-Men* (based on mutant super-heroes with special powers enabled by the X-Gene who fight against anti-mutant discrimination), and two issues of the *Marvel Swimsuit Special* (1991–1995) (a now defunct magazine-like comic that parodied the *Sports Illustrated* swimsuit edition by featuring Marvel Comic book characters in sexualized swimwear). The story of Amy Cooper, saving Tianna Priest from her adulter-ous ex-husband (despite being-herself the "Other woman" in Martin's life) calls to mind the fictional super-heroes Christian Cooper invents that stand in for what he calls the "gay experience" (as cited in Silberman, 1998). Both

Coopers do things with the heterosexual impasse or with what Lacan calls the sexual non-rapport. Amy Cooper makes a friendship with a man's divorced wife while Christian Cooper creates alternative men.

In an interview with *Wired,* Christian Cooper explains that X-Men look "like everyone else, but they learned a deep secret in adolescence that made them different. They were feared and hunted by society, but they just wanted to make the world better" (cited in Silberman, 1998). While genetic females have XY sex chromosomes and genetic males have XX sex chromosomes, the X-Men are unlike non-mutant females and males. The single sex chromosome gives them, counterintuitively, an X-factor (a little bit extra in Lacanian terms). There is not one, but multiple series of *X-Men.* Titles include Giant Size X-Men, Uncanny X-Men, New Mutants, X-Factor, Excalibur, X-Force, Generation X, X-Men Legacy, Astonishing X-Men, All-New X-Men, Amazing X-Men, Extraordinary X-Men, and X-Men Gold.

The X-Man sub-species (originally created by Jack Kirby and Stan Lee in 1963) is not only aligned with non-mutant men but animals. They fight for equality, and this includes, on occasion, queer, feminist and anti-racist battles with anti-mutant and demonic others in futuristic landscapes. Anti-mutant characters, like white (racist) Americans in the present-day Anthropocene, are an ever-present threat to the those of mutant genetic heritage. X-Men, unlike the vilified Martin Priest (who betrays Tianna Priest and Amy Cooper), hold the tyranny of the non-mutant Other to account. Let us remember that the X-Men series is (not only) popular because the comics feature sexy, white, conventionally attractive men, but because the characters lack.[11]

Amy Cooper's fantasy, relating to an African American man threatening her life is, in the language of science fiction, out of this world. But unlike Christian Cooper's fantastical superheroes who challenge anti-black racism, her fantasy (enacted) puts black lives at risk. Christian Cooper's interest in science fiction and fantasy may be inspired by the question of how to be not-all in the Anthropocene replete with homophobia and anti-black racism. Amy Cooper confronts an analogous problem relating to sexism in late-stage capitalism. But she turns to the Other of the Law (the police, lawyers, etc.) to impose punishments whereas Christian Cooper creates another parallel scene at the level of fantasy through his fiction, and in reality, through his anti-racist activism.

A Real-live Beating

What is unusual about the Central Park case is that it is Amy Cooper, not Christian Cooper, who gets punished. Not only was Amy Cooper banned from Central Park upon mayor Bill de Blasio's request but the American multinational holding company who employed her tweeted: "Following our internal review of the incident in Central Park yesterday, we have made the decision to terminate the employee involved, effective immediately. We do not tolerate racism of any kind at Franklin Templeton." Pardoxically, the company logo of Benjamin Franklin's face appears alongside the tweet. The Founding Father of the United States was both a slaveholder and, later, an abolitionist. His image sits, ironically, if not mockingly, alongside the anti-racist sentiment.[12]

The New York City Commission on Human Rights investigated Cooper for having issued a false report against a member of a protected group (African Americans). She was issued a desk appearance ticket to appear in criminal court. But the charges against Amy Cooper were dropped without a trial or guilty plea largely because Christian Cooper declined to participate in the proceedings. In psychoanalytic terms we might say that he does not want to beat Amy Cooper (as she tried to beat him). From a socio-political perspective, Christian Cooper does not want to collude in a racist justice system that systematically incarcerates, murders, and enables violence, against large numbers of African American men. Nor does he wish to align himself with a legal authority, be that authority a police officer, a lawyer, or a judge. Although the District Attorney said that "We are strongly committed to holding perpetrators of this conduct accountable," Christian Cooper remains un-swayed. He does not seem to think that accountability for anti-black racism can be established through legal means. In a statement given to the *New York Times*, Christian Cooper said, "if the DA feels the need to pursue charges, he should pursue charges. But he can do that without me" (Ransom, 2020, para 3). Believing that Amy Cooper has already suffered enough, Christian Cooper reasoned in an interview with CNN: "if the fear [on the part of African Americans who want me to testify] is that the police would have done me harm [following the fraudulent police call] then the solution is to fix policing" (Sanchez and Joseph, 2020). Amy Cooper tapped into what Christian Cooper calls a "deep vein of racial bias that keeps cropping up." He knows and is, in fact, quoted as saying "It's not about her" (Nir, 2020, para. 11).

Christian Cooper knows that the problem of anti-black racism is not reducible to Amy Cooper and that it is a structural (not an individual) problem. In Lacanian terms, he also seems to offer a commentary on the non-existence of the Other, not the actual other of Amy Cooper as a person (who taps into a racist vein) or the actual other of a police officer (who may be violent), but upon the tyranny of the Other as it applies to him in the racist beating fantasy.

There is, in Lacanian terms, no Other of the Other and, by this, he means that there is no essential or inevitable support for whatever tyranny may be perpetuated by particular (individual) others. Likewise, Christian Cooper understands that the racism underlying Amy Cooper's racially motivated police call is not founded upon anything that is true or inevitable like, for example, racial difference. Race is a dangerous fiction that can be overwritten by new, creative, emancipatory fictions. He also seems to know something about a significatory, as opposed to a legal, injunction. As an African American writer, he knows that the racism and aggressivity of others must be symbolically leashed. This is not the same as saying that racist aggressivity must lead to police arrest, fine or imprisonment. Christian Cooper recognizes the difference between a significatory leash (like a sign) and the tyranny of legal agents, the latter of whom do not typically act in the interests of African Americans as a group and reinforce existing (white) power structures. Etymologically speaking, "leash" derives from the Latin word "*laxa*" meaning thong or a loose cord. Its feminine form is "*laxus*" and means loose. Not only was Henry-the-dog unleashed but so to was Amy Cooper's fantasy relating to an African American man threatening her life and her dog. The leash, not unlike a Lacanian signifier, has some give (slack). It is tightly held but affords room to play. The Law, by contrast, is exacting and leaves no room to maneuver. It also reinforces the power of the Other (as agent of the law), part of what must be disarmed to ameliorate anti-black racism. Cooper knows that the law, let alone policing, will not end anti-black racism. But more than this he, like the Lacanian analysand who completes a successful analysis, makes a passage to the act. In essence, Christian Cooper leaves the scene (of trauma) and acts in a way that disregards and disarms, if only in his science fiction, the racist tyranny of the Other. In so doing, Christian Cooper does not lend support or give consistency to the logic of racism and redemption through the law which does not emancipate but largely criminalize African Americans.

Conclusion

Amy Cooper, by contrast, does not escape the law. She was ordered by the courts to complete an educational and therapeutic program on racial identity. The prosecutor said that the therapy-education program is "designed not just to punish but to educate and promote community healing" (as cited in Bromwich, 2021, para. 5). The order involved five therapy sessions at the Critical Therapy Center in Manhattan dealing with racism and identity. According to the prosecutor and reported in *The New York Times*, Amy Cooper's therapist reported that the sessions were "a moving experience" and Amy Cooper "learned a lot." But the president of the Critical Therapy Center acknowledged that they cannot "end racism in five sessions" (as cited in Bromwich, 2021, para. 25).

They cannot end racism in five sessions because it is a structural problem tapping into desire and *jouissance*, thereby involving a Real excess that cannot be easily defused. Like the beating fantasy, racism is structured in such a way that the one having the racist fantasy occupies the position of victim (child being beaten) while the one subject to racism (at risk of an actual beating) occupies the position of aggressor. What the structural logic of the beating fantasy reveals is that racism cannot be remedied by policing (as Christian Cooper knows) or by instruction-oriented psychotherapy (education). Racism is a Real problem that concerns being, and the (*jouissant*) excitation is, in the contemporary case, animated by and channeled through animals. What Christian Cooper teaches us is that we can create fantasy-solutions (fiction and animation) that are sinthomatic (curative and creative knots). New fantasies involving characters like X-men and Northstar are needed to reconfigure the socio-Symbolic tied as it is to the Imaginary and to the Real. It is the signifier, not the letter of the law, that will denote (scansion) anti-black racism in the Anthropocene.

Aknowledgements

I wish to Sheldon George and Derek Hook for organizing the Lacan and Fanon stream of the Psychology and the Other conference where this chapter was originally presented. I also thank Caitlin Janzen for valuable feedback relating to the conceptualization of this chapter.

Notes

1 The fraudulent call for help in Central Park follows the actual deaths of Michael Brown who was grabbed by the neck and then fatally shot by police officer Darren Wilson in Ferguson, Missouri; Eric Garner who was also killed by a police officer, Daniel Pantaleo, after being put in an illegal chokehold in Stanton Island (for allegedly selling single cigarettes from packages without tax stamps); Ahmaud Arbery shot to death by Gregory McMichael and his son, Travis McMichael in South Georgia (because he allegedly resembled a house break-in suspect but was actually just out for a jog); and Amadou Diallo who was killed by forty-one bullets shot by four plain-clothed police officers who misidentified him as a rape suspect.
2 In 1978, Richard Totten "Dick" Button, a figure skater (who twice won gold at the Olympics and is a world champion five times over, also) was, along with five other men, brutally assaulted by a gang of young men with baseball bats intending to target gay men cruising in the park.
3 Anthony said in 1869 that "if intelligence, justice and morality are to have precedence in the government, let the question of women be brought up first and that of the negro last."
4 Their sentences were vacated after Maties Reyes confessed to the crime.
5 Donald Trump who was then a real estate financier bought an advertisement in the *Daily News* that called for a return of the death penalty. The advertisement was believed to have swayed public opinion against the six teens which led, in part, to their wrongful conviction. When it became clear that the teens were prejudicially accused and wrongfully convicted protests were held outside the Trump Tower asking for an apology (which was not given).
6 It is worth noting that cocker spaniels and birds have, like Amy Cooper and Christian Cooper, an adversarial history dating back, at least, to the fourteenth century. Cocker spaniels were bred as bird-hunting or "gun dogs" in the United Kingdom. Their job was to launch birds hiding on land into flight (to be shot),

and then to retrieve the gunned-down bird with a "soft mouth." The "cocker" (a phallic signifier) originates from the Eurasian woodcock that they were trained to hunt in the United Kingdom and later, the American woodcock, they hunted in the US.

7 Christian Cooper is a Harvard graduate (with a degree in political science), senior editorial director for *Health Sciences Communications,* and an award-winning comic book writer. He has such an impressive following that he is called upon to endorse political candidates (democrats) like, for instance, Ritchie Torres, who is openly gay and Latino, to represent the south Bronx in Congress. Even Barak Obama makes favorable references to Christian Cooper.

8 https://ecojustice.ca/environmental-racism-in-canada/.

9 Amy Cooper claims the firm suspended her without having done a proper investigation. She sued Franklin and Templeton for wrongful dismissal and claimed that a proper investigation was not done into the incident because of her gender and race. Her attorney, Matthew Litt, wrote that "Franklin Templeton perpetuated and legitimized the story of 'Karen' vs. an innocent African American to its perceived advantage, with reckless disregard for the destruction of Plaintiff's life in the process" (as cited in Stieb, 2021).

10 https://www.nytimes.com/2020/06/14/nyregion/central-park-amy-cooper-christian-racism.html.

11 Due in no small part to the Christian Coopers of the world, X-Men are becoming more bio-genetically, culturally, and sexually diverse. Cooper was the first out gay writer and editor at Marvel Comics and introduced one gay and one lesbian character in the series. He was also associate editor for *Alpha Flight* which includes a gay character named Northstar who marries his lover in *Astonishing X-Men.* Northstar was a member of the Canadian super-team featured in the comic (first appearing in X-men). Interestingly, Northstar (created by Christ Claremont and John Byrne) was, like Amy Cooper, of Canadian origin. Unlike Amy Cooper, Northstar has extra-human powers and can fly at nonhuman speeds and send photonic energy blasts out into the universe. While Amy Cooper's fraudulent police call had the effect of a photonic energy blast and did circulate on social media at non-human (virtual) speed, it was caught (by video-recording) and exposed (as counter-factual prejudice).

12 The mutual fund company was named after Benjamin Franklin because of his conservative, frugal, and prudent approach to finance.

References

Bromwich, J. E. (2021, February 16) Amy Cooper, who falsely accused black bird-watcher, has charge dismissed. *The New York Times.* https://www.nytimes.com/2021/02/16/nyregion/amy-cooper-charges-dismissed.html.

Cacich, A. (2020, June 17) New wave of backlash hits woman who called cops on black birdwatcher. *Distractify,* https://www.distractify.com/p/did-amy-cooper-get-her-dog-back/.

Cleary, T. (2021, December 18) Amy Cooper: New York woman calls police on black man who asked her to leash dog. *heavy.com.* https://heavy.com/news/2020/05/amy-cooper-video-new-york/.

Comedy Central. (2020, June 1) Trevor Noah on George Floyd, Amy Cooper & racism in society [Video]. Youtube. https://www.youtube.com/watch?v=Jb4Bg8mu2aM.

Davies, B. (2020, April 15) Freud At Home with His Dogs. Freud Museum London, https://www.freud.org.uk/2020/04/15/freud-at-home-with-his-dogs/.

Freud, S. (1955) A child is being beaten: A contribution to the study of the origin of sexual perversions. In J. Strachey (Ed. & Trans.) *The standard edition of the complete psychological works of Sigmund Freud, Volume XVII (1917–1919): An infantile neurosis and other works*. Hogarth Press, pp. 175–204.

Giovannetti, M. D. F. and Slotkin, P. (1997) The scene and its reverse: Considerations on a chain of associations in Freud. In E. S. Person (Ed.), *On Freud's "A child is being beaten"*. Yale University Press, pp. 95–111.

Gupta, A. H. (2020, August 6) For three suffragists, a monument well past due. *The New York Times*. www.nytimes.com/2020/08/06/arts/design/suffragist-19th-amendment-central- park.html.

Los Angeles Times. (2020, May 27) Amy Cooper apologizes after Central Park confrontation [Video]. YouTube. https://www.youtube.com/watch?v=iUQWd4q3tjA/.

Mercado, M. (2022, January 6) Childless man says not having kids is "selfish." The cut. *New York Magazine*. https://www.thecut.com/2022/01/pope-francis-choosing-pets-over-kids- selfish.html.

Nir, S. M. (2020, June 14) How 2 lives collided in Central Park, rattling the nation. *The New York Times*. www.nytimes.com/2020/06/14/nyregion/central-park-amy-cooper-christian- racism.html.

Quaglia, S. (2019, October 23) Cracking the bronze ceiling: The US has fewer than 400 statues of women – but that's changing. *Quartz*. qz.com/1732974/new-york-citys-central-park- will-get-its-first-statue-of-women/.

Ransom, J. (2020, July 7) Case against Amy Cooper lacks key element: Victim's cooperation. *The New York Times*. www.nytimes.com/2020/07/07/nyregion/amy-cooper- central-park-false-report-charge.html?searchResultPosition=12.

Romano, A. (2020, July 21) How "Karen" became a symbol of racism. *Vox*. www.vox.com/21317728/karen-meaning-meme-racist-coronavirus.

Sanchez, R. and Joseph, E. (2020, July 15) Black birdwatcher Christian Cooper says prosecuting Amy Cooper "lets white people off the hook". CNN. www.cnn.com/2020/07/15/us/christian-cooper-central-park-op-ed/index.html.

Silberman, S. (1998, December 29) Can Miss Thang save Earth? *Wired*. www.wired.com/1998/12/can-miss-thang-save-earth/?fbclid=IwAR3iEjyOmx-   OGot3VBzWz cUVRvey1E7nKano-bHvLn4wi_QHX5zfWK28B4E. Accessed 29 Dec. 2021.

Small, Z. (2021, December 21) Historians raise concerns over Central Park's suffragist monument. *Hyperallergic*. hyperallergic.com/514079/historians-raise-concerns-over-central-parks-suffragist-monument/.

Stieb, M. (2021, May 26) Amy Cooper didn't learn much from her time as "Central Park Karen". Intelligencer. *New York Magazine*. nymag.com/intelligencer/2021/05/amy-cooper-didnt- learn-much-from-being-central-park-karen.html.

The Centre for American Progress. (2021, July 21) The nature gap: Confronting racial and economic disparities in the destruction and protection of nature in America. CAP.org. www.americanprogress.org/issues/green/reports/2020/07/21/487787/the-nature-gap/.

Vera, A. and Ly, L. (2020, May 26) White woman who called police on a black man bird- watching in Central Park has been fired. CNN. www.cnn.com/2020/05/26/us/central- park-video-dog-video-african-american-trnd/index.html/.

Viñar, M. N. (1997). Construction of a fantasy (trans. P. Slotkin). In E. S. Person (Ed.), *On Freud's "A child is being beaten"*. Yale University Press, pp. 179–188.

Weiss, B. (Host). (2021, August 3). The real story of 'the Central Park Karen. (No. 256) [Audio podcast episode]. In Honestly with Bari Weiss. www.honestlypod.com/p odcast/episode/256bac0b/the-real-story-of-the-central-park-karen. Zupančič, A. (2017) *What is sex?*MIT Press.

Chapter 9

Colonial Pathologies

Revisiting the Puerto Rican Syndrome

Patricia Gherovici

My clinical work as a psychoanalyst employed first as a psychotherapist, and later as a clinical director, in two inner-city mental health clinics in the heart of the poverty-ridden, racially segregated, so-called "Hispanic" community of North Philadelphia, made me come across a mysterious diagnosis I never heard of before – the Puerto Rican syndrome. I purposely use here the label "Hispanic," a controversial racialized designation noting that most of my patients were of Puerto Rican origin and lived in an area of language-demarcated boundaries identified primarily as belonging to "the Puerto Rican race" rather than as Hispanic or Latino. "Hispanic" is a problematic construct conflating categories of language (a Spaniard, for example, is not Hispanic), of race (there is no unique ethnic group identifiable solely as Spanish-speaking), and of class (a rich Hispanic, away from the ghetto, loses most of the characteristics associated with being Hispanic).

Coming myself from a country like Argentina, where the middle class is slowly disappearing and poverty keeps increasing, where one often finds in a European-looking city like Buenos Aires, barefoot children begging for food and entire families of litter-pickers pushing carts full of the found trash that they will try to sell (*cartoneros*), I was expecting to find in a rich, developed country like the United States a more egalitarian situation. In fact, I found comparable levels of hardship and scarcity. The reality of life in the "barrio" introduces the Third World at the core of the US mainland. As for the clinics like the ones I worked at, they are not just mental health treatment centers but locations for social buffering. The prevailing model is pedagogical, proposing heavy medication combined with behavioral orthopedics in order to straighten up what is seen as deviant, maladaptive conducts. To adjust as quickly as possible is the treatment goal, an objective that given the realities of life in the ghetto means adapting to an oppressive situation of need. My experience with clinical work in Philadelphia's barrio has proved that psychoanalysis can be effectively conducted in settings not considered "traditional" in the United States. Psychoanalysis, thanks to its power of actualizing otherness, can reveal its emancipatory potential with populations

DOI: 10.4324/9781003394327-10

marginalized by race, class, gender, or sexuality. Furthermore, psychoanalysis is not only possible but much needed in the so-called Hispanic ghetto.

Not only was I shocked by the poverty in the barrio but also taken aback by the diagnosis of "Puerto Rican syndrome," which was a novelty for me. This diagnosis attached to a nationality, is a suggestive, symptomatic label for a community that still lives in a semi-colonial situation. It describes a group of striking and seemingly inexplicable symptoms: attacks of anger, eccentric seizures with no organic origin, anxiety, and fear in a choleric battle with an imaginary enemy, suicidal gestures, hallucinations, amnesia. Labeled "Puerto Rican syndrome," all these manifestations confirmed an uncanny return of the somatic grammar of classic hysteria. As I was going to learn, the "Puerto Rican" syndrome would involve complex symptom formations bringing together clinical and political issues.

Historical Context

What is remarkable about this syndrome? This baffling psychiatric label applies uniquely to Puerto Ricans identifying a pathology affecting nationals living in an unresolved semi-colonial situation, since Puerto Rico is not an independent country having gone from being under Spanish colonial power to falling under US control after the Spanish-American war, and more than a century later it continues caught up in a complex dependence from the United States. Thus, this diagnosis links nationality, cultural phenomena, and psychiatric disease. It is strikingly similar to the extravagant behavior of classical hysterics who rendered the invention of psychoanalysis possible. This group of varied manifestations has also been described as "hyperkinetic seizure," *nervios* (nerves), *mal de pelea* (disease of fighting), and *ataque de nervios* (which means attacks and nerves, respectively, and could be translated as nervous breakdown). The re-appearance of such noteworthy, almost "old fashioned" form of hysteria is even more surprising at a time when the mere use of the word "hysteria" in clinical practice seems an anachronism. Although hysteria has its place of honor in the history of psychoanalysis, the diagnosis quickly disappeared from the standard psychiatric nomenclature during the 1950s. Ironically, the semantic suppression of the diagnosis of hysteria took place at the time that the Puerto Rican syndrome was identified. Besides its theatrical characteristics, what is most startling about this syndrome is that is allegedly a mode of disease uniquely Puerto Rican, reminding us that its symptoms knot together clinical, racial, gender, and political issues.

That diagnosis was coined in the 1950s, when US Army doctors in the Veteran administration noticed a cluster of strange symptoms in some Puerto Rican soldiers, all participants in the Korean War. That conflict began on June 25, 1950 when communist North Korea (Democratic People's Republic of Korea) invaded territories of South Korea (Republic of Korea) supported by the United States. In the context of the cold war, the conflict quickly became internationalized, since North Korea had the support of the communist bloc made up of China and the Soviet Union while South Korea was defended by the United Nations, which at that time brought together a coalition of nineteen countries allied to the interests of the United States. In fact, most of the troops that participated in the battle were from the United States. There was one very special units among those sent by the United States to the Korean front lines, a regiment renowned for its bravery and battlefield prowess: the 65th Infantry, the only section of the US Army made up almost exclusively of Puerto Ricans. The "65" was also known as the "Borinqueños" regiment, a designation calling up the pre-Columbian name for the island of Puerto Rico – Borinquen. The participation of Puerto Rican soldiers in the Korean War was enormous – between 45,000 and 65,000 Puerto Ricans fought in Korea. Many of those soldiers were part of the "65." The fact that the regiment was almost exclusively Puerto Rican was an exception since US armed forces had already been desegregated in 1948. This war ended with a precarious cessation of hostilities on July 27, 1953, after the signing of an armistice in Panmunjom that established the 38th parallel as the line of separation between the two Koreas, that is, returning to the same territorial situation that existed before from the war.

The active participation of Puerto Rican soldiers who fought under the US flag, not only in the Korean War but also in other armed conflicts, disappeared from collective memory.[1] For the historian Silvia Álvarez Curbelo, the figure of the Puerto Rican soldier embodies the transition from the plantation colony "to an autonomous pact among equals" under US domination (Álvarez Curbelo, 2008b, 220). A Puerto Rican soldier fighting for the United States in the Korean War was in an ambiguous position marked by the many contradictions in the political relationship between Puerto Rico and the United States.

The Puerto Rican syndrome was diagnosed in soldiers whose participation in the Korean War took place at a time of enormous historical significance for the island. Those "disturbed" soldiers played a role in a war that exposed and exacerbated the tensions and paradoxes of the colonial status of a Puerto Rico in the process of rapid modernization. This was a process that involved "violent psychological and spatial displacements". Nearly 250,000 Puerto Ricans emigrated to the United States between 1947 and 1953. This migration process devastated agriculture and rural life on the island.

The participation of Puerto Rican soldiers in the Korean war as first-line troops was expected to "help Puerto Ricans to come out of their complexes of insularism, and erase the marks of inferiority, which are the byproduct of hundreds of years of colonial type regimes" as asserted in San Juan's *Periódico El Mundo* in an editorial published on October 12, 1950 also known as "The day of the race," the celebration date of Columbus "discovery".

The expectation was that the participation of Puerto Rican fighters in the Korean war even though in a still segregated all-Hispanic regiment would prove that they were equal to the mainland soldiers. The complexity of the position of a Puerto Rican soldier is illustrated by the statement of 65th Corporal Ruiz:

> We are proud to be part of the United Nations Forces, and we are proud of our country. We feel that too many people do not know anything about Puerto Rico; they think that we are all natives who climb trees... We are glad for the chance to fight the communists and also for the chance to put Puerto Rico on the map. It will be a great accomplishment if we can raise the prestige of our country in the eyes of the world.
> (Harris, 2001)

Álvarez Curbelo notes that the regiment's ethnic homogeneity was the reason for its heroic commitment and strong performance in the front battles. The action of the "Borinqueños" in Korea was undoubtedly extraordinary. In the summer of 1951, peace talks gave hope for a swift end of the conflict. These were days of glory for the "Borinqueños," a regiment that considered Puerto Rico their homeland. When the first troops returned from the Korean front, the Puerto Rican government declared a holiday and the entire island celebrated their soldiers as heroes. During the first year of the war, the 65th had quite a lot success despite few setbacks. However, with the stalemate in the peace talks, the morale of the troops began to falter.

In May 1951, because of the rotation system, the regiment lost its skillful commander. Colonel William Harris was relieved of his duties, along with most of the elite soldiers who comprised this unit. They were replaced by less trained officers. The new soldiers were not volunteers and, unlike their predecessors, hardly spoke English. At the beginning of the armed conflict in Korea, the soldiers sent to the front were bilingual and highly trained career military members. But the longer the war lasted, many more inexperienced, Spanish speaking-only soldiers joined the regiment. The newcomers were placed under the orders of less senior officers. Letters sent by the soldiers to their family and friends describe an increasingly desperate situation. From the island, Luis Muñoz Marín, who had been newly elected governor of the freshly-minted Puerto Rican "commonwealth" (in English) and Estado Libre Asociado (Freely Associated State, in Spanish) urged his compatriots to fight in Korea for freedom and democracy (exactly the same motto used in 1898 when the United States took control of the island and started its colonial rule). To relieve tensions and reinforce the patriotic message, Juan César Cordero Dávila, a Puerto Rican and a friend of the charismatic governor, was appointed head of the regiment. The pessimism of the soldiers was not alleviated.

The need to choose a Puerto Rican leader in the US military reveals the complexity of the situation of the "Borinqueños" and the contradictions inherent in the political relationship between Puerto Rico and the United States in the 1950s. A few years earlier, in 1948, Puerto Rico had elected its first governor and as the Korean War began, the country's constitution was being drafted. In 1952, after more than half a century of American occupation, the Puerto Rican flag and national anthem were decriminalized. The soldiers were encouraged to express their patriotism, and it was only natural that Puerto Rican flags should be sent to Korea, where the Puerto Rican soldiers planted them proudly on conquered territories.

What was known as the Battle for Outpost Kelly, in which dozens of Puerto Rican soldiers died, was a misdirected operation. According to some military personnel involved, the botched action was motivated by Commander Colonel Cordero's wish to conquer Kelly and give an emblem of the loyalty of Puerto Ricans to the United States, that is in fact a tribute of blood (Álvarez Curbelo, 2008a). Following this failed operation, which entailed the highest loss in human lives among all military actions carried out during the Korean War, Cordero was relieved of his duties. He was replaced by a new commander, the "continental" Colonel Chester De Gavre, an American from Wisconsin who showed mostly contempt for the Puerto Rican national pride of the regiment.

De Gavre found himself at the head of a regiment of bearded and badly dressed soldiers looking more like Che Guevara than US marines. They were using handkerchiefs under their helmets, for instance. De Gavre felt that he had to reinforce the disciplinary policy, which entailed a swift and drastic "Americanization." In addition to demanding a military salute, haircut, shoe polish, regular maintenance of the uniform, equipment and weapons, he forbade soldiers to wear a mustache "until they demonstrated that they were men" (Villahermosa, 2009, 239). The order to shave the mustache was tantamount to an emasculation for a Puerto Rican male in the 1950s. The measure raised serious objections; De Grave's questioning of a soldier's virility was perceived as humiliating and insulting. Three chaplains of the regiment tried to mediate, but Colonel De Gavre persisted: "The chaplains came to me and told me that if I maintained this order, Iwould be assassinated within twenty-four hours. But I've stood firm, and I'm still alive" (Villahermosa, 2009, 240). In fact, the order was ignored as long as possible; some soldiers resigned themselves to shaving their mustaches only under threat of court martial.

De Gavre also changed the regiment's diet: Puerto Rican rice and beans were replaced by American dishes like potatoes and hotdogs. There was also an order to erase the name "borinqueños" from the regiment's jeeps. Obviously, the morale of the troops deteriorated even more. The intensive training ordered by De Gavre increased their frustration because of supply problems in Korea that prevented it from being done efficiently – there was not sufficient ammunition.

A month later, faced with increasingly intolerable conditions and an incompetent, tyrannical command, indifferent to the regiment's idiosyncrasy, the Puerto Rican troops rebelled on Jackson Heights Hill. In the testimonies collected by the court martial, the soldiers declared that they refused to obey the orders simply because they were inapplicable. Not only they felt that it was a suicide mission, but the commander himself was unable to clearly define the objectives. Of the almost two hundred soldiers arrested for "deliberate inaction in the face of the enemy" and "disobedience to the orders of a superior," ninety-two soldiers and an officer appeared before the court martial. The Puerto Rican government did not publicly oppose the trial of its nationals and tried to silence the story. At the end of 1952, the incidents were made public in a local newspaper, which had been made aware of the events by letters sent by the detained soldiers to their families.

The incidents that occurred in Korea are "a highly intricate process in which subordination and resistance mechanisms are intertwined," observes Álvarez Curbelo. If by the end of the year 1950, the Puerto Rican soldiers were "perfect colonial subjects," both for the military authorities and for the local elites, two years later, while on the battlefield, this project was in a downward spiral with "hundreds of soldiers dead to defend a piece of barren land; their otherness exposed in broad daylight with fierce force, and the 65th returning home dishonored." For the Puerto Rican people, who had been so proud of their "Borinqueños," the main issue was dignity; the courage and initiative of its soldiers were perceived as fundamental elements of their cultural identity.

These military operations of 1952 that caused the dissolution of the 65th Regiment and which today are a footnote in the history of the Korean War, show complexities and antagonisms that are inherent in all colonial rapports. While studying the transcripts of more than ninety testimonies and depositions presented during the court martial of the soldiers accused of desertion, Álvarez Curbelo identifies a recurring tendency: the infantilization of the Puerto Rican soldiers, whose capacity to speak and to understand was put in question, or simply denied. All the defendants were found guilty and sentenced to five to sixteen years of forced labor. They were dismissed from the army. Eventually, they were rehabilitated as a result of secret negotiations between the governments of the United States and Puerto Rico.

For Álvarez Curbelo the position of Puerto Rican soldiers in the Korean War illustrates a foundational asymmetry sustained by more than one hundred years of colonial domination while showing the ambiguity of the position of a "colonized" subject in response to imperial projects, all the while remarking that ethnicity can function both as a mechanism of adaptation and resistance. Álvarez Curbelo interprets the role of the Puerto Rican soldiers in Korea as a paradoxical collective affirmation of identity in the face of military irrationality, defined by a wish to enforce order at the cost of tactical success.

As Sophie Mendelsohn suggests,[2] the project of producing an integration of the indigenous male population through the army and within the framework of an imperialist conflict (the war in Korea as a war of influence during the Cold War) could be considered as a paradoxical means of achieving a colonized masculine pride that would be the counterpart of the Puerto Rican syndrome, which both exposes colonial humiliation in the feminine (and perhaps that can only be sustained in the feminine) and attacks the imposture of masculine pride in a colonial context.

Indeed, there seems to be a clear structural homology between the appearance of the symptoms grouped in the diagnosis "Puerto Rican syndrome" a diagnosis invented by US Army doctors evaluation Puerto Rican soldiers involved in the Korean war and two minor military operations in the Korean war that included incidents of insubordination culminating in a court-martial trial for ninety-two soldiers and an official, which also provoked the dissolution of the famous Borinqueños 65th Infantry.

What struck me was that by inventing the diagnosis, the US Army doctors had kept alive the memory of what was a forgotten chapter in American-Puerto Rican history. In fact the same symptoms had been called *ataque de nervios*, and have been considered a common occurrence in Puerto Rican culture for a long time prior to the invention of the syndrome. One can see an example of this ubiquity in the novel *Candle in the Sun* written in English by Edith Roberts (1937/2018). The story immerses us in the experiences and vicissitudes of a young American newly-married woman, who follows her husband to the island and thus discovers the ins and outs of life in an American colony, which despite not being directly named, is obviously Puerto Rico. The author of the novel was a true connoisseur of the island, a prolific writer that under different aliases published numerous books on Puerto Rico.[4]

The Novel of Colonialism

I will further develop here the discussion of the novel in *The Puerto Rican Syndrome* (Gherovici, 2003) so as to highlight aspects of gender, race, and colonial domination touched upon too briefly in the book. The problematics of race are a determining factor not only in the plot but also in the ideological positions represented by the main characters.

The *Candle in the Sun*'s protagonist is Avery Carpenter, an educated, independent feminist, who, fascinated with the promise of romance and adventures with a gallant Puerto Rican man, marries "precipitously", that is, in the United States, away from both families and bypassing the religious ceremony. Her husband is Hernán Colón y Cortés, a young lawyer, freshly graduated from Harvard. He belongs to a traditional and powerful family of politicians, who boasts of being descendants of Christopher Columbus and whose father is the figure in command of the "federals," one of the two parties that dominate the island's local political arena. Avery abandons her college studies and follows her husband to the island, and is quickly immersed in the new and opaque, agitated and oppressive world of the "inner island" represented by the imposing Colón and Cortés family.

Maybe to give authenticity to the account while accentuating the exoticism of the location, the author reveals a typical and everyday occurrence. Roberts begins her novel with a detailed description of the *ataque* of Doña Concepción. In a dramatic contrast of styles, Avery's parents, Charles Carpenter, a university professor and an anthropologist, and his wife Helen, receive in the privacy of their home a telegram with the news that their daughter is the brand-new "Señora de Colón" and they respond with contained emotion. They express little of their feelings beyond a few tears and they quickly comfort themselves by speculating that the colonial status of the island will protect her. The "Island" is a territory of United States and therefore they trust the island's authorities because the governor is an American citizen appointed by the president of United States. Their daughter may be in a hurried marriage but she will be safe.

In the island, Doña Concepción, the mother of the brand-new husband, reacts with intense drama and crumbles "as a mountain of sand in an earthquake" (Gherovici, 2003, 10) and "collapse[s] in rage under the shock", not without first having boisterously expressed her pain and displeasure at the news of the marriage through a severe nervous breakdown whose epicenter is her bedroom but quickly expands throughout the neighborhood by summoning numerous onlookers, all fascinated witnesses to her desperate crisis. Here is the description:

> Doña Concepción was having an *ataque*. The four-poster rocked with it. The whole house vibrated to it. A purple and gilt image of Mary hanging against the blue wall at the head of the bed was particularly agitated. It seemed likely to fall and smash at any moment.
>
> When two hundred and ten pounds of irrational femininity burst into hysterics, reverberations are apt to reach even the public. Thus in the street a little bony *negresse* paused in the hot June sunshine and stood open mouthed without removing from her head a wooden tray piled with a snowy mountain of laundry. She was joined by an itinerant vendor of live lobsters. These two formed a nucleus for the quite large group of passers-by soon staring into … Doña Concepción's bedroom where a considerable number of persons could be discerned milling about.
>
> (Gherovici, 2003, 9)

The situation of Puerto Rico in the late 1930s is a time of transition for the island that until then had been administered as a large dependent sugar plantation. At the time, an educated and progressive native elite emerged and played a key role in politics, under the populist leadership of Luis Muñoz

Marín. This situation is part of the narratological structure of the novel that describes at length the cultural shock experienced by the American young woman, but the reference to this political background is not as precise as the description of discriminations based on race, class, and gender. All this is seen through the naïve gaze of the protagonist, who examines with astonishment the lives of the "others."

Already the opening scene of the *ataque* disturbs us with the stereotypical description of the young girl's brown skin in stark contrast with the "a snowy mountain of laundry" piled over her head. Unlike this girl who witnessed the *ataque*, Avery cannot remove from her head the heavy weight of her white privilege. Her distance and estrangement as an "other" herself as a non-Catholic American is only slightly mitigated over time, before a great crisis that is produced when the protagonist discovers with great surprise that she has given birth to a lesser "other" since his eldest son, Juanito, has a physiognomy that reveals the presence of black ancestors in the husband's maternal lineage. Avery is disturbed by this discovery and experiences this fact as an "injustice" pondering how her youngest daughter could look so much like her while her first-born would have "colored blood" (Roberts, 1937, 270) whose otherness is evidenced

> not so much in pigmentation nor in the snowy softly curling hair, but rather in an indefinable cast of countenance, in a molding of features so subtly as to defy description. You couldn't, in a word, tell *how* you knew but you immediately *knew*.
>
> (Roberts, 1937, 271)

Avery operates under the colonial libidinal economy but represses its "unsayable", which corresponds to the reality of her racism even if she denies to herself that there is any difference between her children. At the same time, she worships her daughter's light skin, blue eyes and blond hair. "Avery deliberately planned to live a lie. That was the paradoxical price placed upon happiness by convention" (Roberts, 1937, 388). What is the "convention" Avery accepts?

The plot explores the Oedipal rivalry between mother-in-law and daughter-in-law and the attendant clashes between the Puerto Rican and American cultural models. I want to highlight that Avery's resistance to the pressure of "the Puerto Rican Family" to make her convert to Catholicism and adopt a subservient role may also imply a resistance to a return of the repressed of heterosexist and racist "conventions." Her husband turns out to be a *machista* and a philanderer. Avery ends up finding love outside her marriage in the arms of a fellow white American, Curt Baring, who is also in a tense inter-racial marriage. The self-effacing third person narrator makes tangential reference to the political background. Nonetheless, politics are a main character in the story: Avery's in-laws belong to the "Federals" whose "*cacique maximo*" is her husband's father. There is also repeated mention of anti-American feelings among the Family. Her being the *americanita* invites all kinds of political attacks from the opposing party to the Federals, the Progressives. Despite all this, it is only in brief and almost ironical tones that Avery thinks explicitly of the colonial status of the island. A few pages before the end, Avery comes to another cocktail party and chats with an American economist. The "Important Expert" appears more concerned with cocktails and picking up the local beauties than with discussing politics; Avery teases him with uncharacteristic impertinence until he is moved to ask her opinion. Then Avery drops the word "independence," but then alarmed, she corrects herself: "I didn't mean independence for the Island," she says quickly. "I just mean independence from busybody 'experts'" ... . For a few moments Avery considered the possibility of such a political upheaval, which would put in the shade everything that happened up to now. But not for long. National problems, however great, faded into a dim perspective before the towering shadow of her personal trouble (Roberts, 1937, 387).

With some interpretive effort, one may recognize references to the real events behind the imaginary characters and situations in this book. Let us take a look, for example, at the very ending of the novel:

> As she stopped before the country house, she saw that it was blazing with lights. A quite large cluster of peasants, numbers of whom were always passing along the busy highway, were staring across the hedge towards the dwelling from which poured the unmistakable sounds of Doña Concepcion's hysteria ... Pushing by the gaping peasants who murmured "*La Americanita*," as she passed, she hastened to join the Family.
>
> (Roberts, 1937, 391)

In Avery's decision "to join the Family," we can easily recognize an allusion to *La gran familia puertorriqueña* (the great Puerto Rican Family), a slogan stressing unity that played a key role in the cultural discourse of the *autonomistas* movement of the turn of the nineteenth century. In this last scene, the *campesinos* (peasants) who stare across the edge represent the impoverished working class witnessing the decline of the now disenfranchised upper class matron Doña Conception whose husband first loses the elections and then ends up in shameful poverty. Throughout the novel, Doña Conception, a devoted Catholic, opposes the claim for women's rights upheld by Avery in open confrontations. According to Mariano Negron-Portillo, these two features – Catholicism and opposition to women's rights – defined the *unionistas,* a nationalist organization in the Puerto Rico of the 1930s (Negron-Portillo, 1997, 50–51). The Federals and Progressives of the novel call up the two main political parties that dominated Puerto Rican life. The "growing figure of the Laborite, Lorenzo Gomez...that gentleman, with his rolled-up shirt sleeves" (Roberts, 1937, 384) evokes

Pedro Albizu Campos, the leader of the newly founded pro-independence *Partido Nacionalista*. Since Albizu Campos entered politics as a member of the Unionist party, and later, of the Alianza, it is quite likely that Doña Conception's defeated husband, Don Sancho, would have been displaced within his party by the emerging Albizu Campos who, like Don Sancho and like most actors in the long elitist nationalist tradition, defended the Catholic Church and invoked concepts like *La Raza,* claiming Hispanic ancestry based on Spanish soul, language, customs, and idiosyncrasy (Negron-Portillo, 1997). The main character is constantly reminding us of Puerto Rican animosity towards her as an American, for she is perceived not just as a foreigner but as an antagonist.

On many occasions, however, Avery criticized the arrogance, naiveté and lack of goodwill of Washington-appointed bureaucrats, the "just-at-the-moment-unoccupied Experts ... aware that the hitherto obscure territory tucked away among the Indies had a PROBLEM." If this novel gives voice to a political critique of the colonial situation the heroin observes, it is obliquely. Just like Avery, who as we have seen, glimpses momentous "National problems" but allows them to fade "into a dim perspective before the towering shadow of her personal trouble." If Avery blurted out "independence" as the only solution when she faced a US expert, her statement is immediately undercut by what appear as annoyance at American arrogance.

The context of this outburst should not be downplayed: the young American wife, also a young mother, is having an affair with a handsome white American man soon to leave the island. The last chapter evokes the final nights of intimacy and her sadness after he has left. Another male American friend tried to teach her to disguise her feelings in order to avoid a full blown scandal. Still full of the memories of intense love-making, Avery returned to fetch her kids at her mother-in-law's and this is when she discovered that the latter was having an *ataque*. No clear reason for the outburst of hysteria is given, the reader is left to surmise its causes. Has the family heard of the affair? Has a new political event happened? Is it to be blamed on Dona Concepcion's cycles of mood changes? More than any reason given to these ominous fits, what stands out as very revealing is that the book opens and closes with Doña Concepcion having an *ataque*.

This narrative twist reveals the *ataque*'s function: more than the exposition of a "native malady" it is a paradigm of how the colonizers see the "other" as other. The "incoherent screams" constitute a message addressed to the Other. The *ataque* – a precursor of the Puerto Rican syndrome – epitomizes the view of the outsider who is surprised by such strange manifestations. Most importantly this novel exemplifies the fact that the *ataque* always intertwines personal dilemmas and political upheavals. One could not fully understand the *ataque* just by focusing on the symptoms. In order to make sense of Doña Concepcion's *ataques* one must take into account the intense, explosive emotions triggered by a context determined by colonial politics, sexual betrayal, racial oppression, and divided allegiances.

Ultimately, Avery accepts her new homeland, more resigned than adjusted, and with it she agrees to a life in a place where prejudices reign along deplorable racial lines. This predicament torments her and that in a moment of despair she considers committing suicide during her second pregnancy and also killing her first child. Avery takes shelter in the prerogatives of her upper-class new family but she does not avoid feeling stranger everywhere: "She would never really belong in any place but the Island. She was, by an inexorable fate, an exile". Indeed, "an alien" who "barely suppressed hysteria", Avery could only appear as an "exile" (Roberts, 1937, 265–266).

Lacan on the Father and Families

In order to make sense of Avery's position as an "exile" in Puerto Rico's colonial context, let me backtrack in this last part of my essay. In 1938, one year after the *Candle in the Sun*'s publication, Jacques Lacan explored the evolution of the Western family and predicted a decline in the role of the father (Lacan, 2001). More than eighty years later, we can wonder whether our contemporary situation shows an aftermath of this decline and whether race has intervened as a symptomatic new marker of difference. Lacan's 1938 article for the *Encyclopédie Française*, "The Family complexes in the formation of the individual" develops the notion of the "decline of the paternal imago." Lacan mentions that the decline of the father's figure in modern times had created the "appearance of psychoanalysis itself"[4] but also "economic concentration" and "political disasters" (totalitarian states, heterosexism, the "conjugal dialectic" and "matrimonial requirements" of "American Life") (Lacan, 2001). Juan Pablo Lucchelli (2017) has argued that Lacan owed some of these ideas to thinkers of the Frankfurt School, in particular to Max Horkheimer. Horkheimer in his contribution to the collection *Studien Über Autorität und Familie* ([1936]1974) quotes a Catholic author, Le Play, and refers to a "decline [*Verfall*] of paternal authority [*väterlichen Autorität*] (...) as the cause of unease in Modern Times" (Horkheimer [1936]1974, 49 quoted in Lucchelli, 2017, 85). Lucchelli notes that Horkheimer criticizes the sociologist Le Play but he agrees with him on a specific point: "From his anti-liberal perspective, Le Play has grasped the situation very precisely. The same can be said of the current totalitarian states" (Horkheimer, [1936]1974, 49 quoted in Lucchelli 2017, 86). These quotations make evident that Horkheimer's contention is followed by Lacan in the "decline of paternal authority" not only to explain the origins of "the neurosis of modern times" but also when making the reference to "totalitarian states" as linked to the "decline of the fatherly imago".[5] There is no bibliography in Lacan's "Les complexes Familiaux" encyclopedia entry itself but Lucchelli (2017) found in an annex to the encyclopedia that lists the general bibliography a reference to a collection co-edited by Horkheimer, Marcuse, and Fromm. *Studien Über Autorität und Familie* ([1936] 1974).

is a formidable collection of some 800 pages exploring the problem of authority and the family. It contains essays by Horkheimer (a historical and theoretical sketch of the recent role of family authority in the maintenance of our social order), E. Fromm (the psychological dynamics of submission to authority, making use of Freudian concepts such as ego, super-ego, and sado-masochism as dependent on the family and society), and H. Marcuse (conceptions of freedom and authority prevalent in the history of western European thought). The second section reports results from several extensive empirical surveys about attitudes, activities, and living conditions, questionnaires filled out by 700 German skilled workers and clerical employees in 1930–31; questionnaires about post-war changes in sexual morality filled out by 245 German medical men; questionnaires about family relationships filled out by thousands of young people, and 589 experts in several European countries from 1933 on; and finally, two investigations of the unemployed in Europe and in the United States. The third section contains long summaries of the recent literature on authority and the family, and a number of individual essays and abstracts pertaining to specific theoretical or bibliographical aspects of the general problem of the family.

What kind of declining father is Lacan invoking in his substantial study of the family complexes? In the era of Erdogan, Bolsonaro, Trump, Putin, is his father the fascistic father that the Frankfurt school deplores, the one that creates a totalitarian state? What about the father as a function, as someone or something that intervenes as the representative of the law, the law to which they are subjected and of which they are an effect?

One may reproach Lacan for not having yet made a careful enough reading in 1938 of Freud's (1913) *Totem and Taboo* (the function of the symbolic father is not just the force of the paternal threat; a father is not a Master); one key link here is provided by hysteria, an issue that had not been perceived by the proponents of the Frankfurt school. I take hysteria here not as a pathology but in a broader sense, as a structure that offers a privileged access to how and why in front of paternalistic discourses (or Master's discourse) the hysteric resists identification with the Master while challenging the Master. This mode of interaction can be clearly illustrated even in the clinical setting. Let us think of someone with strange theatrical symptoms: foaming at the mouth, screaming, biting, kicking, crying uncontrollably, shaking in seizures, and fainting. Making the physician in the emergency room in a New York hospital a witness to such impossible pain, the patient's suffering urges the doctor to give a name to his illness. The physician answers with a diagnosis: "Puerto Rican syndrome." Totally recovered in a matter of hours, the hysteric harshly criticizes the doctor. He is not cured at all, the illness persists; this time the pain has moved and a leg and an arm are paralyzed, leaving the patient unable to walk. Let us not neglect a consideration of the political dimension of hysteria; hysteric subjects are always ready to sacrifice themselves to expose power and debunk false knowledge. The hysteric protests the Master discourse.

Lacan, however, would suggest in the 1970s that the hysteric props up the father: "the hysteric is sustained in her cudgel's shape by an armor (which is distinct from her consciousness) and that is her love for her father"[6] (Lacan, 1976–1977, my translation). Freud elevated Sophocles' *Oedipus Rex* tragedy to a universal model of psychic organization, giving the father a main but complex role not only in the family but most importantly, in the family romance. But this father is someone who lays down a law, be it of sexual difference, the law of the prohibition of incest, or the laws of language, a father that is not a tyrant but rather works as a diplomat, as an agent of a metaphor. This father is not a person or a gender but a position, an agent of separation (what psychoanalysis calls castration); father is what separates the child from the mother (or main care-taker), the mother from the child, and what represents an order that also subjects them. The father is the knot that fastens drives and cultural conventions.

In "The Family complexes in the formation of the individual," Lacan provided a short summary of his earlier views on hysteria, connecting the "organ-morphic symbolism" of hysteric symptoms with the experience of the fragmented body of the mirror-stage (Lacan, 2001, 75). Lacan concludes this brief section on hysteria by saying that in hysterical subjects one sees the pathetic images of humans' existential drama.

In the case of Avery, her existential drama is about class, race, parenting, love, women's rights, colonialism. Let us recall that the novel opens with an *ataque de nervios* and closes with another one, "the unmistakable sounds of Doña Concepción's hysteria" (Roberts, 1937, 391). What are those sounds expressing? Is the message of Doña Concepción's *ataque* the *conceptio per aurem*, like that of the Virgin Mary who conceived through her ear at the instant of hearing the angel's heavenly message? The last paragraph reads:

> As these incoherent screams smote upon Avery's ear, something suddenly seemed to right itself in her throbbing head, as when in one of those aggravating glass-covered puzzles the little balls all at once click into place. Pushing by the gaping peasants who murmured "*La Americanita*", as she passed, she hastened to join the Family.
>
> (Roberts, 1937, 391)

What clicked into place for Avery? As we know, the etymology of the word "family" derives from Latin *famulus* "servant, slave". So what is this "f" word, the Family with a capital F? Can one pluralize the family complex and talk not about families but about fami-*lies*, which can correspond with Freud's joke borrowed from Heine about a millionaire who treats him famillionaire*ment*. Highlighting a similar concept of the unconscious as *une-*

bévue or one-blunder, Lacan takes some distance from the Freudian idea that hysterics suffer from memories. When he talks about the unconscious as *une-bévue*, the one-blunder, he introduces the dimension of error, an error that one can trace back to Freud's early notion of the hysterical *proton pseudos*, for the term means both logical error and lie (Rabaté, 2007, 260–277). Hysterics are caught between deception and wayward thinking, between simulation and flawed logical reasoning, all along telling the truth with a lie.

Language cannot lie even if it can never tell the whole truth. "Avery deliberately planned to live a lie" (Roberts, 1937, 388). Here is how Doña Concepción's *ataque* fulfills the hysteric's passion: she wants to expose the truth at any cost. However Avery's lie also reveals a truth. Let's call Avery's lie a tool, a lever that undermines from within the racist, heterosexist, patriarchal, and colonialist *proton pseudos*. Only a hysteric will show that an excess of truth exerts political power, which will call into question previous lies, the lie of the patriarchal order underpinning a racist colonial exploitation.

Notes

1 I had addressed this important historical event that adds a new dimension to the psychosocial overdeterminations of the invention of the label "Puerto Rican syndrome" in my chapter "Psychoanalysis of Poverty, Poverty of Psychoanalysis" in *Psychoanalysis in the Barrios: Race Class and the Unconscious* (pp.227–231). Some passages from this chapter include modified sections from this 2019 essay.
2 Personal communication. See Livio Boni and Sophie Mendelsohn, eds. *Psychanalyse du reste du monde: Géo-Histoire d'une subversion*, Paris: Éditions La Découverte, 2023.
3 She wrote this 1937 novel with the same pseudonym that a decade earlier she used for three books: *Tales of Borinquén (Porto Rico)* (1928), *The Hurricane* (1929) and *Tropical Tales (Porto Rico)* (1929). Under the name Elizabeth Van Deusen Roberts she published *Porto Rico: A Caribbean Isle* (1931), a book she wrote alongside Richard James Van Deusen, and as Elizabeth Kneipple Roberts, she published a poem dedicated to Puerto Rico, the sonnet "Borinquén Sunrise Across Candado Bay" which appeared in the anthology *Puerto Rico in Pictures and Poems* compiled by Cynthia Pearl Maus (1941).
4 "…social decline of the paternal imago. A decline conditioned by the recurrence in the individual of the extreme effects of social progress, a decline that marks itself above all these days in the collectivities most marked by these effects: economic concentration, political catastrophes. […] Such that the future will follow, this decline constitutes a psychological crisis. Possibly it is with this crisis that it is necessary to relate the appearance of psychoanalysis itself. The sublime chance of genius may not be the only explanation of what happened in Vienna-at that time the center of a state which was the melting-pot of the most diverse familial forms, from the most archaic to the most evolved, from the last agnatic groupings of peasant slaves to the most reduced forms of petit bourgeois homes and to the most decadent forms of unstable coupling, in passing through the feudal and mercantile paternalisms-that a son of a Jewish patriarchy imagined the Oedipal complex. Be that as it may, these are the forms of neurosis dominant at the end of the last

century which reveal that they were intimately dependent on the conditions of the family" (Lacan 2001, 60–61, my translation).
5   Lucchelli's discovery of a direct influence of the Frankfurt school in Lacan's work, specifically Lacan's reference in the 1938 "Family Complexes" to Max Horkheimer's 1936 essay "Authority and Family" is mentioned by Slavoj Zizek in *Incontinence and the Void*, MIT Press, 2017, p. 302.
6   "…l'hystérique est soutenue, dans sa forme de trique, est soutenue par une armature. Cette armature est en somme distincte de son conscient. Cette armature, c'est son amour pour son père." Unpublished seminar.

References

Álvarez Curbelo, Silvia (2008a) Sangre colonial: La guerra de Corea y los soldados puertorriqueños. *Caribbean Studies*, 36(1), January–June, pp. 219–223.

Álvarez Curbelo, Silvia (2008b) War, Modernity and Remembrance. *Revista: Harvard Review of Latin America*, Spring. https://revista.drclas.harvard.edu/war-modernity-and-remembrance.

American Psychiatric Association (1952) *Diagnostic and Statistical Manual of Mental Disorders (DSM-I)*. American Psychiatric Association.

Gherovici, Patricia (2003) *The Puerto Rican Syndrome*,.Other Press.

Harris, William (2001) *Puerto Rico's Fighting 65th US Infantry*. Presidio Press.

Horkheimer, Max ([1936]1974) Autorität und Familie (trans. C. Maillard and S. Muller). In *Théorie traditionnelle et théorie critique*. Gallimard. (New ed. 1996.)

Lacan, Jacques (2001) Les complexes familiaux dans la formation de l'individu. In *Autres écrits*. Seuil, pp. 23–84.

Lacan, Jacques (1977) Séminaire XXIV: "L'insu que sait de l'une-bévue s'aile à mourre": unpublished seminar.

Lucchelli, Juan Pablo (2017) Lacan, Horkheimer, et le déclin du père. In Lacan, J. *De Wallon à Kojève*. Michèle, pp. 81–90.

Negrón-Portillo, Mariano (1997) Surviving Colonialism and Nationalism. In Frances Negrón-Muntaner and Ramon Grosfoguel (Eds.) *Puerto Rican Jam: Essay on Culture and Politics*. University of Minnesota Press, pp. 39–56.

Rabaté, Jean Michel (2008) *The Ethics of the Lie*. Other Press.

Roberts, Edith (1937/2018) *Candle in the Sun*. Henry Holt.

Villahermosa, Gilberto (2009) *Honor and Fidelity: The 65th Infantry in Korea, 1950–1953*, United States Army Center of Military History.

Chapter 10

White Panic and the Rhetoric of Exposure

Confronting the Uncanny in our New Racial Times

Sam Binkley

In 1989, an article by a professor at Wellesley College brought to light a dimension of personal life that had hitherto remained hidden to many in the post-civil rights era. Peggy McIntosh's "White Privilege: Unpacking the Invisible Knapsack" focused new attention on the shadowy presence of a habitualized inequality etched into the everyday routines of American culture (McIntosh, 1989). As political manifestos go, its topic seems rather banal. It describes the managed ignorance that shrouds whiteness, and all those mundane, undeclared benefits which flow to whites as a consequence of their participation in daily structures of racial inequality (Mills, 1999). Such accomplished apperception is detailed in a list that extends across a spectrum of unremarkable assumptions: "I can go shopping alone most of the time, pretty well assured that I will not be followed or harassed," "I can swear, or dress in second hand clothes, or not answer letters, without having people attribute these choices to the bad morals, to poverty, or the illiteracy of my race" – everyday advantages packed into an imperceptible knapsack whites carry about with them. The contents of this knapsack, though unseen for its over-familiarity, comprise a supplemental comfort afforded to white people, a protective cocoon insulating them from the suffering of others while veiling their own complicity in deeply rooted patterns of inequality. But it is precisely through the invisibility of these privileges (to whites and in many cases to others), that the piece acquires its resonance. The piece gives language and focus to a growing need to expose a toxic malevolence, a hidden white racism, many sense circulating just beneath the surface of everyday white racial civility. Moreover, the knapsack's invisibility establishes a certain trope through which the critique of whiteness was made to operate and continues to function today: whiteness is bound to the problem of visibility and concealment, and a critical intervention into a white supremacist racial order is one that is bound to the dynamic of a certain rhetorical strategy of exposure. Since the publication of McIntosh's article, the white racial condition has emerged as a topic of public commentary in film and popular media, and as the focus of a broad program of white self-examination and reconstruction implemented broadly across a range of professional, corporate and educational settings.

DOI: 10.4324/9781003394327-11

(Wise, 2011; Ahmed, 2007; Coates, 2015; DiAngelo, 2018; Oluo, 2019, Yancy, 2012) Today white knapsacks are being openly discussed and exposed, and white people themselves are being asked to reflect on the unthought and unacknowledged habits that guide them through social space. Particularly during the months of global demonstrations following the police murder of George Floyd and the "summer of racial reckoning," calls to make visible those hidden dimensions of white comportment that had previously remained concealed resonated across a range of public conversations. (McWhorter, 2020) At the center of these discussions is the wish to draw out an object – an attribute of white psychic life thought to operate just under the surface of white skin. White privilege must be exposed. (Rothenberg, 2004) To understand this rhetoric of exposure that underpins current critiques of whiteness, we must grasp the perceptual shift through which the ordinariness of white privilege is made to stand out, an epistemic reversal that derives from an inversion of traditionally defined ways of understanding power and inequality. While everyday accounts of oppression focus on the exceptional disadvantages experienced by minority and oppressed groups, the critique of white privilege implies a perceptual shift, a transposal, or a figure-ground reversal through which the long concealed advantages undergirding normal civility are given a unique positivity (like an exposed backpack), made to stand out and to admit their operation. Phrases such as "less fortunate" or "disadvantaged" foreground the exceptional conditions of the poor, people of color and so on. These are phrases used by dominant groups to place the problem "out there," and by doing so to distance themselves from their complicity with deeply structured inequalities. They presume a standard against which exceptional cases of oppression might be consigned to the outside, as unauthored effects of faceless systems, or tragic events of nature that befall only those exceptional groups. Where privilege remains in the background, those possessing privilege are allowed to declare their general disdain for inequality. As privilege foregrounded, however, the normal is made the exceptional, as silence is made to speak, to admit its function not only in sustaining these very forms of domination but in obscuring these functions behind the façade of a benign neutrality (Schwartzman, 2016). I read this figure-ground inversion as the moment of a certain exposure: hidden truths are drawn to the fore, with the effect of an at times excruciating panic.

Robin DiAngelo demonstrates this shift of perspective with the example of Jackie Robinson, the first African American accepted into major league baseball. Popular accounts of Robinson attribute his accomplishment to his own efforts, to his perseverance and resolution in the face of challenge. What they don't do is blame the whites who, up to that point, had conspired so cynically to exclude blacks.

> Imagine if instead, the story went something like this: "Jackie Robinson, the first black man whites allowed to play major-league baseball." This version makes a critical distinction because no matter how fantastic a

player Robinson was, he simply could not play in the major leagues if whites – who controlled the institution – did not allow it.

(DiAngelo 2018)

Foregrounding that act of camouflage through which the violence of whiteness is made to disappear, not just in the eyes of those against whom it is mobilized but more strikingly in the very self-awareness of whites who view the cherished contents of their own knapsacks as only the benevolent effect of universal racelessness, constitutes the aim of a new racial sensibility, a new critical attitude directed at the cultural authority of whiteness.

In this way, strategies of exposure can be understood as analogous to efforts to disturb states of sleep, and to bring the subject around to new states of wakefulness. As normal, whiteness becomes a somnambulistic life, asleep to itself and to the world it produces. The exposure of white privilege and the "call out" culture through which white somnambulism is jolted into wakefulness brings about a unique and distinct set of responses from white subjects. Sleep, and the dreams it brings, is thought to be more pleasant than the waking world, and the emergence into wakefulness is necessarily an unpleasant one. As "woke," the everyday rights and the entitlements of "normal" civility are made plain for what they are: implicit, if soft habits of a racial domination that would have preferred to remain concealed, banished to the realm of a great racial unseen. White people must be awakened to their own condition by being plunged into the icy waters of a reality which they may not be fully prepared to face. They must be led out of their self-willed immaturity and from the sleep of a certain childhood into a world of harsh truths whose callousness is only compensated by veracity (Magee, 2019). Though whites know in their hearts of the necessity for this awakening, they often lack the will to undergo treatment, balking when the medical instruments are drawn from the doctor's bag. White normativity provides a zone of racial comfort, a safe buffer zone through which feelings of superiority in relation to others bring a sense of ontological security upon which whites themselves have developed an almost infantile dependence (Mills, 2007). The prospect of being led out of this blindness elicits powerful spasms of anxiety and defensiveness at the merest suggestion that the comforts of whiteness might be taken away. This characterization of the sick as fundamentally reluctant to participate in their cure is a belief that is central to the

therapeutic logic upon which call-out culture depends – a belief that can be traced to Freud's comparison of the neurotic patient to the man with a tooth ache, whose consuming pain becomes the exclusive focus of attention, indeed a sort of love object, to the exclusion of all other possibilities, including that of the cure itself (Freud, 1991, 12.)

Robin DiAngelo has used this therapeutic logic to interpret the fear and resentment that grips her white informants at the first hint of attention to vulnerabilities and sensitivities they have inherited from lifelong habits of racial privilege. She reads this as a display of "white fragility," an ambivalence or hostility reflected in the attitudes of participants in her anti-racist workshops: "anger, fear, and guilt, and behaviors such as argumentation, silence, and leaving the stress-inducing situation. These behaviors, in turn, function to reinstate white racial equilibrium" (Di-Angelo, 2018, 57). Similarly, Eduardo Bonilla-Silva, through a series of ethnographic interviews with white college students describes the odd conversational quirks that afflict his white research subjects as they attempt to reconcile conflicting commitments to an egalitarian stance with regard to issues of race while at the same time preserving deep seated feelings of superiority with regard to people of color (Bonilla-Silva, 2003). On the question of whether he would marry a person of another race, one respondent answers:

> I mean, personally, I don't see myself, you know, marrying someone else. I mean, I don't have anything against it, I just I guess I'm just more attracted to, I mean, others. Nothing like, I could not and I would never, and I don't know how my parents would – just on another side, I don't, like, if my parents would feel about anything like that.
>
> (Bonilla Silva, 2006, 68)

In the chapter that follows, the specific dynamic of this exposure will be considered. Drawing on perspectives deriving from psychoanalysis and affect theory to phenomenology and the sociology of emotion, the unique structure of this exposing operation will be traced and examined for the affective content it induces and the resonances it shares with wider understandings of intimacy and the privacy of subjective life as a function of civil society and public life. Whiteness, it will be argued, and the new racial critique through which it is problematized, has attained immense influence and brought about important transformations in the American racial order by tapping into key assumptions about race, subjectivity, private life and the threat of exposure. Some of the complex responses some white people have exhibited to this exposure can be better understood when considered through a broader understanding of exposure and its effects. Toward that end, I will make the following points: in the first part of this chapter, I will consider the dynamic of racial exposure as it is manifested as habitual life is exposed before a critical, public gaze. Such a gaze, long brought to bear on the racial subaltern, is today, through a series of tactical reversals, now directed against the habitual life of whiteness itself, with the effect of a certain traumatic exposure. Next, this dynamic of exposure is read against the backdrop of a certain shame at the prospect of the invasive breach of private life, which, when conducted thoughtlessly, it is argued, diminishes shame's moral potential. And finally, in the third part of this essay, exposure is understood for the trauma it induces. Through a reading of Freud's notion of the uncanny as the unique affect of white racial exposure, an explanation is offered for the fragility and panic of white racial being.

Unseemly Habits and White Panic

The shock brought on by the call-out no doubt exposes the white subject, bringing hidden racism to the surface, but it also disrupts the naturalness of the habitual life that it exposes, holding those habits up to the unfriendly scrutiny of hostile spectators (MacMullen, 2009; Ngo, 2017; Sullivan, 2006, 2015). Indeed, the intensity of the call-out's exposure can be understood in relation to the psychic and social functioning of habitual life: under any circumstances, habitual conduct is a sensitive and vulnerable aspect of social life, as evidenced in the ensemble of unthought habits that accompany us in all of our interactions and endeavors, not just those linked with practices of racial domination. Any shock to that organized latticework of habit so essential to our social and existential equilibrium is bound to bring ripples of shock.

In our habits we are only half aware of what we do. Habits reveal the helplessness of our sovereign intentions before the sheer inertia of our own embodiment. To have one's habitual character called out, or held up for public scrutiny is to be exposed for a state of unawareness and dependence through which our actions appear not as the effects of conscious intention but as a consequence of the layering of accumulated, half-thought actions and movements whose memories are stamped on the very mattering of our flesh. The exposure of our habits, as such, brings feelings akin to shame: habits sit between self and world, between the ideality that constitutes our sovereign, conscious intentions and the materiality of our bodies, things of the world. The exposure of our habits, which grow on our daily conducts like barnacles on the side of a ship, is an experience that threatens to draw us into a startling state of denigrated self-discovery the mere thought of which makes us bristle with apprehension. The realm of the habitual, as Pierre Bourdieu has written, is essential to the naturalness required for comfortable sociability, though such habits must be naturalized, remaining on the level of the inconspicuous, invisible not just to those around us but to ourselves as actors. Indeed, the suppression of awareness that comes with habit is essential to the flow of social conduct, to the embeddedness of the actor within a given field. Bourdieu calls this the *habitus*, the unthought seat of sedimented routines of conduct by which social dispositions are established and social life is reproduced (Bourdieu, 1977). A sure fire way to trip someone up, to derail their flow in any situation, is to make them suddenly aware of their habitual nature. Habits reveal the dependence underpinning our presumption of autonomy and are in this way unseemly: we typically look away from other people's hair-twirling, change-jingling and other tics of habitual behavior for fear of igniting in them an unwelcome flash of self-consciousness, one that will quickly spread to others and to ourselves. The fleeting sense of shame we feel in the grip of habitual life is the grist for practical jokes that induce light touches of shame by playfully exposing the unthinking way we walk into our offices or sit on cushions (Tangney, Price, and Dearing, 2002; Tomkins, 1995).

But what is at issue here, and what the present chapter will attempt to address, is not just the social ontology of habit and its relationship to shame but the development and dissemination of a framework, a way of seeing or an epistemic stance through which habits thought to be attributable to white racial dispositions are made to stand out, and the shame associated with habits is read and experienced as a uniquely racialized shame. Habits always carry the glint of a certain shame, deriving from the half aware state in which we enact habitual life. Moreover, in habit, we are always in a tense relationship with ourselves, like a rider embarrassingly trying to control a resistant horse. Habit's shame is intensified as the contrary movements inscribed in habit are marked as expressions, not just of any corporeal existence, but of uniquely racial being, and of the contrary movements and interests that are implied by the very idea of racial domination. While every habit wears a halo of aversion, appearing as a thing from which we are compelled, by the very norms of civility, to avert our eyes lest we provoke embarrassment, what we think of as our white racial habit brings its own obscenity and unique dread of exposure. That the habit in question is a racial habit only doubles the shameful sense of exposure that this implies, although the racial stigmatization of habit is not, I contend, an effect restricted to whites but one that attaches to race more generally. That race is thought to reside ultimately in habits that remain concealed to the actor but are only too obvious to others gives race its unique sense of shame (Scheff and Retzinger, 2001).

To understand this, we must consider the more general way that the critique of everyday white racism is imagined as a gesture of exposure, of the examination of a habitual life, understood as a kind of sleep, that most of us would prefer to confine to the background of social awareness, and whose emergence brings us into a stark and unsettling awareness of ourselves as strange and unnatural. My answer to the question of white shame, white rage and white fragility comes with this sense of our habits and their exposure, with the trauma of a sudden awakening. Such an exposure, I will argue, presumes a breach in the hidden realm of what we consider intimate: in the privacy of our habitual life, we are at home, and we sustain a certain personal relation with ourselves that must be veiled from public view (Dyer, 1988). It is in the half-aware state of habit that, for example, I wash myself, prepare my food, and conduct other functions of a sheltered, domestic life. But as that realm is opened up to the public examination of the strangers, to the gazes of a newly diversified public sphere, the intimacy of our privacy appears to us a suddenly strange thing. In habitual life we are at home with ourselves. We are our most intimate with ourselves when we let our bodies move us in ways that don't require us to think or to act with the kind of intentionally we exercise in public life (Schneider, 1977). To be suddenly awakened from habits of domestic self-intimacy is a disruption that brings a certain shock of estrangement. For the habitual to suddenly stand out in relief induces a moment of uncanny shock – a sudden strangeness of the familiar which hangs over the phenomenon we have heard described as white fragility, white rage and white panic.

Exposure and The Racial Gaze

The sense of being looked at by people we don't already know is as existentially unsettling as it is indispensable to our formation as subjects of civility. The public gaze is something we admonish our children to consider as part of their formation as adults with the belief that it will give them some bearing, an audience for whom to perform good character. But the look of strangers is two sided: it lifts us up, bestowing wholeness and desirability on celebrities and public figures but also devastating disgrace on those whom it singles out for ridicule and opprobrium. Even in our quietest moments, an awareness of the ubiquity of the public gaze brings a vague sense of unease and estrangement, and perhaps a dull feeling of shame (Crozier, 2000). A scientific term appeared in psychological literature of the turn of the century to describe this feeling: scopaesthesia designated this new sense of publicity conveyed in the experience of being stared at from an unknown source. As described by the psychologist Edward Titchener, the term designates a common feeling, a tingling sensation in the nape of the neck usually occurring in public spaces such as church or in the theatre. Following a series of experiments with his students, Professor Titchener characterized this sensation as "'uncanny,' a feeling of 'Must,'" reported by his subjects who felt the compulsion to turn and to search the room for the source of this anonymous gaze in order that a certain tension might find relief (Titchener, 1898, 897). Though the theory of scopaesthesia turned out to have no basis in actual science (people can't, it is now believed, physically sense the stares of others), the Must and the uncanniness that Titchener discovered continues to resonate with people's experiences, imagined or real, of being looked at, earning the condition a venerable place in the archives of folk psychology. In fact, scopaesthesia's uncanniness, and its feeling of "Must" is, I would argue, a constitutive feature not only of civic life, but of racial subjection – a dynamic element that has come to the fore of recent phenomenological accounts of racialization in public spaces, and which is deeply intertwined with the function of shame in the production of racial being.

The imbrication of race and public exposure is a fact long noted by those that suffer most the psychic violence of the racial order. To appear "raced" in public space is already to stand out, to appear conspicuous, as a threat to public order and in a sense as exposed to an anonymous public gaze. In the years following the rise of social media and with the proliferation of smart phones equipped with digital cameras, the real extent of everyday racial exposure, to the unfair bias directed towards people of color in public inter-action, has itself been subjected to media scrutiny as never before. Cell phone videos depicting spectacular instances of police violence epitomized by the strangling to death of Eric Garner for selling cigarettes on a public sidewalk and the shooting of Michael Brown whose death sparked violent demonstra-tions in Ferguson, Missouri and ultimately led to the establishment of the #Blacklivesmatter movement, all changed the tone and intensity of the con-versation on race in America. But beyond these more spectacular instances of racial exposure, what has also come to light in recent years are the mundane moments of everyday racism that people of color encounter as part of their daily round – small disputes with law enforcement and squabbles with stran-gers, in which petty racial suspicions and resentments normally pushed to the margins of popular awareness are suddenly thrust into the public view.

For example, in April of 2018 a white woman in Oakland, California called the police on a black family for barbecuing in a public park. The stop by the police and the ensuing exchange was captured on video and posted to You-Tube, where it was quickly viewed more than two million times within a few days. Backlash against the incident, which built on similar occurrences on college campuses, in department stores, and more famously at a Starbucks in Philadelphia, was quick and passionate, leading to a "BBQing while black" festival at the site of the incident attended by several hundred participants and including food vendors, DJ's and a speech by Angela Davis (Holson, 2018). That black people in America experience public space under radically different conditions of public visibility and surveillance, relations that intrude so rudely into realms of life that should be kept private, is a fact that is today increasingly difficult for white audiences to ignore.

The phrase "– while black" is one that began to circulate in the 1990s to describe the undue attention brought to bear on black drivers by highway police (abbreviated to DWB, a play on DWI or "driving while intoxicated"), though later the phrase came to apply more broadly to a range of everyday activities shaped by the quasi-criminal status affixed to black behavior in general. Dining while black, learning while black, shopping while black, etcetera, came to describe heightened levels of police attention and popular anxiety directed at people of color, and a creeping sense of public danger implied simply by the presence of black people undertaking regular activ-ities. As such, the criminalization of blackness in public space is nothing new (Alexander, 2012). Jim Crow legislation imposed not just a strict judi-cial code but an informal culture of suspicion, drawing law enforcement and the white population together in the policing of a set of vaguely articulated criminalities (vagrancy, indecency or simply the very condition of being suspicious itself – a tautological status which says as much about the one holding suspicion as it does anything else) under which any form of conduct undertaken by a Black person might be readily subsumed. But central to all of these concerns is the very phenomenological condition of visibility and exposure to which people of color are consigned. Black people are made to stand out against the backdrop of a white civility that is often mobilized against their very presence. To do anything "while black" is to do so conspicuously, as a potential threat to public safety. Numerous studies have confirmed racial profiling as a ubiquitous feature of public life whose repercussions range from the erosion of trust in law enforcement amongst targeted communities to the traumatic effects on the psychological wellbeing of individuals held at arms' length from white civility by the constant suspicion of an intrinsic, essential criminality. Indeed, a growing psychiatric literature on race-based trauma has detailed the emotional impact of a perpetual and permeating public stigma that leaves subjects resentful and afraid. These are the more innocuous effects of the criminalization of blackness that fly under the radar of more spectacular, traumatic episodes of police violence but nonetheless lodge themselves in the everyday textures of the emotional lives of black people.

In two of the most broadly influential accounts of this process, W. E. B. Dubois and Frantz Fanon have studied the effect of the racial look as it is brought to bear on the non-white subject in European or American settings. Objectification, in both cases, implies the coerced identification of the raced subject with the subject of this racializing gaze, and with the overpowering compulsion to view oneself through the eyes of a normalizing whiteness. Fanon's account of his response to the words "Look! A negro!" uttered by a white child in a train station relates an intense sense of dislocation and loss: "the corporeal schema crumbled, its place taken by a racial, epidermal schema... I discovered my blackness, my ethnic characteristics; and I was battered down by tom-toms, cannibalism, intellectual deficiency, fetishism, racial defects, slave-ships..." (Fanon, 1967, 112). In a related way, Du Bois' discussion of "double consciousness" describes a "sense of always looking at one's self through the eyes of others, of measuring one's soul by the tape of a world that looks on in amused contempt and pity" (Du Bois, 1994, 2). For Du Bois and Fanon, the assumption of this gaze involves a coerced, and perverse identification with and internalization of the look of the other that is both chronic and episodic, both the slow process of adult socialization but also prompted by jarring moments of self-discovery. Du Bois recalls his earliest experiences of a racializing self-exposure: as a child he participates in a school exercise in which children deliver greeting cards to each other, though when his is rejected by a white girl, "peremptorily, with a glance," he is struck by a revelation: "then it dawned upon me with a certain suddenness that I was different from the others... shut out from their world by a vast veil" (Du Bois, 1994, 10). Elsewhere, in an essay entitled, "On Being Ashamed of Oneself: An Essay on Race Pride," Du Bois extends the revelatory moment of this bifurcated self in a framework more readily readable as shameful (Du Bois 1995). Recalling his grandfather's indignant rejection of an invitation to attend a "Negro picnic," Du Bois reflects on the racialized class anxieties of the "upper colored group," who avoid mingling with lower class negroes because of their desire to accommodate the racial judgments of a white spectator. "This exaggerates, at once, the secret shame of being identified with such people and the anomaly of insisting that the physical characteristics of these folks which the upper class shares, are not stigmata of degradation" (Du Bois, 1995, 251). Both of these accounts assess the racial glance or stare as an effect of the generalized conditions of anonymous civility one finds in public spaces, and presumes from these encounters a more lasting resonance, an enduring afterglow that carries the broader consequences of a racial subjection.

Within such moments, the raced body is experienced as a body "out of place," available to the specular consumption of strangers – in some cases as an object of licensed staring, in others under a mandate to look away or to look through, but more often as a body that is at once noticed but not acknowledged. Sarah Ahmed, describing the experiences of non-white bodies in white spaces, relates the precarious condition of this visibility: "Such bodies are made invisible when we see spaces as being white, at the same time as they become hyper-visible when they do not pass, which means they 'stand out' and 'stand apart'" (Ahmed, 2007, 159). The experience of living while black, however, is paralleled in the shifting experiences of other racial groups and of white people in particular, for whom some measure of racial conspicuousness is becoming an ever more apparent feature of public life. To claim that white people today are becoming more self-aware, that the cloak of invisibility that has long imbued whiteness with a normative authority as the racially unmarked and thus universal standard for civic conduct, is necessarily to describe a process of reversal: the same brutal regimes of exposure long trained on people of color are now, with some justification, brought to bear on white people themselves. In a passage from the introduction to his anthology Look, A White! George Yancy offers a play on Fanon's famous iteration, a flipping of the script through which whiteness is made the object of public scrutiny – a strategic reversal summarized in a remark by James Baldwin speaking to a white audience: "I give you your problem back. You're the 'nigger', baby; it isn't me" (Yancy, 2012, 5).

Invitations to this exposure are alternately embraced and reviled by different white demographics, although the effect of a white exposure is a more or less common experience. The same viral videos that show black people's subjection to the prying eyes of strangers also hold a mirror to the gaze of white people themselves, whose shock is no doubt also a shock of recognition. As much as white audiences are moved by the experiences of people of color for the invasive scrutiny to which they are subjected, they also no doubt recognize their own paranoid glances and stares in these videos, and greet with reluctant familiarity the objectifying eye that these videos depict. With every new story of public racial surveillance, white people encounter their own habits of indecent scrutiny, their prying exposure and intrusion into the hidden place where others cultivate their dignity. In other words, in these videos, the power to impose public exposure long wielded by whites in public spaces is itself revealed as a shameful thing. That a white stare can quickly and easily transform even the simple act of barbequing (not to mention sleeping in a student commons or waiting for a friend at a Starbucks) into a shameful act, an act originating in the criminality of one's contaminated racial flesh, is itself a capacity of shameful provenance. The eye is, after all, an organ of flesh, and thus exposed, the white gaze becomes a flesh for which the white spectator feels shame. With so many exposures come so many shames, both new and old, not least of which is a new shame attached to an exposed whiteness that cannot escape itself and has nowhere to hide – a whiteness whose prurient fears and resentments, whose infantile dependence on unearned entitlement and willed self-delusion is increasingly laid bare for all to see. Such is the feeling of the "uncanny Must" of scopaesthesia, experienced as a dull, ongoing satiation habit of the racial flesh. To better understand the nature of this uncanny exposure of white habits, we must take up the very dynamic character of exposure itself, which, I will argue, operates between the veiled, protected realm of the private realm, and the distanced regard of the public stranger.

Privacy and Exposure

White racial affect, understood as a relation sustained through a certain dynamic of exposure, must be understood for its historical specificity. As a panicked response to the exposure of white racial habit, the sense of violation that many whites express emerges in relation to a uniquely Western conception of interior life, wherein a sense of personal dignity is sustained through the demarcation of a boundary between public and private existence. This distinction between public and private spheres, that cleavage which Norberto Bobbio referred to as "the great dichotomy," constitutes the organizing scheme through which Western modernity sustains its political and moral self-understanding (Bobbio, 1989). The public-private dichotomy implies a splitting of the social world into complimentary zones whose mutually constitutive exclusion is consolidated, I would argue, around the feeling of shame. Shame's pain reminds us of the need to protect certain realms of experience from illicit exposure before the eyes of strangers, and that the failure to do so results in a radical diminishment of personal life (Schneider, 1977; Levinas, 2003) The obligations, performances and roles one assumes in public take a certain priority and enjoy a certain dignity over those adopted in private: the public constitutes that arena of political life in which individuals display themselves before others through collective, shared and valorized conduct in which human beings engage in the mutual work of shared governance and rational deliberation. Life in the polis, or the public life of the city state, summons individuals to their highest moral and intellectual capacities as participants, through the rhetoric of persuasion and acts of civic commitment, in the practice of just rule. As such, the public realm became, for the Greeks and in the tradition of normative political theory that claims their legacy, a sphere of freedom shaped by the presumption of the equality and autonomy of all participants in the pursuit of greatness achieved through the assessment of one's peers. Indeed, the public sphere is, for the ancients and moderns alike, a sphere of appearances and judgments: through publicity, one shows oneself to others and makes oneself available to their scrutiny, criticism, and their collective assessment. The private sphere is typically recognized as a residue, or as the exclusion from this arena of public visibility of all those elements and activities that make the public possible. As the antithesis to all that is public, the private sphere is that realm of everyday practice through which individuals attended to the personal needs of bodily life and physical reproduction and to the bare necessities of brute existence. If the public sphere is the place of freedom and ideas, the private is that of necessity, of one's enslavement to one's body and to what Agamben calls bare life (Agamben, 1995). If one is one's most human in public, in private one's concerns are with those aspects we share with animals. It is in privacy that one engages in the work of the oikos and of economy more generally, where the family comes together to prepare food, to raise children and to cope with the mundane trials of daily existence through a set of relationships that are not necessarily egalitarian but shaped by the sometimes violent necessity of just getting by. As such, the private sphere has traditionally been understood as a subordinate realm to that of the public, though it is a realm that, in its subordination, remains outside of public view, hidden from the scrutiny and from the view of strangers by a veil of decency and opprobrium.

Yet the sphere of privacy has also served as the site for the production of a certain kind of subjectivity, an individuation centered on the autonomy of introspective thought and on the elaboration of a realm of interiority through which existential questioning takes up significant problems of meaning and purpose. It is in privacy that we develop relations of intimacy and self-authenticity not possible in a public domain defined around observable performance and visibility before others. Hannah Arendt, who makes no secret of her admiration for the public sphere as the privileged site of the political, nonetheless holds out the significance of the private as that place in which an escape from public scrutiny brings the opportunity for the cultivation of richer, more human traits, and of the necessity of maintaining the private sphere as a space visually sequestered from the gaze of strangers. The sacred character of the oikos derives, in part, from its association with processes of birth and death, events that are not only exterior to the performative identity of publicity, but irreducibly mysterious owing to the unanswerable question of human origins and mortality that they pose: "It is hidden because man does not know where he comes from when he is born and where he goes when he dies" (Arendt, 1998, 63). In order that the unknowable character of the private sphere be preserved, "the darkness of what needs to be hidden against the light of publicity" must be sustained, and the gaze of strangers must be deflected from certain areas of life:

> The four walls of one's private property offer the only reliable hiding place from the common public world, not only from everything that goes on in it but also from its very publicity, from being seen and being heard. A life spent entirely in public, in the presence of others, becomes, as we would say, shallow. While it retains its visibility, it loses the quality of rising into sight from some darker ground which must remain hidden if it is not to lose its depth in a very real, non-subjective sense
>
> (Arendt, 1998, 71).

That said, the great dichotomy has proven remarkably mutable over the course of its existence, particularly in recent years with the onset of such structural transformations as the postmodernization of the economy, the dissemination of new digital media, the rise of flexible and emotional labor, and the increasing incorporation of public medical and psychological discourses in public and personal life – changes which have brought a dedifferentiation of public and private with mixed consequences for each. Of course, there is much in this traditional separation that we should be glad to see go, such as the function of the private realm as a zone of the less-than-human, a place to which certain bodies could be consigned to the status of the permanently pre-political. Such has for a long time been the fate of women and sexual minorities. Yet the increasing porousness with which public is divided from private brings other effects. Richard Sennett is perhaps the author most recognized for the analysis of the effects of this erosion: public statuses are, Sennett has argued, increasingly presented today in terms that would have seemed indecently personal to an earlier generation, and public issues are increasingly debated in terms of a criteria of personal authenticity originating in the private realm with the effect of undermining both the intimacy of private life and the capacity to make public displays characteristic of civil society (Sennett, 1992). Where the boundary between the public and the private erodes, or where it erodes thoughtlessly and without reflection, something is lost which is difficult to replace. An opportunity to be alone with oneself, or to be together with others in something other than shallow ways, presumes the maintenance of some screen for the deflection of the gazes of strangers.

Importantly, what sustains this great dichotomy, the diminishment of which is in part tied to its weakening, is precisely the social and subjective function attributed to the affective field of shame. Shame is what reminds us and others of what needs to be kept private and what can be brought into the realm of the public. Shame's toxicity is what makes intimacy, both in relation to oneself and to others, a serious undertaking, what makes it a struggle, what gives it its intensity and its quality of a rupture with the everyday, and thus what makes the contents of private life powerful enough to warrant seriousness. Carl Schneider has argued for the indispensability of shame as the hallmark of authenticity in intimate relations, and as that which, as Arendt argues, gives depth to a life that is withdrawn from the public scrutiny of strangers (Schneider, 1977). In intimacy, exposure before others with whom we share a bond of love is a sought after and managed relation between individuals, one that is forged through the confrontation with and surmounting of shame feelings. In the course of this struggle to expose oneself, intimates form a closeness that derives from the depth of the other's subjective experience. As such, shame "conceals and reveals at the same time" (Schneider, 1977, 65), and it is only by overcoming shame, together, in a relation of intimacy, that any meaningful revelation of the self becomes possible. Without shame, self-revelation in intimacy loses all tension and meaning. Max Scheler, in an early phenomenological reflection on shame, tells the story of a female model who, in the course of posing nude for a male painter, senses in him the stirrings of an erotic appreciation (Scheler, 1987). This awareness brings about a shift of focus in which she perceives the presence of her body in this scene not as the object of abstract aesthetic contemplation but of a baser animal investment, causing her to recoil in shame. Shame, therefore, emerges as a means by which she preserves her uniqueness as human against this violent reduction to the animal, to the flesh, in the very moment of the turning from one to the other. Had the model remained as she was, an object of artistic rendering, or if she had simply succumbed to the position of the object of erotic desire, shame would have had no role. Thus, the suspension of shame is itself a means by which private experience is subjected to the effects of what Arendt referred to as a certain shallowing. Of course, to be freed of shame is, in a sense liberating – as many women, queers, transgender, and other people can attest. Shame, as an instrument of violence, hurts, and to be shamed is a rending public experience that, when leveraged violently, leaves subjects decimated. But at the same time, shame is also the condition of our autonomy, and to be denied shame entirely, or the right to shame, is itself an insidious form of everyday violence, akin to the denial of privacy or subjective intimacy with oneself. This self-intimacy is not by itself a productive relation, an occasion for the elaboration of developmental self-change. But it is an important precondition.

Public racialization under the gaze of strangers brings the consequence, not just of shaming, but of the denial of shame. "Look! A Negro" is a statement that presumes a subject with no use for the defenses shame provides. This denial operates today in the recurring return of a curious phenomenon: white people fondling the hair of black people with whom they are not acquainted, and without any solicitation of permission for doing so. Accounts of this habit vary: a black woman with "natural" black hair takes her children to a public swimming pool where a white woman, also there with her children, approaches from behind and pokes and caresses her hair, exclaiming of its beauty and novelty. Waiting in line at a fast food restaurant, an older white woman standing behind a younger black woman runs her fingers through her long dreadlocks, smiling and commenting on its beauty – both instances which drew shock and indignation from the object of their fondling, and a panicked effort to reclaim some private space. Indeed, hair touching has become something of a flashpoint for feelings of racial objectification: a song by rapper Solange and a book by comedian Phoebe Robinson detail the awkwardness of such public encounters, particularly as they involve not the direct hostility of white people, but a sort of spontaneous curiosity or fetishization of black beauty, even without the traditional regard for the sanctity of private space that normally safeguards the surfaces of human bodies in public (Solange, 2016; Robinson, 2016). Though these intrusions are often brushed off politely, for many critics they are more disturbing, experienced as a lingering trace of the right to the appropriation of black bodies under slavery and to more mundane forms of the criminal racialization of black people, which also involves the suspension of the privacy the body is typically allowed in the company of strangers. The fondling and stroking of hair is, in short, something reserved for intimates, and for pets and animals for whom shame is a useless emotion. And it is the reduction of this zone of privacy to the status of the animal, and to an animality that does not possess the right or the capacity to give or deny consent to its own touching, that makes this pattern stand out. The tragedy of this episode is not just that these women were threatened with the shame of being treated like animals, but also, and inversely, that they were threatened with the denial of the very possibility of that shame. Less friendly intrusions implied by racial violence, cat calling and harassment at least confer upon their victims the original dignity of a private body, albeit a privacy that is offered only in the moment that it is forcibly taken away, leaving the victim to suffer in shame. What is striking about these more benign acts of intrusion is that the subject is not even granted the capacity for shame itself, with the argument that one's body is a novelty available to a fondling for which one should feel no shame. The indignant response of one white woman to a black woman's pulling away from her probing fingers, "What? Are you serious? I can't touch your hair?" conveys this presumption of shamelessness with regard to a person thought to have no interiority and to keep no secrets (LosAngelista, 2009). In the course of being admired for their beauty, their shame is taken from them, the right to feel the shame that comes with the inability to deflect the gazes of strangers and with it the relation with themselves in their own bodily intimacy.

Looking and fondling define modes of racial exposure that breach the boundary of the public and the private in ways that diminish the meaning of intimacy itself, and it is surely here that we find the roots of at least some of the psychic violence of racial civility itself. Exposure "shallows" our relation to ourselves. Indeed, for the white subject, newly held up to such an exposure, the denial of shame brings its own unique sense of panic. Exposure of white racial habit induces an odd effect as the intimacy of one's habitual life suddenly emerges strange – an effect we can trace to what I term the white racial uncanny.

The Racial Secret

Within the phenomenological tradition, the look is a force that imposes a powerful effect on its human objects, one capable of sending forceful tremors through the body. To be seen by the other is to disrupt that fit with the world that Merleau-Ponty referred to as a "natal pact," a state of ordinary equilibrium between the body and its surroundings in which the body itself attains a state of invisibility to the subject herself (Merleau-Ponty, 1964, 6). In those moments in which this equilibrium is disrupted, such as with a fall or an accident, awareness of the body suddenly surges to the forefront of consciousness as we are revealed to ourselves in our determination by a materiality we thought we had overcome. Luna Dolezal, citing Drew Leder, attributes such moments to the effect of a "dys-appearance": "the body appears as a thematic focus, but precisely as in a dys state – dys is from the Greek prefix signifying 'bad,' 'hard' or 'ill'" (Dolezal, 2016, 28). Dys-appearance entails the manifestation of the hard, ill or bad body as "other," as an alien presence to the self. This is a body that appears as a thing in the world, an object inscribed with a base existence that marks its externality to the freedoms of the conscious self – a point famously elaborated by Jean Paul Sartre in his account of the "look" that comes to bear upon a person (presumably Sartre himself) who discovers themselves being spied upon by another (Sartre, 1993). Sartre's scene has often been retold: a man, moved by jealously or vice, bends down to a keyhole to spy on his lover, whom he suspects of infidelity. (Sartre, 1993, 340–400) Consumed in this act of voyeurism, the man's body is invisible, subsumed in the flow of this illicit action. Yet, all at once, footsteps can be heard down the hall and the voyeur is himself caught in the act of spying, spied upon by a stranger in this despicable act. "I see *myself* because *somebody* sees me," a moment of intense self-discovery as the shamed subject recognizes something of himself in his exposure before the gaze of the other:

> Pure shame is not a feeling of being this or that guilty object but in general of being an object; that is, of recognizing *myself* in this degraded, fixed, and dependent being which I am for the Other. Shame is the feeling of an *original fall*, not because of the fact that I may have committed this or that particular fault but simply that I have "fallen" into the world in the midst of things and that I need the mediation of the Other in order to be what I am.
>
> (Sartre, 1993, 288–289)

The loss of freedom that Sartre describes is enough to elicit intense feelings of shock and fright, even horror, precisely for the sense of inevitability that is prescribed by the very condition of objectivity in which one discovers oneself.

Since I can only be what I am through the other, I am dependent on the other and what the other sees of me. The sense of the "uncanny Must" experienced by the scopaesthesic, who cannot escape the feeling of being looked at is like this: it shows us how incapable we really are of transcending ourselves, of being any more than what we are compelled to be. The look of the other leaves us trapped in a pattern of compulsive repetition of our basic, fleshly natures the full determination of which we ourselves cannot fully grasp (though we feel the other knows only too well). In modern life, as I have argued, such feelings of exposure, feelings of being stared at, compose the backdrop of our everyday existence, inscribing a shameful sense of the inevitability of our conduct, reducing us to a determination of the creatures that we are and that the other knows us to be. Such feelings of shame induce a sense of the uncanny, a simultaneous refusal of and resignation to this inevitability. The "degraded, fixed and dependent thing," the sense of our being that resides somewhere between self and other, living tissue and inanimate matter, spirit and flesh – this thing that the other knows us to be is one that elicits in us a special sense of horror. Like being trapped in a house with a killer from whom we cannot escape, this inevitability is something we are desperate to transcend yet to which we find ourselves inextricably bound. For this we feel unbearable shame, and this is a shame that is deeply constitutive of racial effect.

In his autobiography, Malcolm X recalls his encounter in 8th grade with his English teacher, Mr. Ostrowski, whom he recalls as a "rather reddish white man," a "natural-born 'advisor'" who seems to have the capacity to direct his students in everything from literature to career choices (X and Haley, 1965). It is with regard to the latter that Ostrowski approached Malcolm, as one of his top students, with some advice: "Malcolm, you ought to be thinking about a career. Have you been giving it thought?" Though he had not, he hesitantly suggested "I've been thinking I'd like to be a lawyer." Malcolm recalls the response of his teacher who, leaning back in his chair, folding his hands behind his back and with a half-smile, responds:

> Malcolm, one of life's first needs is for us to be realistic. Don't misunderstand me, now. We all here like you, and you know that. But you've got to be realistic about being a nigger. A lawyer – that's no realistic goal for a nigger. You need to think about something you can be. You're good with your hands – making things. Everybody admires your carpentry shop work. Why don't you plan on carpentry? People like you as a person – you'd get all kinds of work.
>
> (X and Hayley, 1965, 41–42)

Malcolm recalls the impact this exchange had on him as these words began to settle on his conscience. "The more I thought afterwards about what he said, the more uneasy it made me. It just kept treading around in my mind"

(X and Hayley, 1965, 42). This sense of unease would prove to be pivotal in Malcolm's unfolding understanding of his predicament as a black man in racist America, and of the future trajectory his life might take. "It was then that I began to change – inside," withdrawing from exchanges with white people and becoming increasingly intolerant of the appellation n–.

The sense of having someone, a stranger, assess one's future by probing the most private of private realms – the realm of one's intellect, conviction, perseverance and the very ingredients of one's soul – is an experience that brings violation, a cheapening of the self, and some evanescent moment of shame. That the other might see some pattern in you to which you are beholden, compelled, against your best effort, to repeat; that your freedoms could be shown to be illusory and you are in fact lashed to forces that remain invisible to yourself but apparent to others – all this brings an estrangement from self that is, I contend, satiated with shame, and that operates at the heart of the affective field of race itself. The affect with which Malcolm confronted this moment, and in which he began his inner work, was, I would propose, an exposure that brought on the uncanniness of a certain racial shame.

Freud's (1919) essay "The 'Uncanny'" is perhaps one of the most widely read of his short works. The insight he proposes into the uniquely unsettling presence associated with such objects as lifelike dolls, corpses and simple mundane coincidences has been taken up in a range of cultural and literary fields, as well as in popular understandings of the aesthetics of horror. (Freud, 1919) The uncanny describes an odd mixing of alien and familiar, of a feeling of intimacy that is offset and made frightening by a vague sense of the radically foreign. In the uncanny, the familiarity we bring to things we know and with which we feel at home, becomes somehow strange, novel and foreign: comfort is discovered as alien, its strangeness greets us in a surge of novelty. Typically, the uncanny takes up residence in those objects that straddle the animate and the inanimate: the wooden doll, described in the story *The Sandman* by Hoffmann, at once lifelike while clearly inanimate, produces a creepy feeling as we encounter in it both the familiarity and comfort of a doll along with the unexpected novelty of human life (Hoffman, 1991). In this sense, there is, at the heart of the uncanny, a sense of a return to the familiar, a feeling of repetition, of coming back to a familiar place, while at the same time discovering that this place has been transformed in some subtle way. The word uncanny is a translation of the German "unheimlichen," or unhomely, the opposite of heimlichen, a word whose precise meaning is itself complex and traversed with contradictions. Heimlichen connotes, as Freud puts it, "'familiar,' 'native,' 'belonging to the home, not strange, tame, intimate, comfortable and homely" (Freud, 1919 220), conveyed by the pleasures of domesticity and the enclosed space of private life: "concealed, kept from sight, so that others do not get to know about it, withheld from others... secret." Heimlich is at once convivial and intimate, warranting trust, but also secret and sheltered from the view of strangers. At the same time, Heimlich derives from privacy an element of the sinister: that which is secret in heimlich is also conducted behind the backs of others, deceitful and malicious, like a criminal conspiracy or the dark sorcery of a magic art. It is at this point, Freud argues, that heimlich and unheimlich, while ostensibly opposed in meaning, seem to converge on a shared designation of concealment, understood both as a condition for intimacy but also as a shadowy, hidden world of potential evil. The hidden quality of the home is one that generates intimacy and warmth, but also hints at something malicious, ghostly, "uneasy, eerie, bloodcurdling: 'These pale youths are unheimlich and are brewing heaven knows what mischief'" (Freud, 1919, 223).

Examples of the reversibility of heimlich and unheimlich are not difficult to conjure: the too life-like doll, the obsequious greeter at the door of a Wal-mart, the sinister clown or the department store Santa on whose knee a child, only moments ago bubbling with excitement, suddenly bursts into tears of fright. In all these cases, the familiarity of the smiling face brings a shiver of repugnance as one senses the movement of some concealed element, some deep malevolent force. Freud explains this inversion as a re-encounter with the primordial experiences of comfort and belonging experienced in infancy. Coddled and stroked, the pleasures of infantile helplessness are reexperienced at the edges of adult consciousness as something vaguely familiar or reminiscent of this earlier sensation, but this time edged not just with the sense of a familiar comfort, but with something frightening, threatening and unsettling. After all, such pleasures have to be disowned if one is to grow out of childhood helplessness into mature autonomy: a sense of dependence, which Freud would elsewhere describe as an oceanic feeling, a state of blissful continuity with the world, would have to undergo repression through the developmental process if the adult were to emerge from the child. For this reason, the reencounter with these feelings is at once pleasant, yet steeped with a sense of the horrific, of a threatened undoing of the subject that fears being cast back into the murky pleasures from which it came – a sort of death. The uncanny signals a sense that freedom, the adult autonomy one attained by repressing the infantile state is slipping away, that one is in fact trapped within a pattern of compulsive repetition, compelled to return, in one's undoing, to the place from which one originated. The conspicuous recurrence of incidental events, such as the appearance of the number 62 over the course of a day in a series of seemingly unrelated contexts ("addresses, hotel-rooms, compartments in railway-trains") induces that same sense of inevitability and helplessness that once brought warmth and comfort, now reencountered as an eerie presentiment of one's approaching death (Freud, 1919, 237). Or, Freud tells us, the commonly experienced dream of being buried alive is an uncanny re-experiencing in adulthood of the same warmth and pleasure known to the child in intra-uterine existence (Freud, 1919, 243).

Freud's notion of the uncanny is, in this respect, helpful in understanding Malcolm's encounter with his teacher, and the experience that spurred him to begin his voyage of self-transformation. But it is also helpful, I contend, in understanding the shame that affixes to racialized subjectivity itself, and in particular those moments which I have described as the exposure of whiteness. To be told that what one is, is what one will always be, that one's future is already written in one's flesh and that this writing is legible to the stranger who peers into one's soul even as it remains inscrutable to oneself, is necessarily to encounter oneself in a racialized version of the shameful uncanny. It is to discover that soul, that most intimate and heimlich of objects, as unheimlich, as strange and malevolent, as foreign to itself, and to experience in the compulsion to repeat the scene of one's own death. Just as, as Sartre pointed out, the look of the other induces a sense of shame in the revelation of our determination before an other who sees the forces (our jealousy, our malice, our voyeurism) that compels us to undertake disreputable acts, so the uncanny reveals to us how locked we are into patterns we cannot escape. Exposure, whether for the one whose comfortable home is suddenly opened to the prying eyes of strangers or for the child who senses the artificiality of Santa's beard, connotes the return of a primordial helplessness, a return to a feeling of continuity with the world the very banishment of which is the condition of the subject's own consolidation as sovereign. As such, the uncanny, through the mechanism of repetition-compulsion, invites a certain paranoid, frantic search for those hidden forces, those concealed agencies that animate us from within, lurking behind what might otherwise be viewed as haphazard events.

The uncanny is always a moment of discovery, one which resonates with the startling novelty of that which is disclosed, though this discovery is never complete. The object of uncanny discovery is always elusive, always partial and always a little obscured, like a prognosis delivered in an expert language which one only partially understands, but also in the stare of the stranger in a public setting who quickly looks away. Sensing the uncanny, we often become paranoid, and search for a more complete picture of what frightens us most. Hearing a noise at night which suddenly makes our comfortable home feel weirdly haunted, we strain to hear more until every creak and rustle seems to confirm our initial impression of uncanniness. The uncanny invokes a compulsive suspicion of subterranean forces with the power to command common events, a wariness and mistrust of surfaces that masks hidden forms, concealing but not entirely concealing a cryptic ordering of things. We direct this sense of phantasmagoric paranoia at bodies – at the bodies of others and at our own bodies, and specifically at the abnormal body. Referring to an earlier article by Ernst Jentsch, "On the Psychology of the Uncanny" (Jentsch, 1906), Freud invokes Jentsch's account of the uncanniness associated with the epileptic seizure. While in ordinary encounters with ordinary bodies, Jentsch argues, we prefer to believe in the "relative psychical harmony" of the other's mental state. However, with the uncanniness of the epileptic's seizure we are reminded that "not everything in the human psyche is of transcendental origin, and that much that is elementary is still present within even our direct perception" (Jentsch, 1906, 14). The seizure brings on a sort of shock in the observer, a "dark knowledge... that mechanical processes are taking place in that which he was previously used to regarding as a unified psyche." What is exposed is "not from the human world but from foreign and enigmatic spheres, for the epileptic attack of spasms reveals the human body to the viewer... as an immensely complicated and delicate mechanism" (Jentsch, 1906, 14). For Freud, Jentsch's claim crystalizes the effect of this paranoid view of the uncanny, here applied to the physical manifestation of an abnormal body in social space, and the manner in which the movement of hidden life forces binds that body to a compulsion to repeat. Freud writes:

> The ordinary person sees in [epilepsy] the workings of forces hitherto unsuspected in his fellow-man but which at the same time he is simply aware of in a remote corner of this own being.... Indeed, I should not be surprised to hear that psychoanalysis, which [is] concerned with laying bare these hidden forces, has itself become the uncanny of many people for that very reason.
>
> (Freud, 1919, 243)

Conclusion

Race in general, and whiteness in particular, is satiated with this sense of the uncanny that derives from its exposure. This uncanny is evidenced in the hands of strangers that fondle the hair of black women and in the indifferent school teachers who claim insight into the futures of promising young students. In recent years this sense of an uncanny exposure had seeped into the racial experiences of white people themselves, with highly combustible effects. That white people explode at the suggestion that their whiteness might be discussed, that they exhibit the effects of a certain fragility, an extraordinary sensitivity and a surging need to flee the discussion, is evidence that a new white uncanny has emerged as an increasingly common theme in American popular culture. Jordan Peele's 2017 film *Get Out* represents only the most obvious instance of this tendency, thought there are many more. For those interested in the prospect of working through the problem of their own whiteness, for subjecting the unexamined effects of white habit to moral scrutiny and committing their efforts to the work of a broader anti-racist reconstruction of their own white habits, some confrontation with this uncanniness is in order, and this confrontation, I would argue, can only begin once the very normative character of white racial exposure itself has been understood. Such a confrontation today seems remote, as the white uncanny far more often operates through a fumbling, awkward avoidance, or a violent investment, than through any form of moral seriousness.

I would like to close this discussion, perhaps, on a rather uncanny note. I would like to turn to a figure that perhaps has hovered for too long on the fringes of this conversation, yet who, I would argue, embodies important and intense manifestations of white uncanniness, perhaps far more prevalent than those of the white panic or white avoidance. This is the uncanniness of the unapologetic white racist, for whom the white uncanny is less an expression of inner panic than of outward white racial contempt: a sardonic grimace like that which Freud attributes to the uncanny dead. In January of 2019, the spectacle of this deathly white uncanny erupted into the public eye and resonated across the American conversation on race. A group of students from Covington Catholic High School, an all-boy's school in southern Kentucky, travelled to Washington D.C. as part of a school trip, and were soon caught up in an incident that briefly became the center of the national conversation, driven largely, I would argue, by the image of a deeply uncanny smile. As a large group of mostly white young men donning red MAGA hats, the students formed an imposing presence on the lawn near the Washington monument, and in the course of their visit became involved in a confrontation with a larger group of participants in a march for Native American heritage. During the confrontation, name calling and provocations erupted from both sides, which was caught in several video clips that went viral. One image from the event drew a swift response: it was that of a young white student, Nick Sandmann, in a close staring match with a native American activist, Nathan Phillips. As Phillips stood chanting and drumming, and taking slow steps into the group of high school students, Sandmann stood his ground directly in front of Phillips, leering forward within inches of Phillips' face, wearing a broad, mocking grin with deadpan eyes. His affected expression was, in my view, unmistakably uncanny: seemingly, but only superficially convivial, he smiled as if to declare the falseness of his own geniality, and in doing so to gesture toward a deeper, darker force, the moral death of his own racism. "I was not intentionally making faces at the protester." In an interview, Sandmann seemed to depict his smile as friendly and welcoming: "I did smile at one point because I wanted him to know that I was not going to become angry, intimidated or be provoked into a larger confrontation" (Williams and Grinberg, 2019). But this explanation is impossible to accept for anyone who has seen the smile, though also impossible to contest, as smiles themselves cannot be readily reduced to falsifiable claims. As I read it, Sandmann's smile was an allusion to the speciousness of smiles themselves, and an invitation to Phillips to sense the reality of the cold, racialized death swirling beneath. As such, Sandmann's smile gives me the creeps. It is like an epileptic seizure: its contortion betrays the tempest of a racist rage, the rage of a shamed white flesh, coyly curled up inside a civility it would be only too happy to explode. Sandmann is in love with his racial uncanny, in a bad way. One only wonders of the intensity of the shame that made it necessary for this young man to transform himself into such a monster, for him to perform the strangeness of his own flesh in this murderous smile. A creepy smile like Sandmann's brings many important meanings beyond the shame from which certain forms of white racialization derive. It testifies to the frozen nature of a white self-intimacy that encounters itself as irreducibly strange. It is a strangeness that, ironically, is shared with those other modes of whiteness that operate at the other end of the political spectrum, which seek to expunge the kernel of their own privilege in a flesh they perceive as equally uncanny. Sandmann's self-intimacy is not the intimacy from which it is possible to confront oneself and envision oneself transformed, the self-intimacy from which creative work is derived and which shame protects. It is the estranged intimacy of a shame transfixed by the creepiness of its own flesh, one that chooses instead to project this creepiness out, onto others. Sandmann's smile is the essence of the white racial uncanny made over into an erotics of murder.[1]

Note

1 A widely circulated still from the viral video of Nicholas Sandmann's confrontation with Nathan Phillips can be discovered through a google image search of "Nicholas Sandmann", or by visiting the wikipedia page entry for "2019 Lincoln Memorial confrontation".

References

Agamben, Giorgio (1998) *Homo Sacer: Sovereign Power and Bare Life* (trans. Daniel Heller-Roazen). Stanford University Press.

Agamben, Giorgio (2002) *Remnants of Auschwitz* (trans. Daniel Heller-Roazen). MIT Press.

Ahmed, Sarah (2007) A Phenomenology of Whiteness. *Feminist Theory*, 8(2), pp. 149–168.

Alexander, Michelle (2012) *The New Jim Crow: Mass Incarceration in the Age of Colorblindness*. The New Press.

Arendt, Hannah (1998) *The Human Condition*, 2nd ed. (trans. Margaret Canovan). University of Chicago Press.

Bobbio, Norberto (1989) *Democracy and Dictatorship: The Nature and Limits of State Power* (trans. Peter Kennealy). Polity.

Bonilla Silva, Eduardo (2003) *Racism without Racists: Color-blind Racism and the Persistence of Racial Inequality in the United States*. Roman & Littlefield.

Bourdieu, Pierre (1977) Outline of a Theory of Practice. Cambridge University Press.

Coates, Ta-Nehisi (2015) *Between the World and Me*. Speigel & Grau.

Crozier, W. R. (2000) Blushing, social anxiety and exposure. In W. R. Crozier (Ed.), *Shyness*. Routledge, pp. 154–170.

DiAngelo, Robin (2018) *White Fragility: Why It's So Hard For White People To Talk About Racism*. Beacon Press.

Dolezal, Luna (2016) *The Body in Shame: Phenomenology, Feminism and the Socially Shaped Body*. Lexington Press

Du Bois, W. E. B. (1994) *The Souls of Black Folk*. Gramercy Books.

Du Bois, W. E. B. (1995) On Being Ashamed of Oneself: An Essay on Race Pride. In Fred L. Hord, Jonathan Scott and Lee Amherst (Eds.) *I Am Because We are: Readings in Black Philosophy*. University of Massachusetts Press.

Dyer, Richard (1988) White. *Screen*, 29(7), pp. 44–64.

Fanon, Frantz (1967) *Black Skin, White Masks* (trans. Charles Lam Markmann). Grove Press.

Frankenberg Ruth (1993) *White Women, Race Matters: The Social Construction of Whiteness*. University of Minnesota Press.

Freud, Sigmund (1919) The Uncanny. In *The Complete Psychological Works*, Vol. XVII (trans. Alix Strachey). Hogarth Press.

Freud, Sigmund (1991) On Narcissism: An Introduction. In Joseph Sandler, Ethel Spector Person and Peter Fonagy (Eds.) *Contemporary Freud: Turning Points and Critical Issues*. Yale University Press.

Hoffmann, Ernst Theodor Amadeus (1991) *Sandman* (trans John Oxenford). Virginia Commonwealth University. https://archive.vcu.edu/germanstories/hoffmann/sand_e.html.

Holson, Laura M. (2018) Hundreds in Oakland Turn Out to BBQ While Black. *New York Times*, May 21. https://www.nytimes.com/2018/05/21/us/oakland-bbq-while-black.html.

Kendall, Frances (2012) *Understanding White Privilege*. Routledge.

Jentsch, Ernst (1906) On the Psychology of the Uncanny (trans. R. Sellars). *Angelaki: Journal of the Theoretical Humanities* 2(1997): 7–16.

Levinas, Emmanuel (2003) *On Evasion/De L'evasion*. (trans. Bettina Bergo). Stanford University Press.

LosAngelista (2009) No You Can't Touch My Hair. blog post, September 13. http://www.losangelista.com/2009/09/no-you-cant-touch-my-hair.html.

MacMullen, Terrance (2009) *Habits of Whiteness: A Pragmatist Reconstruction*. Indiana University Press.

Magee, Rhonda A. (2019) *The Inner Work of Racial Justice: Healing Ourselves and Transforming Our Communities Through Mindfulness*. Tarcher Perigee.

McIntosh, Peggy (1989) White Privilege: Unpacking the Invisible Knapsack. *Peace and Freedom Magazine*, July/August, pp. 10–12.

McWhorter, John, (2020) The Great Awokening. The Weeds podcast, July 31.

Merleau-Ponty, Maurice (1964) *Primacy of Perception* (ed. J. Edie, trans. A. B. Dallery). Northwestern University Press.

Mills, Charles (2007) White Ignorance. In Shannon Sullivan and Nancy Tuana (Eds.), *Race and Epistemologies of Ignorance*. SUNY Press.

Mills, Charles W. (1999) *The Racial Contract*. Cornell University Press.

Ngo, Helen (2017) *The Habits of Racism: A Phenomenology of Racism and Racialized Embodiment*. Lexington.

Oluo, Ijeoma (2019) *So You Want To Talk About Race?* Seal Press.

Robinson, Phoebe (2016) *You Can't Touch My Hair: And Other Things I Still Have To Explain*. Penguin.

Rothenberg, Paula S. (2004). *White Privilege: Essential Rreadings on the Other Side of Racism*, 2nd ed. Worth Publishers.

Sartre, Jean Paul (1993) *Being and Nothingness* (trans. Hazel E. Barnes). Washington Square Press.

Scheff, Thomas (2003) Shame in Self and Society. *Symbolic Interaction*, 26(2), pp. 239–262.

Scheff, Thomas and Suzanne Retzinger (2001) Shame as the master emotion of everyday life. *Journal of Mundane Behavior*, 1(3), pp. 303–324.

Scheff, Thomas J. (2014) The Ubiquity of Hidden Shame in Modernity. *Cultural Sociology*, 8(2).

Scheler, Max (1987) The Location of the Feeling of Shame and Man's Way of Existing. In *Person and Self-Value: Three Essays* (trans. Manfred Frings). Nijhoff.

Schneider, Carl (1977) *Shame, Exposure and Privacy.* Norton.

Schwartzman, Paul (2016) Why some whites are waking up to racism. *Washington Post.* https://www.washingtonpost.com/local/social issues/why-some-whites-are-waking-up-to-racism/2016/08/03/5f2c2386–5051–11e6-aa14-e0c1087f7583_story.html.

Sennett, Richard (1992) *Fall of Public Man.* Norton.

Solange (2016) "Don't Touch My Hair, featuring Sampha" *A Seat at the Table*

Spelman, Elizabeth (2007) Managing Ignorance. In Shannon Sullivan and Nancy Tuana (Eds.) *Epistemologies of Ignorance.* SUNY Press.

Sullivan, Shannon (2006) *Revealing Whiteness: The Unconscious Habits of Racial Privilege,* Indiana University Press.

Sullivan, Shannon (2015) *Good White People: The Problem with Middle-class White Anti-racism.* SUNY Press.

Tangney, June Price and Ronda L.Dearing (2002) *Shame and Guilt.* Guilford Press.

Titchener, Edward B. (1898) The Feeling of Being Stared at. *Science. American Association for the Advancement of Science. New Series*, 8(208) (December 23), pp. 895–897.

Tomkins, Silvan (1995) Shame-Humiliation and Contempt-Disgust. In Eve Kosofsky Sedgwick and Adam Frank (Eds.) *Shame and its Sisters: A Silvan Tomkins Reader.* Duke University Press.

Williams, David and Emanuella Grinberg (2019) Teen in Confrontation with Native American Elders says he was Trying to Defuse the Situation. *CNN*, January 23. https://www.cnn.com/2019/01/19/us/teens-mock-native-elder-trnd/index.html.

Wise, Tim (2011) *White Like Me: Reflections on Race from a Privileged Son.* Soft Skull Press.

X, Malcolm and Alex Haley (1965) *The Autobiography of Malcolm X.* Grove Press.

Yancy, George (2012) *Look, A White!: Philosophical Essays on Whiteness.* Temple University Press.

Yancy, George (2016) The Elevator Effect: Black Bodies/White Bodies. In *Black Bodies, White Gazes: the Continuing Significance of race in America.* Rowman & Littlefield.

Chapter 11

Being-At-The-Intersections

Dwelling in Ambiguity, Vulnerability, and Responsibility

Robin Chalfin

Introduction

In this chapter, the feminist philosophy of intersectionality is explored phenomenologically as a language and praxis of possibilities, illuminating that which is in plain sight yet simultaneously unknowable and irreducible. As a metaphor, "intersections" name the deadly crossroads where the minoritized are rendered invisible; "intersections" name seamlessly interlocked systems of oppression where privilege and power are effectively concealed; and finally, "intersections" name the unsettling ambiguity and complexity of human beings themselves which resists dichotomous categorizations.

This discussion addresses the question of being-in-between – of dwelling at intersections, drawing on the spatial and temporal metaphors of the intersectional analytic. This paradigm aims to make visible not only the obscured workings of interlocking systems of power-over but also our unwitting participation in or power in reinforcing these structures of domination – invisibilized dwellings, we could say – not only formed and fashioned in the material sociopolitical dimension, but lived and embodied in our thoughts, imagination, and our very bodily gestures such that it is hard to be, to think otherwise. Yet, we must, as the consequences are severe.

The transformative potentiality of intersectional theory attends to the precarity and complexity of the human being situated in inter-connected systems of power and oppression. However, this prevailing analytic, adopted across academic discourses and activist projects, has become so accessible and applicable across disciplines that it has at times ironically trended toward institutionalized and depoliticized applications and buzzword statuses (Davis, 2008). Amidst the dilution, an ever more rigorous attention to power and embodied resistance to reductive thinking is called for in the conceptualization of the human subject in its irreducible ambiguity, vulnerability, and responsibilities. Attending to the vivid and evocative metaphors and language of intersectionality born out of black and women of color feminisms, re-situates the theory and praxis in a vital and radical lineage which resists the whitewashing and reductive pull toward additive modes of theorizing the

DOI: 10.4324/9781003394327-12

human subject. Indeed, the possibility of the intersectional analytic is to hold rigorous critique of structures of power whilst opening a conceptualization of the irreducible ambiguity of lived embodiment as the very condition of dwelling in the world. By attending to the particular ambiguities of dwelling-in-between social categorizations of race, gender, and sexuality, this discussion foregrounds the tensions in dwelling in the necessary tensions of vulnerability and responsibility.

Embodied Intersectionality

The intersectional lens seeks to bring to the foreground hierarchical and categorical systems that cannot be understood in isolation, but rather intersect and compound one another within matrices of power, privilege, and oppression. Further, the intersectional analytic resists the logic of singular categories such as race, gender, class, sexual orientation, or disability, and the predominant discourses that perpetuate sociopolitical erasure and psychological fragmentation. Intersectionality, a theory of spatial metaphors, not only makes visible the often-obscured workings and disavowed impact of structural violence but also our *participation* in it – in its doing and its undoing. This is the realm of the implicit, and as a feminist, phenomenological, psycho-analytically oriented therapist and educator, I am interested in this implicit dimension – the unconscious, the background, the social constructs and givens of our existence, and how we access and act on this dimension. Indeed, intersectional praxis requires an embodied engagement with the theory. As intersectionality points to obscured social injustice, we are already complicit in its perpetuation. Given this embeddedness, it is not surprising that engaging in intersectionality risks recapitulating the very hierarchies it seeks to subvert.

Within the habitus of life, it is difficult to actually *see,* and thus a central challenge to *feel* such things, and without feeling, our perceptual capacities are quite limited. Think of the colloquial saying "I feel you," which means "I see you" (here, in my body) – "I see what you are saying" and "I get it" or "I get you." At the same time, it is particularly hard to feel (in here) when we lack perceptual clarity. When we attest to understanding something that has been hard to grasp within ourselves or in another individual, we say (often after a hard conversation) "I can see that," which is to communicate that I can now feel what you are saying. This circular process of feeling and seeing (not surprisingly) is of particular interest to me as a psychotherapist, and also as a teacher to counselors in training and practice. To see (in here and out there) – to develop perceptual awareness (through both, psychological and critical consciousness), I will argue – requires that we see from a specific embodiment (an embodied vulnerability and responsibility rather than care-fully avoided fragility). How each of us does this depends on tarrying with the questions of "who and where we are," which implies differential and intersecting responsibilities. In this regard, I will speak from my own experience – where I find, feel, see myself – and will also draw on experiences helping other teachers and therapists to *feel* and wrestle with that which is difficult for them to *see*.

Not only do we easily become disembodied (from what we feel and thus can understand), but specifically, the way we theorize becomes disembodied – *dislocated* – where the academic and professional languages we use elude that which we purport to understand (in here and out there). Our learning communities and therapeutic spaces reproduce structural violence through reductive and defensive positions, distortions, and erasure. Indeed, the practice of intersectionality has proven to be both transformative of and caught up in this very problem.

When we exist outside and between social categories, as feminist and critical race theorist Kimberly Crenshaw (1989) famously analogizes, it is like standing unprotected in a traffic intersection. Deadly collisions and cumulative injuries are not accidents. However, when one is inevitably harmed at this intersection, the injury is regarded as unintentional at best, or worse, a fault of one's own. Furthermore, single-issue movements – and even anti-discrimination laws – fail to protect the injured as they are conscripted into divisive and essentialist positions wherein persons are categorized as *either/or*, never *both/and*, or certainly not recognized as *beyond or betwixt* these mutually exclusive constructs. Such calcified thinking reinforces bodies into safe conformity, or precarious, expendable, and exploitable *others*. Indeed, alterity is dangerous, deadly even, and yet, it is the conditional possibility of our living. How do we relinquish the protection of privilege or the pursuit of protection for precarity?

I have long been interested in what we learn from explicitly living between the protected and legible categories of being. One can see that this betweenness evokes questions and requires living in questions – it certainly brings us as practitioners to consider the particular ontological and urgent dimensions of this work. While this can wear and tear the material fabric of being, might this also not hold open the possibility of being toward our own potentialities? Indeed, we approach the question of what it means *to be* at all – to dwell at all – between language and body, self and other, hope and fear, pleasure and pain, and how the literal positioning *in-between* lights up the imperative of dwelling in our indivisible and multiplicitous situatedness. The phenomenological philosopher and therapist Eugene Gendlin aptly observes that dwelling involves the material situatedness of being-in-the world all the while reconstituting the conditions of our living. Gendlin writes of this tension between conditioned and creative living that "[d]welling is in the built forms yet beyond them" (Gendlin, 1988, 149). Dwelling – owning our embodied living – must then involve the acute awareness of our respective vulnerability and responsibility. First and foremost, this concerns dwelling in and between privilege and oppression, between and in protected, precarious, and polarized categories of being and affiliating in the world.

When we inhabit a protected social position – enjoying the support and shelter of belonging – we face not a deadly, but a dead*ening* effect. Rather than the vulnerability of an exposed intersection, normatized living occurs in the flow – the momentum – of systematically organized traffic. When we are on the road and going places, we implicitly know and follow the signs and signals, and we are safe to stay in our lane; we can relax, even go on autopilot. We do not notice how our ease makes the existence of others more precarious. We are insulated from the viscerality of human finitude. There is a numbing, and yet when we critically engage the conditions of our corporal reality – we find cracks, curves, and contradictions that undo and yet animate our living. As Beauvoir aptly observed: "It is in the knowledge of the genuine conditions of our life that we must draw our strength to live" (Beauvoir, 1948, 1). This reckoning can be difficult when we feel threatened and reach for shelter.

Dwelling-Between

One of my shelters is feminism, yet where the production of emancipatory practices emerges, so does the reproduction of exclusionary practices, resulting in continual tension. In this case, we can see that the most radically relational discourses emerge outside the margins of the severing singularities of White feminism, with intersectionality growing out of multiple genealogies of Black feminism, women of color, and queer feminist activism from the earliest periods of suffrage, to the contemporary "say her name" movements (Crenshaw et al., 2015). Intersectionality has, in my opinion, become a formidable dwelling of its own across movements and academic spaces – since my undergraduate Women's Studies readings of Lorde, Lugones, Collins, Anzaldua, Moraga, Min-ha, hooks, and other Black, indigenous, women of color, and queer visionaries offering sense-making capacities born out of the precarious prescient places in between the sheltering norms of Whiteness, imperialism, and heteropatriarchy. However, even intersectionality must be held in continual living tension to avoid systematizing and institutionalizing reductive modes.

I find myself dwelling in tension, particularly as I move in the world with so much privilege—I live and work in my first language, and I look like a middle-aged, White, heteronormative, conventionally-feminine, married, able-bodied, and cis-gendered woman. Benefitting from these social registries means that I enter normative spaces with ease. However, this access eventually involves disruption, as I also live by a queer orientation and my family embodies multiple nonbinary identities. My spouse identifies as lesbian, although the younger generation might claim her as a genderqueer. My two children, with varying brown skin tones and coiled hair textures, alternately identify as Black and biracial. My partner, my children's stepparent, is White. My children's father is Black. We are a blended family in multiple ways. Depending on who I am standing with at any given time or collaborating with regarding the parenting tasks at hand, I can be *perceived* as being in a heterosexual interracial relationship with biologically biracial children. At another moment, I may be seen as a lesbian, in a same-gender marriage, with transracially adopted children. The ambiguity of our identity as a family disrupts the deeply held notions of purity and biology surrounding kinship, and the invisibility of my identity in particular, produces a phenomenon of "passing" in and out of minoritized spaces where my bisexuality disrupts both heteronormative and homonormative expectations. Rather than standing at a deadly intersection, I "pass" and weave through traffic, and this movement gives me an appreciation for the paradoxical experience of being both invisible and visible, yet unseen (Chang et al., 2021). My particular location informs not only my interest in the ambiguity of identity and the illusion of singular and essentialized categories, but also the simplistic demarcation between privilege and oppression, and the particular accountability required for living at the crossroads of a normatized and minoritized social positioning.

Dwellings and Metaphors

Heidegger's familiar, yet specifically challenging metaphor of "dwelling" evokes shelter, hearth, harmony, home, even as *being,* is defined by its awareness of its own precarity and finitude. Thus, *da-sein,* meaning *there-being,* emerges from dwelling not in illusions of safety but rather in the authentic tension between longing for one's place, and always *being-displaced* toward our own death – toward the unknowable. Crenshaw also offers familiar and visceral metaphors to conceptualize being-in-the-world, in this case, *with-out* actual shelter and *with-in* the literal and disproportionate imminence of death. She analogizes, in her temporal "basement" metaphor, a structure of entrapment fashioned across generations of walls and floors enclosing movement, wherein the only hope of "rising up" to gain protected ground involves crawling and contorting oneself, or climbing on the backs of others (Crenshaw, 1991). From a privileged point of view, we rarely *see* this suffering underground, nor do we feel our structural implications within it.

Further, wherever we stand – basement or glass ceiling – we may bury our deep-seated consciousness that might threaten hard-earned personal or social solidity. No one wants to be among the "down and out." It is interesting to look at this repudiation of alterity, between and within, in relation to Crenshaw's relational praxis metaphor of "coalition," which typically refers to political bridging across distinct groups, but in this context is a call to allies exiled or tokenized, or those denied visibility *within* "home" or "affiliation" groups. This opening of a space for otherness, precisely where we most want to feel familiarity, is challenging, yet the metaphor goes even further. Not only must we recognize our very own affinity groups as a coalition, but we must also reckon with our individual identities as coalitions (Crenshaw, 1991). The coalition metaphor challenges the protective function of otherizing, and orients attention toward alignment with the dimensions of our humanity that we are taught to deny, repress, or even eradicate. Bringing together the aspects of one's identity that have been falsely and often forcefully separated, both within the institutions of dominant society and within single-issue movements, allows space to authentically connect and align with the self and other (Lugones, 2003). Thus, genuine movement out of the dangerous psychic and social intersections, the suffocating basements, and all the places in-between occur through relational coalitional modes of being that resist, both literally and figuratively, capitalizing on the other.

Holding these three metaphors of intersections, basements, and coalitions fully requires embodiment – a seeing and feeling that is uncomfortable and yet deeply engages our capacity for being in and with the world. This is not easy. We can sense through these spatial, temporal, and relational metaphors - not only implicit biases and structural violence but also our involvement within where we censor our history, ourselves, and one another. Fortunately, we see not only the cost of these social and psychic structures, but also constructive or modes of being cultivated on intrapsychic, interpersonal, and collective levels. Anna Carastathis articulates these intersectional modes of discourse, practice, and being as "simultaneity, complexity, irreducibility, and inclusivity" (Carastathis, 2016, 235). Indeed, these ontological structures are urgently needed and broadly applicable from the consulting room to the classroom.

Holding together the costs and constructive possibilities of engaging our positionally can foster critically needed consciousness, but is continuative and may be most readily accessed through embodied practices. For example, in one of my counseling courses on gender and sexuality, I utilize an experiential exercise that asks students to embody their social positioning visibly. I recite a series of simple statements: "The part of my identity that I am most aware of daily is…, least aware of is…, was most emphasized growing up…," and so forth. The students answer by standing under one of several identity signs on the classroom walls (presently, Zoom boxes), representing predominant social categories of race, gender, class, sexual orientation, ability, and immigration status. This is not a complete list and represents a part of the identarian problem – students must wrestle with the wrenching sensations surrounding the dilemma of where to stand, which may feel imperfect, reductive, or even fracturing.

Students with visibly minoritized racial identities often find themselves standing alone. One student spoke from this experience, saying, "This feels different. I am painfully aware of being the only person of color in the classroom, but I am usually the only one dealing with that fact. Yes, I feel bad standing alone, but it's also a relief to see all the White students standing across from me looking at reality." Another student standing alone in her Black identity observed a shift within herself in making other people – White people – comfortable by way of "code-switching" and how different it felt standing with "no filter."

When asked, "What part of your identity was most emphasized while growing up?", a White student spoke from the center of the room – from the center of her privilege, saying "I feel empty and strange…sad. I do not think I have anywhere to stand, but here in the center. I am not connected to anything…anything but this idea that we are just regular, just normal." At this moment, her privileged position became visually and viscerally strange to her. Tolerating the distress of this disorientation, she paradoxically experienced unprecedented groundedness, which became the basis for critically accounting for the costs of her privilege and consciously engaging with her world. Students with invisible otherized embodiments related to sexuality, socioeconomic status, and disabilities often express feelings of vulnerability in standing openly within these truths, simultaneous relief in finding themselves standing with others, and unexpected sensations of collective strength that had often already been foreclosed through self-censure and silence.

Paradoxically, the practice of standing in embodied relations to power, and the process of speaking from alterity, generates presence or what one student describes as "feeling really here" – we could say *dwelling here* not because it is easy or promises protection, but rather that embodying the truth of where (or *that*) we stand shifts the energy from illusions of protection to possibilities in living, for where one stands is never a complete reflection of who one is. Often, students are deeply pained as they choose where to stand, but beginning from these material conditions, they can speak of their conflicts and complications. These coalitions within the self and collective are counterintuitive and involve consciousness, creativity, and courage in owning one's complexity and complicity within the systems that produce and reproduce our very ways of being in the world. This counterintuitive inner work calls for an existential dialectic – as *movement* (Chang et al., 2021) – movement through and within deeply held conflicts with neither transcendence nor synthetic resolution – finding in its place an open, indeterminate space that holds and harnesses the energy produced by polarization, toward a more complex expression of being. Black scholar, poet, and activist Audre Lorde writes: "Difference must be not merely tolerated but seen as a fund of necessary polarities between which our creativity can spark like a dialectic" (Lorde, 1981, 100). Indeed, many dialectics arise in an intersectional praxis. In this paper, I focus on one aspect.

Vulnerability and Responsibility

This tension evokes the binary of the powerful/powerless – of the strong and weak aligned along those who are valued as prototypical humans and otherwise. While this violent asymmetry is tremendously impactful, its functions remain largely invisible. We are typically uncomfortable with having power because it implies responsibility, which is often terrifying. Simultaneously, we cling to power over others, as power feels like the absence of vulnerability, and instinctually, vulnerability is also to be avoided. However, this polarity does not just perpetuate behaviors of dominance and control over or against, but also a sense of ongoing victimhood and disavowal of agency because powerlessness is also a release from responsibility and shame. With polarized positions of power over or powerlessness, authentic responsibility and vulnerability are equally disavowed. Thus, this polarity produces fragility on all sides.

Retreating from responsibility and vulnerability often get expressed in regard to the work being "too difficult," "someone else's responsibility," and feelings of helplessness around "doing it right" – we will often say we are constantly "stepping on toes" or unintentionally "pushing buttons." Then, with resentment, we say, "I feel like I have to walk on eggshells." These physically cringe-inducing metaphors evoke the depth of responsibility that is required for intersectional consciousness – we must be responsible not only for obvious or intentional harm, but much more importantly, for *un*intentional harm – for that which we cannot yet see, feel, or hold in our awareness. Responsibility goes so much further than what we can control and anticipate – rather, it is to be responsible for what we do not know and did not intend, and as such, responsibility is to ask to be disoriented – to be vulnerable. Perhaps we could consider the sensation of walking where the ground is tender, is living, and feels our presence.

As this intersectional analytic disrupts the simplistic divisions between the powerful/powerless, or victim/perpetrator, it calls for a nuanced account of vulnerability and responsibility implicated in our interrelatedness. Indeed, owning responsibility requires us to resist illusions of separateness, relinquish defensive control, be disoriented – to be vulnerable. However, when vulnerability is held open, even in difficult situations, and a desire to connect and be known is expressed, then we are present, we are *in* presence, we are *dwelling* in relation, we are dwelling-in-between; it is to address the other; I am here – see me in my living, hear me in my language, in this place, this situation. It is challenging to stay in this vulnerable desire, which allows for the messiness and mattering of human connections.

Being-Between

All this makes me think about family vacations and the immersive intimacies and intersections with others (families and hospitality service workers) oriented toward creating a sense of belonging wherein we collide with a background of assumptions and microaggressions, misrecognition, erasure, tokenization, sensationalizing, and reductive and repetitive questions such as "Are these your children?", "When did you adopt?", "Is your husband joining you?", "Is this (referring to my spouse) your sister?", "How do you get their hair to do that?" (while patting or pulling my children's curls). Indeed, traveling has become a potent ground for engaging with the tension between vulnerability and responsibility. For example, during winter vacation in 2019, just before the pandemic-induced lockdown, we travelled north to a lodge on a large lake that was cleared for skating. Here, we predominantly found White, working-class, testosterone-fueled families obsessed with ice hockey – an *almost* perfect fit with my partner's upbringing and one of my daughters' burgeoning interest in hockey. We were, most strikingly, the only multiracial family and the only queer family in sight.

Following our first day of festivities, we went to the common dining hall to be seated for dinner. This venture quickly comes to a standstill, as our hostess, while looking around, asks whether we would like to wait for the rest of our party before being seated. "Oh, no, we are all here," I say. After another pause, the hostess asks if we would "be sitting together or dining separately." We then realize that she does not see us, or that she sees us as fragments. I exhale. "Yes, we are together, and this is all of us, thank you." I feel the sting of invisibility, and I feel her startle in disorientation. I take another breath, stay open-minded, and appreciate that she looks at us a little longer, and then starts to linger as she waits on us through the evening. I like that she is curious and keeps moving through her disorientation, all whilst trying to connect with us. That night, we learnt so much about her. She is from South America and loves the North woods, where she has made great efforts to transplant her family. She lit up when my partner conversed with her in Spanish. Subsequently, we reveled in her company every night during our vacation. Thus, it may be said that we were dislocated, thrown together, and found a place *within* difference, to be questioning beings together.

This incident however felt very different from one that transpired later on in the hot tub, where I was soaking with two other vacationing mothers, while the kids swam nearby in the pool, and my partner received some coveted downtime. Here, we discover that we are all social workers through training. There is a palpable ease among us – strangers with a shared language. One of them asks questions about my practice and what I teach. When I tell them about my counseling of sexual and gender minorities – my LGBT course – conversation stops. My presence has muddied the waters – disrupted the presumption of normativity – these women have now retreated to silence. I keep talking and offer a bridge – I share more about how outstanding my students are, and how much they value the curriculum. My fellow social workers still do not engage, and the conversation comes to a complete halt. The story stops here, but does not have to. Intersectionality calls for us to bear the discomfort we feel and cause in others; it calls for an awkward encounter with alterity rather than careful avoidance of fragility. While we can certainly do this uncomfortable work, it is counterintuitive.

Indeed, even with the strongest intentions, we must prepare for failure. Our energies can get so tied up in being responsible, in "getting it right," which constricts us. I am led to think of a patient in therapy who relayed an intense commitment to critical consciousness work that required, in his mind, to be "in control" at all times. When he mis-stepped in an unwitting enactment of silencing and speaking for his female co-activist and friend, he was horrified to learn that he must have let down his guard and reacted by renewing his resolve to be in "better control." When I invited him to pause with me and reflect on this imperative to control, correct, and constrict, he became perplexed, receptive, and was finally able to touch base with his vulnerability. As we basked in the tension of his precarious positioning as a person of color with the imperative of staying in control, hypervigilance gave way to a vulnerable and responsible experience of relating to himself, his communities, and his allies. There is a reconfiguration of power in knowing our powerlessness; a *response-ability* that emerges. It is the capacity to be shattered out of our presumptive modes, constricted care, and illusions of transcendence that brings us to a threshold of relational accountability, and personal and political growth.

Let us remember my student standing in the middle of the room – standing in the middle of her normativity and recognizing it (seeing and feeling it here) as strange – historically situated for the very first time. Thus, whether dwelling invisibly at a deadly intersection or basement, or in this case, dwelling in the dislocated and fragile center or peak of privilege, critical consciousness begins with a reversal or a refusal of how we typically see, which opens the capacity to feel, to imagine, deconstruct, and reconstruct consciously *being* in the world.

While working on the intrapsychic level, it is common to say that we have "pushed feelings down" or "out of sight," that I "cannot look at that" or "it is buried too deep" to feel. Further, there are often rigid, fragile, and costly personality structures evolved by way of distancing from our own vulnerability. However, this very vulnerability is an essential condition for our conscious existence. That which has been alienated is engaged by any integrative and reparative therapeutic process so that, in embodying the disavowed, we can creatively live our whole and vulnerable selves. This process involves the capacity to spend time in the shadows of the self and to bare threatening truths held in consciousness (Benjamin, 2017; Powell, 2018). This is true whether we are reclaiming parts of ourselves censured in service of the security of belonging within single identity groups, or in service of deflecting shame surrounding the uncertainties of self-worth and crushing guilt born out of unearned privilege.

The metaphor of coalitions is particularly useful here. An integrative therapeutic process is not a synthesis, flattening, or transcendent wholeness of the disparate parts of oneself, but rather a growing capacity to bear tension, difference, and dialectical movement. In the process of growth, the most vulnerable and shameful parts hold critical perceptual truths that are psychically and historically silenced. Our consciousness is dependent on the very process of dismantling that hierarchical polarization and reclaiming the split off parts of ourselves, not by reactively reversing internal conflict, but by developing the capacity to integrate the complexity of our vulnerability and responsibility. This is not only the work of psychological maturation, but also the work of social transformation. To make our intrapsychic and sociopolitical worlds more livable, we must challenge the hierarchical oppositions that relegate and scapegoat aspects of ourselves and our society as deviant and unacceptable. In doing so, we do not wish to eradicate opposition or difference, but rather hope to cultivate the capacity for consciously and creatively living *in* that difference, that very tension.

One of the persistent tensions in intersectional consciousness is that just as we intend to undo oppression, we are doing privilege, and as we undo privilege, we are doing oppression. While cultivating consciousness, we may think we have achieved some understanding, an interpersonal awareness, and a political victory – yet actually, we are simultaneously missing something or reinforcing a power differential, a narrowly defined construct of human beings that further ostracizes or constricts those more marginal than ourselves. While this is inescapable, it is also highly problematic – involving real harm – and hard to feel, and thus difficult to look at directly.

In 1979, Lorde presented her now-famous paper entitled *"The master's tools will never dismantle the master's house."* This phrase is often quoted by White feminists to reference patriarchal oppression at large, but Lorde was speaking *to* White feminists at an all-White feminist conference. Her metaphorical words critique White feminism and its continued failure to see its investment in and reproduction of White supremacy. While Lorde critiqued this forty years ago, we face its devastating costs even today – this failure manifesting as a White feminist movement that has failed to elect a White female presidential candidate. Instead, fifty-three percent of White women voted for a White supremacist sexual predator as the forty-fifth male president (Setzler & Yanus, 2018). These White women embody Crenshaw's image of crawling out of the basements, the desperate dissociation selfhood in service of social protections and status (Crenshaw, 1991). This is the cost of using the master's tools to preserve the master's house. This positioning with patriarchal power is not only on the backs of BIPOC women but   falsely forecloses its possibilities even for White women. Lorde went on to write in this paper:

> Interdependency between women is the way to a freedom which allows the I to be, not in order to be used, but in order to be creative. This is a difference between the passive being and the active being. Advocating the mere tolerance of difference between women is the grossest reformism. It is a total denial of the creative function of difference in our lives. Difference must be not merely tolerated but seen as a fund of necessary polarities between which our creativity can spark like a dialectic.
>
> (Lorde, 1981, 101)

Staying in the polarities of difference requires shifting from survival to creativity. In this dialectic, we may end up undoing oppression only to unequivocally cause harm to something else. However, we cannot easily avoid this harm, and we cannot entirely escape questions of survival; rather, we can face these questions of survival with consciousness and collectivity. Recall that this process begins by looking directly at the conditions of our existence. In considering our existence between structures of power, powerlessness, and agency, I turn also to queer philosopher Judith Butler and her analysis of living this conundrum. In *Gender Trouble* (1994), she illuminates what she calls the performativity of gender, which is to say that just as gender is socially constructed, so too can it be deconstructed or performed consciously and differently – subversively. However, she goes even further in *Undoing Gender* (2004), articulating the nuance – the tension – of freedom and restriction wherein gender is understood as a "practice of improvisation within a scene of constraint," a practice that is always within a social context, and never outside of social norms. In this text, Butler emphasizes the paradoxical tension between societal-mediated survival and individual agency (Butler, 2004, 1). She reminds us that one does not simply author the terms of one's gender because these terms are always negotiated within collective social contexts. As a concrete example, she addresses the tension around the diagnosis of what is now classified as gender dysphoria (at the time of her writing, gender identity disorder). For many clinicians and trans persons, medical classification is used as an economic tool to gain access to funds for gender-affirming medical interventions, such as hormone and surgery modifications, even while recognizing the diagnosis is inherently pathologizing in its conflation of gender nonconformity as a psychiatric disorder. We are never, Butler reminds us, able to remove ourselves entirely from what Lorde termed the "master's tools" but we can with the dominant ideology's norms and systems to subvert their material effects. Indeed, the tension between utilizing norms to survive on a literal level and maintaining a critical distance from norms to survive on a figurative or conceptual level is essential. Butler writes:

My agency does not consist in denying this condition of my constitution. If I have any agency, it is opened up by the fact that I am constituted by a social world I never chose. That my agency is riven with paradox does not mean it is impossible. It means only that paradox is the condition of its possibility...I may feel that without some recognizability I cannot live. I may also feel that the terms by which I am recognized make life unlivable. This is the juncture from which critique emerges, where critique is understood as an interrogation of the terms by which life is constrained in order to open up the possibility of different modes of living.

(Butler, 2004, 3)

This juncture Butler and Lorde articulate is a different kind of intersection wherein the difference is reckoned with deliberately. When we do so, we can see that our efforts toward undoing discrimination result in redoing. As we see, our efforts toward undoing discrimination result in redoing. I feel this very concretely and poignantly with my daughters regarding the recognition of their biracial identity. Hybrid identities are certainly a direct challenge to monistic and essentialized social categories and the divisive terms by which we define human beings. Existing in-between and in ambiguous spaces can be profoundly isolating. The social recognition of hybridity and ambiguity of all kinds, whether racial, sexual, or other, are critical. However, racial hybridity in particular is also taken up in sinister ways by post-identity discourses that inflame colorblind, post-racial, and even explicitly White supremacist narratives. Shortly after my children were born, the US Census, on the heels of tremendous organizing efforts from the mixed-race community, included the self-recognition of multiracial citizens (Abdelal et al., 2009). Now, mixed-race citizens could be counted as human beings challenging both the recent history of erasure into monistic identity groups and an older history of being counted in the census, particularly in dehumanizing and fragmented ways, such as octoroons, half-breeds, or literal percentages and fractions of persons. On the one hand, this self-recognition was heralded as victory for people of multiracial descent. Yet, it was simultaneously experienced as a threat to African Americans and other racial minorities who would lose their numbers and social power/voice/influence as a collective force. Not unlike medical codification, census recognition both affirms a particular existence and fixes it within discourses of pathology and political legitimacy. Such fixity is both liberating and constraining. Every new recognition brings about voluntary and involuntary subjects and erases other subjects. It is not simply semantic, but epistemic, influencing what sorts of identities are available to us and how such constructs are put to use. I want my daughters to be able to grow up and, be "counted" – counted as young women, as biracial human beings, as whole and complex persons who have voices as citizens of this country. However, I also want my daughters to be able to resist the terms by which they count – the terms by which they matter – which includes being cognizant of how our mattering may erase others' mattering.

Counting is caught up in categorization, and categories are formed in the polarities of what is considered human. The transformation of norms, Butler repeatedly reminds us, comes from within an understanding of how one is constituted by them and the question of *survival-based* undoing (Butler, 1990, 2004). There is inescapable tension within constructing and deconstructing our own and others' freedom and constraints. We want to do it right, do it well, and move forward (preferably in a straight line). Rather than offering a sense of knowing, this paper seeks to embrace an uncomfortable, what we often call queer (dis)orientation (Ahmed, 2006), evoking perceptual modes of being toward the limits of our knowing and our capacities, and the responsibilities of our knowing and our abilities. Even as one practices intersectionality, one undoes it – we cannot escape this problem, but rather can be present to it – attentive to it and *accountable* to it. Resisting prejudice amplifies it through the dynamics of avoidance, suppression, denial, etc. It cannot simply be undone, but it can be held with awareness and the tension of owning one's complicity. Thus, we see that doing critical or intersectional consciousness work is much like the psychoanalytic compulsion of working with repetition. It is slippery, repetitive, and always occurring (Benjamin, 2017). Just as you are undoing it, we are doing it again and we must fail to get it right. We must do it to undo it, over and over again.

Conclusion

As we own our responsibilities and vulnerabilities within systems of power, we face the paradoxical movement of doing and undoing power itself. Lorde's words reverberate: "The master's tools will never dismantle the master's house." This is true. Butler further stirs the pot, and the problem: "We will never be able to remove *ourselves* from the 'master's tools'" (Lorde, 1981, 99). The house, the tools, and how we dwell at all come into question, and perhaps in particularly illuminating ways at the intersections of being in the world. Lorde writes that "[t]he house of your difference is the longing for your greatest power and your deepest vulnerability" (Lorde, 2009). Dwelling in this house – this house paradoxically built out of ambiguity rather than mastery holds the possibility of human vulnerability and response-ability. Intersectionality, held metaphorically and materially, can facilitate ways to reconceive identity, subjectivity, collectivity, and (non)belonging that resist the hegemony of power as it constructs categorial, dichotomous, hierarchical logic and as it naturalizes institutions/systems of power. We can then ask: How do we dwell such that we can bear the historical burdens of our identities as a simultaneously constricting and creative starting place for being in the world? What dwellings – places where we are being-in-authenticity – comprise being-at-the-intersections of accountability and ambiguity?

References

Abdelal, R., Herrera, Y. M., Johnston, A. I., and McDermott, R. (Eds.) (2009) *Measuring identity: A guide for social scientists.* Cambridge University Press.

Ahmed, S. (2006) *Queer phenomenology: Orientations, objects, others.* Duke University Press.

Anzaldúa, G. (1990) *Making Face, Making Soul/Haciendo Caras: Creative and Critical Perspectives by Women of Color.* Aunt Lute Foundation.

Beauvoir, S. (1948) *The ethics of ambiguity.* Philosophical Library.

Benjamin, J. (2017) *Beyond doer and done to: Recognition theory, intersubjectivity and the third.* Routledge.

Bernstein, M. and Reimann, R. (Eds.) (2001) *Queer families, queer politics: Challenging culture and the state.* Columbia University.

Butler, J. (1990) *Gender trouble: Feminism and the subversion of identity.* Routledge.

Butler, J. (1993) *Bodies that matter: On the discursive limits of "sex."* Routledge.

Butler, J. (2004) *Undoing gender.* Routledge.

Carastathis, A. (2016) *Intersectionality: Origins, contestations, horizons.* University of Nebraska.

Chang, M., Ri, J., and Chalfin, R. (2021, April) *Dwelling-In-Between: Reification, Rupture, and Resoluteness at the Intersections of Being* [Symposium]. Psychology and the Other Conference 2021.

Chalfin, R. R. (2019) Identity-as-disclosive-space: Dasein, Discourse and Distortion. In D. M. Goodman, E. R. Severson, and H. Macdonald (Eds.), *Race, Rage, and Resistance.* Routledge, pp. 163–179.

Chalfin, R. (2021) The Entanglement of Being: Sexuality Inside and Outside the Binary. *Studies in Gender and Sexuality*, 22(1), pp. 28–39. https://doi.org/10.1080/15240657.2021.1883847.

Collins, P. H. (2000) *Black feminist thought: Knowledge, consciousness, and the politics of empowerment.* Routledge.

Collins, P. H. and Bilge, S. (2016) *Intersectionality.* Polity Press.

Crenshaw, K. (1989) Demarginalizing the Intersection of Race and Sex: A Black Feminist Critique of Antidiscrimination Doctrine, Feminist Theory and Antiracist Policies. *University of Chicago Legal Forum*, 1, pp. 139–167.

Crenshaw, K. W. (1991) Mapping the Margins: Intersectionality, Identity Politics, and Violence Against Women of Color. *Stanford Law Review*, 43(6), pp. 1241–1299. https://doi.org/10.2307/1229039.

Crenshaw, K., Ritchie, A., Anspach, R., Gilmer, R., and Harris, L. (2015) *Say Her Name: Resisting Police Brutality Against Black Women.* African American Policy Forum.

Davis, K. (2008) Intersectionality as Buzzword: A Sociology of Science Perspective on What Makes a Feminist Theory Successful. *Feminist Theory*, 9(1), pp. 67–85. https://doi.org/10.1177/1464700108086364.

Gendlin, E.T. (1988) Dwelling. In H. J. Silverman, A. Mickunas, T. Kisiel, & A. Lingis (Eds.), *The horizons of continental philosophy: Essays on Husserl, Heidegger and Merleau-Ponty.* Kluwer Academic Publishers, pp. 133–152. http://previous.focusing.org/gendlin/docs/gol_2127.html.

Green, B. (2005) Psychology, diversity and social justice: Beyond heterosexism and across the cultural divide. *Counselling Psychology Quarterly*, 18(4), pp. 295–306. https://doi.org/10.1080/09515070500385770.

Grzanka, P. (2020) From buzzword to critical psychology: An invitation to take intersectionality seriously. *Women & Therapy*, 43(3–4), pp. 244–261. https://doi.org/10.1080/02703149.2020.1729473.

Hancock, A. M. (2016) *Intersectionality: An intellectual history*. Oxford University Press.

Heidegger, M. (2008) *Being and Time*. HarperCollins.

hooks, b. (2000. *Feminist theory: From margin to center*. Pluto Press.

Lai, C. H. (2011) Re-writing the subject: The thrownness of being in the multicultural condition. *Canadian Review of Comparative Literature/Revue Canadienne de Littérature Comparée*, 30, pp. 3–4.

Lorde, A. (1981) The Master's Tools Will Never Dismantle the Master's House. In C. Morroga & G. Anzaldua (Eds.), *The Bridge Called Me Back: Writings by Radical Women of Color*. Persaphone Press, pp. 98–101.

Lorde, A. (2009) Difference and survival. In R. P. Byrd, J. B. Cole, and B. Guy-Sheftall (Eds.), *I am your sister: Collected and unpublished writings of Audre Lorde*. Oxford University Press, pp. 201–204.

Lugones, M., (2003). *Pilgrimages/peregrinajes: Theorizing coalition against multiple oppressions*. Rowman & Littlefield Publishing Group.

Moraga, C. and Anzaldúa, G. (Eds.) (2015) *This bridge called my back: Writings by radical women of color*. Suny Press.

Muñoz, J. E. (1999). *Disidentifications: Queers of color and the performance of politics*. University of Minnesota Press.

Nash, J. C. (2008Re-Thinking Intersectionality. *Feminist Review*, 89, pp. 1–15. https://doi.org/10.1057/fr.2008.4.

Nash, J. C. (2018) *Black feminism reimagined*. Duke University Press.

Powell, D. R. (2018) Race, African Americans, and psychoanalysis: Collective silence in the therapeutic situation. *Journal of the American Psychoanalytic Association*, 66 (6), pp. 1021–1049.

Setzler, M. and Yanus, A. B. (2018) Why did women vote for Donald Trump? *PS: Political Science & Politics*, 51(3), pp. 523–527. https://doi.org/10.1017/S1049096518000355.

Tomlinson, B. (2018) *Undermining intersectionality: The perils of powerblind feminism*. Temple University Press.

Trinh, T. M. H. (1989). *Woman, native, other: Writing postcoloniality and feminism* (Vol. 503). Indiana University Press.

Chapter 12

On Approaching Race, Class, and the Unconscious[1]

A Case Study of *Ataque de Nervios*

Christopher Christian

It is fair to say that American psychoanalysis – and particularly ego psychology, the theoretical paradigm in which I was trained – has downplayed, and in some cases completely dismissed, the role of culture in its theories and practice in favor of broad universal claims. One of course could fairly object that this overlooks the important contributions of Erik Erikson – yet, few would disagree that Erikson's work has been sorely neglected and today is hardly referenced in contemporary psychoanalytic works. Nearly twenty-five years ago, Morris Eagle noted that in fact, "Most (italics added) contemporary psychoanalytic theories (as well as psychoanalytic treatment) tend to ignore the role of culture in development and personality functioning" (Eagle, 1997, 337).

In this chapter, I revisit the early history of what has been called "cultural psychoanalysis" in the United States, and discuss how it dwindled, such that by the 1990s, when I began my psychoanalytic training, it appeared to have all but vanished from the psychoanalytic landscape. Candidates entering analytic training during this period faced two pernicious biases that converged into a type of conventional wisdom with a deleterious impact on training: On the one hand there was the implicit belief that any interest by a candidate in cultural issues suggested a less serious interest in psychoanalysis; and on the other, there was the belief that psychoanalysis was simply irrelevant to the suffering of minoritized populations. I will discuss the treatment of a patient presenting with a culture bound syndrome known as *ataque de nervios* to challenge both of these general preconceptions. I conclude the chapter by arguing for a new paradigm of cultural theorizing.

The Vanishing of Cultural Psychoanalysis

The indifferent and sometimes dismissive attitude toward culture that I encountered when I entered psychoanalytic training in the 1990s did not always prevail. In fact there was a period marked by an intense interest in cultural anthropology for its capacity to expand psychoanalysis. Roger Frie writes: "The early history of the field is replete with attempts to demonstrate

DOI: 10.4324/9781003394327-13

the mutual benefit of combining psychoanalytic and cultural perspectives on the human condition, work that became known collectively as 'psycho-analytic anthropology'." (Frie, 2014, 372). The work of the early anthro-pologically minded psychoanalytic thinkers such as Malinowski, Roheim, and Kardiner in the 1930s, 1940s, and 1950s marked a robust interest in a psy-choanalytic approach to the relationship between culture and personality.

Upon reviewing this period, however, we see that for the most part anthropology rejected Freudian principles as a research frame for studying and understanding culture. A critical point of contention was the emphasis placed by Geza Roheim (1950), for example, on the universality of the Oedipus complex – something that was strongly rejected by most anthropologists.

It was Abram Kardiner's neo-Freudian approach that came closest to achieving a psycho-cultural integration. Kardiner was an analysand of Freud and had also been a student of Franz Boas, the founder of American Anthropology. He worked closely with influential anthropologists, teaching an interdisciplinary seminar, first at the New York Psychoanalytic Institute and later at Columbia University.

Nellie Thompson, the Curator of Brill Library at the at New York Psy-choanalytic, shared a syllabus of Kardiner's course. The Seminar was titled, Seminar on the Comparative Study of Cultures, and in addition to Kardiner, featured Ralph Linton, from Columbia, and B. W. Aginsky, from NYU. Notice that the fee for the course was $14, which adjusted for inflation today would be $300.16.

Kardiner's work was more broadly accepted by anthropologists as com-pared to Geza Roheim's. Mainly because, Kardiner rejected libido theory; dropped the emphasis on the universality of the Oedipus complex; and confined his focus to early childhood experiences – such as toilet training, nursing, and weaning – all of which, he argued, contributed to the human acculturation process. Kardiner (1945) developed the notion of a basic per-sonality type. His theorizing rested on the following postulates: (1) early experiences exert an effect on personality; (2) there are similarities in child-rearing practices by culture; (3) members of any given society will have early childrearing experiences in common; and as a result they will have many elements of personality in common. The basic personality type, then, is a personality configuration which is shared by the bulk of the society's mem-bers as a result of the early experiences which these members have in common.

The main criticism of this interdisciplinary enterprise was the tendency for far sweeping generalizations drawing on few specific items of culture. Marvin Harris (2001), in his book, *The Rise of Anthropological Theory: A History of Theories of Culture*, examines this period of cross-disciplinary exchange between anthropologists and psychoanalysts and concludes quite dis-paragingly that the meeting of the two disciplines tended to "reinforce the inherent tendencies toward uncontrolled, speculative, and histrionic general-izations which each in its own sphere had cultivated as part of its professional license" (Harris, 2001, 448).

From the point of view of psychoanalysis one may ask whether any interest in cultural anthropology by the majority of analysts during this period was mainly for the potential that cultural anthropology had to validate psycho-analytic tenets. It seems that when ideas from cultural anthropology (and other fields, for that matter, including research), had the potential to chal-lenge, and lead to revisions of, psychoanalytic principles, they met up against intense resistance.

William Manson (1988), in his study of Abram Kardiner and Neo-Freu-dian Anthropology, writes that for many psychoanalysts, regardless of orien-tation, the period of "excursions into interdisciplinary theorizing" increasingly posed a threat to "an analytic community that was anxious to protect the autonomy of psychoanalysis as a scientific discipline" (Manson, 1988, 112). Kardiner's seminar on Dynamic Sociology at the New York Psy-choanalytic Institute got a lukewarm reception from most orthodox psycho-analysts, and harsh rejections from a few prominent ones. "I have had to work completely alone" Kardiner would remark, "without the benefit of dis-cussion with my fellow psychiatrists" (Kardiner et al., 1945: xix, quoted in Manson, 1988, 61). Eventually, Kardiner's seminar would be moved from the New York Institute to Columbia University's Department of Anthropology. By the end, Kardiner would sound a tone of defeat regarding the future of any collaboration between psychoanalysis and cultural anthropology.

> From my own experience – and I have lived with both disciplines – I can tell you quite confidently that collaboration is impossible. The trained social scientist will not learn a new technique and the trained psycho-analyst regards the social sciences out of his sphere of interest.
>
> (Kardiner, 1961, in Manson, 1988, 26)

Soon, the likes of Sullivan, Fromm, and Karen Horney, were labeled the "cul-turalists" – a term considered a put down. As Blechner (2011) observed "Culture was thought to be superficial, the concern of sociologists and anthropologists, but not the concern of real depth psychoanalysts." And Lionells (2000) notes, "The idea that identity is forged out of variegated social roles and cultural expecta-tions has long been familiar to sociologists and other academics. But analysts thought of these as superficial behavioral enactments, unrelated to the stuff of psychoanalytic interest" (Lionells, 2000, 404). The project of psychoanalytic theorizing about culture would come to an abrupt halt. In 1941 Karen Horney would be demoted from 'training analyst" to "lecturer" at the New York Psychoanalytic Institute by a majority of those voting (Makari, 2008). And, ultimately, the culturalist and their views were exiled from mainstream ego psychology.

Psychoanalysis, or course, has an infelicitous history of expelling critics from its circle and isolating psychoanalysis from other disciplines. Hoffman (2010) wrote that in the United States many psychoanalysts chose to not participate in the American Psychopathological Association because they wished to protect themselves from having to deal with criticisms of psychoanalytic ideas, particularly the concept of infantile sexuality. With the encouragement of Freud, the American Psychoanalytic Association was created in 1911. Adolf Meyer – one of the most influential figures in psychiatry in the first half of the twentieth century – argued that a pressing determinant of the creation of the American Psychoanalytic Association was that leading analysts needed a friendly milieu where, as Nathan Hale put it, "fundamentals need not always be questioned" and where they would not "face continual ridicule and skepticism" (Hale, 1995, 318).

It goes beyond the scope of this chapter to delve into the history of the relationship between the American Psychoanalytic Association, cultural anthropology, and the culturalist. Instead, I will be making some modest claims about how my own analytic training at an institute that by the time I arrived no longer seemed particularly interested in culture, allowed me to conceptualize a so-called culture bound syndrome. Even before I started training at New York Psychoanalytic, and while in a PhD program in clinical psychology in the 1980s, it became clear to me that my growing interest in psychoanalysis and any interest I had in working clinically with Hispanic patients would have to evolve along very separate tracks. Issues of culture, class, ethnicity, and race belonged to the social realm as opposed to the realm of the intrapsychic, which was the "proper" domain of psychoanalysis; and they required interventions that were prescriptive, entailing concrete interventions, and directed at the level of altering the person's environment. Race and ethnicity had become an indication for treatment modality.

During this period, there was very little discussion in the analytic literature about clinical work with Hispanics. It was in this intellectual vacuum, that I came across a paper titled, "The Suitability of Insight-Oriented Therapy for the Hispanic Poor", published in 1990 by Rafael Javier. At that time the words Hispanic and psychoanalysis together in a title were a rarity – and it seemed to me almost subversive. A search on PEP-Web shows that when Javier published his paper, thirty years ago, there were only two other psychoanalytic papers featuring the term Hispanic in the title. Javier challenged the notion, espoused for instance by Sue and Sue (1977) – considered authorities in the field of multicultural psychology – who argued that in clinical work with the Hispanic poor, "reflection of feelings, concern with insight, and attempts to discover underlying intrapsychic problems are inappropriate" (Sue and Sue, 1977, 474).

To give the reader a sense of how class and issues of culture were written about from within psychoanalysis when Javier published his piece, here is an illustrative quote by Judd Marmor. Judd Marmor by all accounts was a progressive and forward-thinking psychoanalyst. He was very much interested in cultural issues and participated in Kardiner's seminar on Dynamic Sociology at the New York Psychoanalytic Institute. He was instrumental in debunking notions that pathologized homosexuality, which is all to say that Marmor's views did not represent overly conservative ideas. Nevertheless, Marmor writes:

> As a rule, blue collar people and working-class people are not as attuned to psychological thinking and uncovering techniques as are the middle class, upper middle-class, and upper-class people. That is to say, the cultural background of the patient sometimes has a bearing indirectly on his or her readiness to work with one technique or another.
>
> (Marmor, 1980, 243)

Here Marmor provides us a fitting illustration of Lacan's statement that in treatment, "There is only one resistance, the resistance of the analyst" (Lacan, 1988, Seminar II, 228).

It is more accurate to say that "the cultural background of the patient has a bearing on the analyst's readiness to work with one technique or another."

Marmor continues:

> in general, clinical experience shows that individuals who are less advantaged culturally are more apt to seek immediate relief by the modification of the stress situation wherever that is possible, then they are to involve themselves in psychodynamic uncovering techniques.
>
> (Marmor, 1980, 243)

From this passage, it is worth noting how Marmor conflates socioeconomic status with culture. As Patricia Gherovici points out in the documentary "Psychoanalysis in the Barrio", in the United States, the term Hispanic has come to mean one thing – poor (Christian, et al., 2016). Marmor's bias is borne out in private practices. In 1999, Richard C. Friedman, Wilma Bucci and I published a paper (Friedman, et al., 1999) where we surveyed the private practice of fifty-seven senior psychiatrist-psychoanalysts who were members of the American Academy of Psychoanalysis. We found that although severely disturbed patients were seen in these private practices – not just the worried-well, few minority patients and certainly few poor patients were being treated privately by these senior practitioners. The average household income for the patients in this sample was $200,000 a year.

In the documentary, "Psychoanalysis in the Barrio", there is poignant scene, where Ernesto Mujica addresses the same issue when he describes a Latino patient, who fears asking if he can use the couch. The patient's timidity in addressing the couch speaks to how even patients are aware of the biases that we thought were only debated in academic discussions about

"The Suitability of Insight-Oriented Therapy for the Hispanic Poor" – to quote the title of Javier's paper. Today, Psychoanalysis is in the midst of a needed reckoning with regard to questions of race/racialization as evidenced, for instance, by the creation of the "Holmes Commission on Racial Equality in American Psychoanalysis" created by the American Psychoanalytic Association (2021) with the stated aim to " identify and find remedies for structural racism that exist within psychoanalysis". It seems to me that the current interest in race and racialization sounds different from the interests in cultural anthropology that I described earlier. Today's interest seems focused on making explicit the structural and systemic racial biases that exists in our institutions and exposing hidden policies of exclusion in our training institutes. Understanding why, as Michael Moskowitz points out, "psychoanalysts of color make up .007% of the profession, far less than in the field of nuclear science" (Winograd, 2014). This focus has less to do with challenging the biases baked into our theories of normal and pathological functioning with information gleaned from other disciplines.

In the clinical material I will be discussing below, I wish to show how clinical practice can go awry because of presuppositions – such as those espoused in the work of Sue and Sue (1977) and others – on how to approach clinical work with a Latinx patient. By way of illustrating the application of psychoanalytic principles to work with latinx populations, I will focus my presentation on a syndrome known as *ataque de nervios* – once labeled with explicit prejudice as the Puerto Rican Syndrome.

Ataque de Nervios and its Relevance to Psychoanalysis

The term *ataques* made its first appearance in the 4th edition of the Diagnostic and statistical manual of mental disorders (DSM-IV, 1994), where it was listed in the appendix – separate from what we presume are not culture-bound syndromes. This "textual out posting" as Ann Lugones (2003) has called it, aptly illustrates a "minoritizing move". Minoritizing discourses, Lugones (2003) argues, attribute to some "specific cultural group, community, or context" (to use the language of DSM-5 (American Psychiatric Association, 2022)) a disorder supposedly uniquely associated with that group, such that symptoms, meaning, and "causes" get affixed to it. This is the case with the Puerto Rican syndrome. In the DSM, the description of *ataques* is accompanied by a list of common features, that include shouting; trembling; loss of muscular control that often leads to falling; heat in the chest rising to the head; dissociative experiences; and a general sense of being out of control often observed in a woman of Hispanic origin.

What becomes obvious to any psychoanalyst encountering an *ataque de nervios* is that the symptoms are indistinguishable from the hysterical attacks that Freud described at the turn of the 20th century. The irony is that the same illness that marked the birth of psychoanalysis a century earlier in

Vienna, is now deemed unamenable to a psychoanalytic approach by analysts in the United States. Yet, we see that Freud had much to say about *ataque de nervios* for they share similarities with conversion disorders and hysteria.

In his paper "The Neuropsychoses of Defence" Freud (1894) explains how repressed contents become manifested in the body, transformed into what he called, "something somatic". Fifteen years later, Freud wrote a paper titled "Some General Remarks on Hysterical Attacks", where he describes the pantomimes of a hysterical attacks as representing an unconscious fantasy. We see that Freud moved away from an explanation of somatic symptoms as physical action meant to discharge a quota of affect, to a psychological explanation whereby, as Laplanche and Pontalis summarize it, "what specifies a conversion symptom (or hysteria) is their symbolic meaning" (Laplanche and Pontalis, 1973, 90).

In time, different psychoanalytic theories of how the mind works would evolve and, in one such evolution, the conception of the mind as a discharge apparatus would be replaced by the conception of mental activity as a set of cognitive functions designed to address intrapsychic conflict by way of compromise formations (Brenner, 1973, 1982, 1994). This evolution is marked by a shift from Freud's conceptualization of emotions as discharge phenomenon to an understanding of the role that emotions play as signals for the purpose of activating defense in the presence of intrapsychic conflict.

With the concept of signal anxiety, we see how a biologically driven impulse is given shape and articulated as a wish by the ego for the ego to determine its fate. That is, to determine how much of the wish needs to be defended against, how much can be gratified, and at what cost. How the biological impulse is articulated, and its fate is determined by a person's cultural context. The outcome of these "ego deliberations" is a compromise formation. That is, an act, a thought, or a symptom, for example, that gratifies as much of the drive derivative (a wish) as possible, without incurring too much unpleasure. From a psychoanalytic point of view, *ataques* can readily be understood, like any other symptom or behavior, as a manifestation of conflict and compromise formation. Specifically, as we will see, *ataques* allow for the expression of aggressive, sexual, and other impulses among women, considering social (morays) in Latino culture that denounce the public expression of such affects. That is to say that what distinguishes *ataques* from hysterical attacks is that the compromise represented in the *ataque* is likely to reflect cultural norms.

Notwithstanding the inclusion of *ataque de nervios* as a culture-bound syndrome in the DSM, it is worth noting that *ataques* are hardly considered a form of psychopathology. One can understand how desire, anxiety, and defense present themselves in an *ataque*, without needing to render *ataques* as a manifestation of psychopathology. This is not a minor issue given a history in psychoanalysis of pathologizing cultural differences. Several authors have aptly shown how cultural differences in relatedness, and the constitution of selfhood, tend to be rendered as immature or unhealthy, while heralding autonomous individuality and the "genital character" as hallmarks of maturity and psychological health. Long before *ataques* ever dreamt of making its way into the pages of psychiatric journals, it was considered a mundane and common idiom of distress among Puerto Ricans. It is safe to say that most homes in Puerto Rico had as a staple Agua Florida (Florida Water), a common remedy for *ataque de nervios*. This body splash made up of a citrus base with spices including clove and lavender water, was introduced over 200 years ago by Robert Murray in New York – in 1808 to be exact (Murray and Lanman, n.d.). Aqua Florida was to *ataques* what aspirin, invented 8 decades later, would be to stress and headaches. In time, Agua Florida gained the status of a magical potion, used in all kinds of spiritual rituals. It was available everywhere. It could be found in the corner bodega or at the local Walgreens (incidentally, in some places, not in the perfume section, but nestled between the Vicks and the Panadol). *Ataques*, thus, had a prescribed home remedy to which agua florida was essential. In my neighborhood, growing up in Puerto Rico, it was not uncommon for an aunt or someone else's relative to have an *ataque*, in which case you knew to first reach for the agua florida. That was the "right" response. The "wrong" response often comes by way of a medical diagnosis. Several decades after the Puerto Rican Syndrome was introduced to American psychiatry, and under the DSM, *ataques* have become a sterile, medicalized terminology, outlining risk factors, and recommendations for treatment plans. The patient, now enlightened by the various expert medical opinions of what ails her, soon begins talking about what she had before simply referred to as *ataques*, now as panic attacks, or nerves, or simply attacks – an ambiguous referent to both an *ataque de nervios*/and a panic attack. Soon, relaxation training, and cognitive restructuring replace the non- evidenced based practice of *sobos con alcolado* (massages with alcohol), prayer, and community support. Lexapro and Xanax replace the Agua Florida and the Vicks in the medicine cabinet; and all of these well-intended interventions culminate in the unintended effect of increased states of self-alienation and misrecognition.

On March 26, 1970 the *New York Times* reported that the rate of first-time admissions for Puerto Ricans with a diagnosis of schizophrenia to the state's mental hospitals was nearly triple that of the general population. In that article, the Rev, Dr. Joseph P. Fitzpatrick, a Fordham University professor of sociology and a long-time student of Puerto Rican affairs; and Dr. Robert E. Gould, chief of psychiatric adolescent services at Bellevue, contended that the "abnormally high" rate of hospitalization of Puerto Ricans for mental disorders in New York State may be the result of "intercultural misunderstanding" (*New York Times*, 1970).

It is important to recognize the performance aspect on an *ataque*. An *ataque* triggers a call-response pattern between a Puerto Rican woman and her community. An important question is what happens to an *ataque* when it is enacted in a foreign land, apart from a community who can understand the language of an *ataque*. For an *ataque* to work adequately it must be performed correctly. *Ataques* are a performance meant to be witnessed. A feature that distinguishes *ataque de nervios* from panic attacks, is that *ataques* have rarely been found to occur when the person is alone (Angel and Guarnaccia, 1989; Guarnaccia, et al., 1989). And, relatedly, there is no such thing as uncued *ataque de nervios*. A precipitant is always present.

Ataques are akin to what cultural anthropologist Victor Turner (2017) described as social dramas, with implied social roles for those involved, and breaches attendant to violation of those roles or norms. *Ataques* are also akin to what linguist John Austin (1975) has described as a performative speech act. Some essential features of a performative speech act, according to Austin include (1) the existence of an accepted conventional procedure; (2) the procedure must be invoked by the appropriate persons and under the right circumstances, and (3) the procedure must be executed by all participants both correctly and completely. "If we sin against any of these rules", Austin warns, "the performative utterance will... not have fully met the criterion for a successful accomplishment, or performance, of an act" (Austin, 1975, 15). Austin's linguistic framework readily applies to an understanding of *ataques*: it is a procedure, invoked by an appropriate person, that needs to be executed correctly or otherwise we have an unhappy ending.

Maria and her *ataques*

In her first session with her therapist, the patient, whom I will refer to as Maria, a young Puerto Rican mother of two children, upon being asked to explain what brings her to treatment, began shaking, fell to the ground, writhing and kicking, in the throes of what appeared to be a seizure. This jarring experience marked the beginning of a two-year treatment. The seizure-like symptoms were recognized as an *ataque de nervios* by the trainee and her supervisor, both Hispanic. In her treatment, Maria would often refer to her symptoms as "my attacks" or my condition, denoting a degree of warmth and even affection for her diagnosis. This attachment to a diagnosis brings to mind what Glover once described as the "inexact interpretation". Glover writes:

> the patient seizes upon the inexact interpretation and converts it into a displacement-substitute. This substitute is not by any means so glaringly inappropriate as the one he has chosen himself during symptom formation and yet sufficiently remote from the real source of anxiety.
>
> (Glover, 1931)

The inexact interpretation, Glover believed, would bring about symptom relief "depending on an optimum degree of psychic remoteness from the true source of anxiety" (Glover, 1931, 400). Not too far off the mark but not spot on either. The diagnosis, like the inexact interpretation, is employed defensively. In the guise of explaining something, it moves the subject away from the wishes, impulses, and conflicts that are at the heart of the subject's anxiety.

The word "attacks" that Maria employed to describe her condition was a hybrid term, straddling two languages meant to capture both panic attacks and *ataque de nervios*. It denoted an in-between state, much like the neo-colonial political status of Puerto Rico, where her family was from. Maria considered herself a hybrid: a Newyorican. She said that she spoke Spanglish – a language denoting a split subject, neither here nor there, yet attempting to bridge disparate and often conflicting aspects of her experience.

When she began therapy, Maria was in an intermittent relationship with the father of her two children, an abusive man. We learned that she experienced her *ataques* only while accompanied by him or other family members. The *ataques* were designed to enlist the other, and the presence of an other was guaranteed by one of her presenting symptoms: an apprehension Maria had of being out alone for fear that she would have an *ataque* without family to assist her. In time, Maria described a family history marked by verbal abuse, poverty, and a personal experience of feeling disempowered in a family of boys. She recalled episodes of being discriminated against, in and outside the home, and witnessing at home marked preferential treatment of her brothers, specially by her father. Maria reported that her father suffered from a "nervous condition" too. He was even psychiatrically hospitalized at Bellevue. She remembers visiting him. She said that, as a young girl, on her way to visit him, she had the frightening image of finding him in a "strait jacket". Now, as an adult, she believes that this image imparted an important message for her: if your nerves are out of control, you can be locked up in a *manicomio* (insane asylum). These fears of being locked up would be manifested in the transference and expressed through several dreams. Her own *ataques* were mimetic representations of scenes (first described by Freud in 1913) in identification with her father.

The precipitant for Maria seeking therapy was a so-called panic attack that ended in a visit to the emergency room. At the time, the attending psychiatrist prescribed antidepressants. However, Maria refused to fill the prescription. The mention of her choice to not take the medication was a point that remarkably could have been handled very differently. Instead, of examining the meaning of medications for Maria, it could have been met simply with psychoeducation about the value of medication-compliance. In exploring the implications that medication had for her, the therapist learned that Maria worried that the pills would no doubt reduce her anxiety – but this in turn would placate a pervasive sense of guilt. And guilt, she explained, served a critical function for her – mainly, guilt helped her counteract an impulse to

have an extramarital relationship. So, we see how one of her presenting com-
plaints – a fear of being out alone – was overdetermined. Her suffering was
the constraint necessary to keep her impulses in check; and the medication
that in her mind would simply wipe away her suffering, was akin to a
recommendation that she need not care so much about constraining these
thoughts.

Over the course of therapy, symptoms were now experienced as telling her
something rather than being aspects of herself that needed to be corrected,
suppressed, or wiped away.

With increasing curiosity about herself, an interest in how she thought, and
a growing trust in her therapist, Maria began examining a longstanding
theme in her sexual fantasies that involved being sexually overpowered. What
became clear over the course of her treatment was that the *ataques* occurred
in the context of a sadomasochistic dream life, marked by fantasies of
aggressive and sexual domination and subjugation. These fantasies replicated
conditions of subjugation and domination in her immediate family but,
moreover, they duplicated conditions manifested in the larger social order,
marked by racial and economic discrimination, and class differences, that
spanned many generations in her family. In time, treatment would elucidate
the complex multiple functions of an *ataque* for Maria that allowed her to
express and simultaneously disavow intense sexual and aggressive impulses
and other thoughts and feelings in the context of an oppressive patriarchal
system. During one episode, in a semi dissociated state, she attacked her
husband. She left scratch marks on his face. In instances such as this, we saw
a rage that was overdetermined. Maria deployed a symptomatic act 500 years
in the making.

As her treatment deepened, there was a growing recognition of how her
own conflicted aggressive and sexual impulses, represented in her fantasies,
were being expressed in her *ataques*. There was an increased sense of agency
in recognizing and expressing her inner life. And with all of this, not surprising to any analyst, we saw a parallel decrease in the occurrence of her *ataques*, such that by the end of her treatment, the *ataques* had dissipated
entirely. In this case, Maria's *ataques* were how she circumvented social conventions that privileged traditional gender roles of obedience, self-sacrifice,
and suffering. Clinicians can unwittingly exploit these same traditional gender
roles in the service of treatment compliance.

Now, we may ask, what made this treatment of an exotic symptom like
ataque de nervios different from the typical psychoanalytically informed
treatment with which we are all familiar? The answer – perhaps a dis-
appointing one – is that the treatment was not so different. And that is precisely my point. In fact, what makes the treatment remarkable is what did not
happen but typically does with someone like her in this setting. The therapist
refrained from adopting an overly active, authoritative approach and
instead privileged the exploration of unconscious content underlying her

symptoms. Yet, we know that reliance on the therapist's authority is not uncommon in approaching work with cultural minorities, who are often deemed, as Judd Marmor puts it: "seeking immediate relief", needing advice, guidance, and emotional re-education. Undoubtedly cultural background determines expectations that patients bring to treatment. This is true of every patient. Every patient has expectations and assumptions when they seek help. It is not the assumptions and expectations of the patient that are problematic, as much as that of the analyst when seeing patients that are not like them. The sensitive analyst will, of course, adjust their approach to understanding the patient, in accord with what facilitates the process with this person. Yet too often when considering work with Hispanic patients we establish a precept regarding the treatment of choice. It needs to be short-term, symptom-focused, or geared toward behavioral change. A focus, for example, on training Maria how to relax, and on challenging the realistic nature of her conscious thoughts, inadvertently, would have reinforced the dynamics of domination that marked the patient's history, now emblemized in the expert judgment of the clinician. A myopic focus on suppressing her symptoms may have even confirmed to Maria that her thoughts and impulses were dangerous and required mobilizing everything at our disposal to quash them, be it medication, strait jackets – as well as other tools made available by managed care, including limiting the number of sessions available to her, to manage how much she could explore such threatening ideas.

Looking Back and Looking Forward

The inattention to considerations of cultural factors in psychoanalysis perhaps can be traced to Freud's own preoccupation that psychoanalysis should not be perceived as what in a letter to Arbraham he called, a "Jewish national affair". It was important for Freud that psychoanalysis have universal appeal, and not be bound by culture. This was the mantle that cultural anthropologist Geza Róheim took on in defending the universality of the Oedipus Complex and concluding that psychoanalysis is not-culture bound. "There can be many types of personality but only one Unconscious" (Róheim, 1950, 491).

Some authors have shown that Freud's wide-ranging cultural interests, notwithstanding, his engagement with intellectual and artistic traditions outside of Western culture was for the utilitarian purpose of propagating psychoanalysis.

Kakar (1995) writes:

> the psychoanalytic encounter with other cultures could not be one of mutual learning and a collaborative inquiry into human existence. The paramount concern of psychoanalysis seems to have been in protecting and gathering evidence in support of its key concepts rather than in

entertaining the possibility that other cultures, with their different world-views, family structures and relationships, could contribute to its models and concepts.

(Kakar, 1995, 441)

Plotkin, in our book "Psychoanalysis in the Barrios" (Plotkin, 2018) makes a similar observation. Plotkin is struck by the fact that when Freud immigrated to London and was forced to pare down his extensive library "33 of the books he took to London were authored by Latin American doctors or intellectuals" (Plotkin, 2018, 15). Yet, Plotkin observes, Freud's interest in Latin American intellectuals was for the most part focused on their role in disseminating psychoanalysis as a system of ideas and beliefs in their part of the world but lacked any serious theoretical engagement. In the analysis of the correspondence Freud kept with some Latin American doctors and intellectuals, Plotkin found that Freud had difficulties in coming to terms with what he perceived as the "exotic world." Plotkin writes: "Freud entered into the depth of the European's unconscious, but it seems that he was not able to totally accept the cultural 'other'" (Plotkin, 2018, 21).

And then there is the unfinished work in Hartmann's theorizing. All fields – in theorizing new constructs – hold some variables constant for the sake of defining other variables. There are assumptions about a fixed ground when defining the foreground. Hartman in seeking to develop a general psychology assumed an average expectable environment and held it as the ground against which he defined the development of primary ego functions. Again and again, Hartman states that the features of normal ego development and functioning that he is delineating assume as background an average expectable environment. We understand that the assumption of an Average Expectable Environment was a heuristic necessary for making some broad claims about how the mind works. In this regard, Hartman put consideration of cultural variations on hold with the assumption of an average expectable environment but clearly the implication was that ego functions might develop differently in non-average expectable environments.

To give you but one example, I will draw on a discussion from Morris Eagle's (2021) book *Toward a Unified Psychoanalytic Theory: Foundation in a Revised and Expanded Ego Psychology*, where he examines the concept of ego capacities for delaying gratification – an executive ego function that develops autonomously in an average expectable environment. Many studies using Walter Mischell's marshmallow paradigm with children (Mischel and Ebbesen, 1970; Mischel, Ebbesen, and Raskoff Zeiss, 1972) have shown that selecting immediate gratification for a smaller reward (fewer marshmallows) rather than delaying gratification to obtain a larger reward (more marshmallows) is predictive of a host of current and future maladaptive behaviors. Yet as Eagle points out in his review, a number of studies argue that:

in an environment of relative scarcity (and, one might add, in an unpredictable environment), choice of immediate gain and gratification as well as a general valuing of the present over the future may be quite adaptive rather than necessarily indicate impairment in ego functioning. On this view, in certain contexts, choice of immediate over delayed gratification may not reflect, or may not only reflect, inadequacy of inhibitory control, but rather a strategy that is adaptive to a particular environment – a sort of take your gains and gratifications now or they will be gone.

(Eagle, 2021, 68)

The problem that I wish to draw attention to is one that arises when we make universal claims made about mental development and functioning that are based on the assumption of an average expectable environment and applied as benchmarks of normal development to populations who have as background very different environments. Hartmann is not explicit about what constitutes an average expectable environment or the effects of non-average expectable environments on the development of ego functions. Picking up on Hartmann's unfinished work and we might rightly ask: How would we define primary ego functions taking into account a background of poverty.

I believe we can revisit the early interdisciplinary study of culture – an effort that goes beyond virtue-signaling, or the quest for self-validation of any field. As Wallerstein (2011) and others have reminded us, it was Freud's hope that training in psychoanalysis include "elements from the mental sciences, from psychology, the history of civilization and sociology, as well as from anatomy, biology, and the study of evolution" (Wallerstein, 2011, 252). The project for a cross-disciplinary psychoanalysis seems to have ended abruptly and we may ask what has changed? I believe a few important things have changed and give us hope for a revitalized ego psychology: We may ask what makes the revisiting of the abandoned project of psychoanalytic anthropology more propitious? Perhaps a few things: First, I believe that psychoanalysis has grown more interdisciplinary and now seamlessly and readily draws on neuroscience, studies of child development, attachment research, and other related disciplines.

Eagle's (2021) most recent work gives us a fitting model for the interdisciplinary exchange that can revive and expand ego psychology. In this book, Eagle evaluates basic tenets of ego psychology against not only competing clinical theories but also, and perhaps most importantly, findings from related disciplines.

Another auspicious and welcomed development is the fact that there is less intra-discipline wrangling. Analysts are more comfortable in drawing on ideas from different psychoanalytic theories in their daily clinical work. An unfortunate outcome of the early theoretical wars is that culture became the province of relational or interpersonal theories. And like code words, the mention of culture would betray some theoretical alliance. We do well to see culture as part of a revised and expanded ego psychology. And, finally, there is a growing discomfort among analysts when recognizing the role of psychoanalysis in perpetuating structural inequities, whether wittingly or not. Freud himself worried about psychoanalysis falling into the clutch of a dangerous elitism as Elizabeth Dantos (2005) phrases it.

Today, many psychoanalysts are not comfortable with a view of the field as generating a type of treatment reserved for the well-to do. Senior analysts, as well as those new to the field, are revisiting the history of Freud's free clinics, and share Freud's aspiration, that there will come a time, as he put it, when "society will awake and remind it that the poor man should have just as much right assistance for his mind as he now has to the life-saving help offered by surgery" (Freud, 1919, 167–168). I would like to think that we are closer to such a time.

Summary

In this chapter, I have reviewed the shifting attention to culture in psychoanalysis and I have attempted to capture how the landscape of psychoanalytic training had changed by the 1990s. The case of *ataques de nervios* helped illustrate misconceptions within and about psychoanalysis. I have concluded the chapter with an appeal for interdisciplinary training through which psychoanalysis and other fields, including linguistics, anthropology, neuroscience, and cognitive science can inform one another and develop a culturally relevant psychoanalysis.

Note

1 Acknowledgement: some passages from this chapter include modified sections from Christian (2018).

References

Angel, R. and Guarnaccia, P. J. (1989) Mind, body, and culture: Somatization among Hispanics. *Social Science & Medicine*, 28(12), pp. 1229–1238.

American Psychiatric Association (1994) *Diagnostic and statistical manual of mental disorders: DSM-IV.* American Psychiatric Association.

American Psychiatric Association (2022) Diagnostic and statistical manual of mental disorders (5th ed., text rev.). https://doi.org/10.1176/appi.books.9780890425787.

American Psychoanalytic Association (2021) Holmes Commission on Racial Equality in the American Psychoanalytic Association. https://apsa.org/commission-on-racial-equality.

Austin, J. L. (1975) *How to Do Things with Words.* Clarendon Press.

Blechner, M. (2011) Interpersonal Psychoanalysis and Sexuality. *Contemporary Psychoanalysis*, 47(4), pp. 571–577.

Brenner, C. (1973) *An elementary textbook of psychoanalysis.* New York: International Universities Press.

Brenner, C. (1982) *The Mind in Conflict.* International Universities Press.

Brenner, C. (1994) The mind as conflict and compromise formation. *Journal of Clinical Psychoanalysis*, 3(4), 473–488.

Christian, C. (2018) The Analyst as Interpreter: Ataque de Nervios, Puerto Rican Syndrome, and the Inexact Interpretation. In Gherovici, P. and Christian, C. (Eds.), *Psychoanalysis in the Barrios: Race, Class, and the Unconscious.* Routledge.

Christian, C., Reichbart, R., Moskowitz, M., Morillo, R. and Winograd, B. (2016) Psychoanalysis in El Barrio. PEP Video Grants 1:10.

Dantos, E. (2005) *Freud's Free Clinics: Psychoanalysis and Social Justice, 1918–1938.* Columbia University Press.

Eagle, M. (1997) Contributions of Erik Erikson. *Psychoanalytic Review*, 84, pp. 337–347.

Eagle, M. (2021) *Toward a Unified Psychoanalytic Theory: Foundation in a Revised and Expanded Ego Psychology.* Taylor and Francis.

Freud, S. (1894) The Neuro-Psychoses of Defence. *The Standard Edition of the Complete Psychological Works of Sigmund Freud*, vol. 3, pp.41–61.

Freud, S. (1909) Some General Remarks on Hysterical Attacks. *The Standard Edition of the Complete Psychological Works of Sigmund Freud*, vol. 9, pp. 227–234.

Freud, S. (1913) The Claims of Psycho-Analysis to Scientific Interest. *The Standard Edition of the Complete Psychological Works of Sigmund Freud*, vol. 13, pp. 163–190. Hogarth Press.

Freud, S. (1919) Lines of Advance in Psycho-Analytic Therapy. *The Standard Edition of the Complete Psychological Works of Sigmund Freud, Volume XVII (1917–1919): An Infantile Neurosis and Other Works*, pp.157–168. Hogarth Press.

Frie, R. (2014) What Is Cultural Psychoanalysis? Psychoanalytic Anthropology and the Interpersonal Tradition. *Contemporary Psychoanalysis*, 50, pp. 371–394.

Friedman, R. C., Bucci, W., Christian, C., and Garrison, W. B. (1999) Private Psychotherapy Patients of Psychiatrist Psychoanalysts. *American Journal of Psychiatry*, 155(12), pp. 1772–1774.

Glover, E. (1931) The therapeutic effect of inexact interpretation: a contribution to the theory of suggestion. *The International Journal of Psychoanalysis*, 12, pp. 397–411.

Guarnaccia, P.J., DeLaCancela, V., and Carillo, E. (1989) The multiple meanings of *ataques de nervios* in the Latino community. *Medical Anthropology*, 11, pp. 47–62.

Hale, N. G. (1995) *The rise and crisis of psychoanalysis in United States: Freud and the Americans, 1917–1985.* Oxford University Press.

Harris, M. (2001) *The rise of anthropological theory: A history of theories of culture.* AltaMira Press.

Hoffman, L. (2010) One Hundred Years After Sigmund Freud's Lectures in America: Towards An Integration of Psychoanalytic Theories and Techniques Within Psychiatry. *History of Psychiatry*, 21(4), pp. 455–470.

Javier, R. A. (1990). The suitability of insight-oriented therapy for the Hispanic poor. *The American Journal of Psychoanalysis*, 50(4), pp. 305–318. https://doi.org/10.1007/BF01254078.

Kakar, S. (1995) Clinical work and cultural imagination. *The Psychoanalytic Quarterly*, 64(2), pp. 265–281.

Kardiner, A. (1961) Psychoanalysis and Anthropology. In *Science and Psychoanalysis*, vol. 4. Ed. J. Massermand. Grune & Stratton, pp. 21–27 .

Kardiner, A. (1939) *The individual and his society: the psychodynamics of primitive social organization.* Columbia University Press.

Kardiner, A. (1945) *The Psychological Frontiers of Society.* Columbia University Press. https://doi.org/10.7312/kard94036.

Lacan, J. (1988) *The seminar of Jacque Lacan (book 2)* (trans. S. Tomaselli). Norton.

Laplanche, J. and Pontalis, J. B. (1973) The Language of Psycho-Analysis: Translated by Donald Nicholson-Smith. *The Language of Psycho-Analysis*, 94, pp. 1–497.

Lionells, M. (2000) Sullivan's Anticipation of the Postmodern Turn in Psychoanalysis. *Contemporary Psychoanalysis*, 36, pp. 393–410.

Lugones, M. (2003). *Pilgrimages/peregrinajes: Theorizing coalition against multiple oppressions.* Rowman & Littlefield Publishing Group.

Makari, G. (2008) *Revolution In Mind: The Creation Of Psychoanalysis.* HarperCollins.

Manson, W. (1988) *The Psychodynamics of culture: Abram Kardiner and Neo-Freudian Anthropology.* Greenwood Press.

Marmor, J. (1980) Crisis intervention and short-term psychodynamic psychotherapy. In H. Davanloo (Ed.). *Short term Dynamic Psychotherapy.* Jason Aronson.

Mischel, W. and Ebbesen, E. B. (1970) Attention in delay of gratification. *Journal of Personality and Social Psychology*, 16(2), p. 329.

Mischel, W., Ebbesen, E. B., and Raskoff Zeiss, A. (1972) Cognitive and attentional mechanisms in delay of gratification. *Journal of personality and social psychology*, 21(2), p. 204.

Murray and Lanman (n.d.) Florida Water. https://floridawater.com.

New York Times (2010, March 26) Hospitalization Rate of Puerto Ricans for Mental Disorders Said to Be High. https://www.nytimes.com/1970/03/26/archives/hospitaliza tion-rate-of-puerto-ricans-for-mental-disorders-said-to.html?smid=em-share.

Pellegrini, A. (2021, September 17–19) *The Return of the Return of the Repressed.* [Talk]. Psychology and the Other. Virtual Conference.

Plotkin, M. (2018) Freud and the Latin Americans: A forgotten relationship. In P. Gherovici and C. Christian (Eds.) *Psychoanalysis in the Barrios: Race, Class, and the Unconscious.* Routledge.

Roberts, E. (1937) *Candle in the Sun.* The Bobbs-Merrill Company.

Róheim, G. (1950) *Psychoanalysis and anthropology; culture, personality and the unconscious.* International Universities Press.

Sue, D. W. and Sue, D. (1977) Barriers to effective cross-cultural counseling. *Journal of Counseling Psychology*, 24, pp. 420–429.

Turner, V. W. (2017) Liminality and communitas. In *Ritual* (pp. 169–187). Routledge.

Wallerstein, R. S. (2011) Psychoanalysis in the University: The Natural Home for Education and Research. *International Journal of Psychoanalysis*, 92, pp. 623–639.

Winograd, B. (2014) Black Psychoanalysts Speak. PEP Video Grants 1:1.

Chapter 13

An Intersectional Feminist Exploration of the Working Lives of Women During COVID-19

Approaching Dignified Work Through a Spirituality of Resistance Framework

Karley M. Gutteres

The Case of Adalia

I met Adalia, a Guatemalan-American single mother of two, in the height of the pandemic. She came in seeking outpatient services due to severe depressive symptoms after being laid off from her job as a preschool teacher. Not only was she worried about the global pandemic and the possibility of infection, but she also had no idea how she would be able to pay next month's rent. Her process navigating the unemployment insurance system was chaotic, unclear, and disorganized and she found herself in an endless loop of phone calls and paperwork, only to be denied on incorrect grounds, and forced to appeal and start the process all over again. At this time, she also took in her younger sister who found out she was pregnant and didn't have the means to support herself. Adalia found herself becoming increasingly worried about her three sons – three young teenagers – who she was starting to recognize were showing signs of increased irritability, anxiety, and depression themselves in the midst of online schooling, and increased disconnection from their peers and regular extra-curriculars. Our work together oscillated between getting Adalia connected to helpful services that could provide some short-term relief, and working to combat the internalization of negative cognitions about herself due to the difficulty of finding work, her feelings of "being a terrible mother" as she watched her kids struggling emotionally, and her worries to make ends meet.

Unfortunately, Adalia's case (which is based on an amalgam of clients that I have worked with) has not been unique during the pandemic recession. Her struggles are emblematic of the experiences of women around the globe who have faced increased burdens of care work as well as the loss of employment that has cost them their financial stability. From a mental health perspective, work plays a central role in life for many. Work can ensure our survival, it can provide a source of personal fulfillment, provide a source of structure, inform our identity, provide us with a source of meaning and purpose, and be a source of social connection (Blustein, 2019). The absence or loss of

DOI: 10.4324/9781003394327-14

work, can therefore be the source of a plethora of psychological, physical, and financial burdens that can drastically impact one's quality of life (Blustein, 2019).

In many ways, the spoke thrown in the wheel of productivity – even momentarily – forced the world to come together, to pause, and to recognize our common humanity and human fragility. However, the COVID-19 pandemic has not simply served to show us our similarities, it has also placed a magnifying glass on inequities in the labor market that existed far before the crisis (Autin et al., 2020). With power and privilege representing major determinants of who has been faced with precarious work, historically marginalized communities have been hit the hardest by this crisis (ILO, 2020).

Both at the outset of the pandemic and longitudinally, it is clear that women, especially racial minority women, have been disproportionately impacted by the devastation in ways that I will explore in this paper. As the world cautiously prepares itself to enter into the process of rebuilding, always with an eye on the possible development of new variants, there are two things that are imperative for consideration. First, it is crucial that the social realities of the most vulnerable are placed at the center of the new way forward. Secondly, during a time when the devastation has proposed major threats to the human dignity of many (or the fundamental agency of human being to apply their gifts to thrive (Lagon and Arend, 2014)), it is of the utmost importance that what has been unveiled during the past year serves as a primary guiding post of envisioning a new approach for the world of work. This is especially important to consider given the possibility that this is not the last global pandemic we may experience (Constable and Kushner, 2021).

Exploring Women and Work via a Spirituality of Resistance Framework

During a time when the understanding of ourselves in relation to the world has become completely disrupted and untethered, an approach that adopts a spirituality – a political spirituality of resistance – may be particularly appropriate. In response to a tragedy of this magnitude, I propose a disposition of resistance that draws from the thought of political theologian Dorothee Soelle. I argue that a spirituality of resistance is an appropriate approach because it can allow one to remain focused on the reality of the suffering other, while at the same time grounding one's work in the principle foundation of human dignity. Dorothee Soelle (1929–2003) offers useful insights to our efforts when approaching devastation and the suffering other because her life and work were deeply influenced by witnessing the atrocities of World War II and growing up in Germany during the years of the Nazi regime (Oliver, 2006, 19).

In her work, *The Silent Cry: Mysticism and Resistance*, Soelle seeks to erase the distinction between the "mystical internal" and the "political external" (Soelle, 2001, 3), the very separation that, according to her, allowed the members of the Nazi party to sleep easy at night, and the very separation that allows each one of us – at some time or another – to create distance between ourselves and the suffering other. Mysticism is, as Soelle writes, "the experience of oneness with God," and as such, "mysticism is the radical substantiation of the dignity of the human being" (Soelle, 2001, 43). In this work, she dialogues the methodology of the process of the mystical journey of resistance today as threefold: (1) "being amazed" of holding a radical openness to wonderment, to awe, and even to horror; (2) of "letting go" of relinquishing false desires promoted by consumerism and egotism, and; (3) of "resisting" or healing through seeking change in the world through compassion and justice (Soelle, 2001, 89). It is this internal process that flows outward that I will demonstrate throughout this paper as a way to approach issues in the field of vocational psychology through a theological lens and with a disposition of resistance.

This chapter will explore the ways that women's vocational – and therefore personal, psychological, physical, and financial – lives have been impacted by the COVID-19 pandemic. It will then explore the underlying interpersonal and systemic barriers that have contributed to this suffering. Finally, I will offer some ways forward for policy, practice, and research informed by what has been revealed by the pandemic, and that resist the negative values and norms that have perpetuated the suffering of the other.

To Be Amazed

The first step along the mystical journey of resistance is to "be amazed." Soelle posits six potential places of mystical amazement, that is, the experience of universal connectedness or oneness; among them are the places of suffering and death – two things we have seen a lot of lately. The process of being amazed, according to Soelle, is the ability to open ourselves to the world, to the option of radical wonderment, to be in awe of beauty, of complexity, and of creation itself. Indeed Soelle posits that the experience of amazement isn't always characterized by bliss. She writes

> Amazement also has its bleak side of terror and hopelessness that renders one mute… Those who seek to leave behind the terrifying, sinister side of wonderment, the side that renders us dumb, take on, through rational superiority, the role of those who own the world.
>
> (Soelle, 2001, 90)

Not only is the experience of amazement one that can be multifaceted, but Soelle argues it is an experience that is necessary for progress and change. She writes

The soul needs amazement, the repeated liberation from customs, view-points, and convictions, which, like layers of fat that make us untouch-able and insensitive, accumulate around us. What appears obvious is that we need to be touched by the spirit of life and that without amazement and enthusiasm, nothing new can begin.

(Soelle, 2001, 90)

Thus, for something new to begin, we must first be amazed by what COVID-19 has revealed about what has been, and what is currently happening for women's vocational lives.

Low Wage and Frontline Jobs

Globally, women earn less, save less, hold less secure jobs, and are more likely to be employed in the informal sector (United Nations, 2020). During the pandemic, these existing realities have only been made more extreme. While regular recessions have historically impacted sectors such as construction and manufacturing which are more male-dominated industries, it became evident early on that the pandemic recession would differ in that it would significantly impact female-dominated sectors such as hospitality and tourism (Alon et al., 2020a).

Women – and particularly women of color – are overrepresented among low-wage workers on the frontline in most developed countries (Bahn et al., 2020; Averette, Argys, and Hoffman, 2018). Yet despite the dominance of women of color in "essential" frontline work, many have lacked job security and being situated in industries hardest hit, many have been furloughed or laid off due to COVID-19 (Bahn et al., 2020; Obinna, 2020). Women who have been able to remain in frontline positions that cannot be done remotely have been placed at greater exposure to the virus that has proven fatal for many.

Indeed some scholars have posited that the pandemic has a predominantly "non-white" female face, arguing that Black women are situated at the nexus of overlapping systems of oppression that facilitate both loss of life and income during the pandemic (Laurencin and McClnton, 2020). Other statistical data revealed that Hispanic women experienced the biggest drop in employment among groups in the labor force at the peak of job losses with a twenty-four percent decrease, while white men – for reference – experienced around a thirteen percent drop in employment (Koeze, 2021).

Not only have women – and namely women of color – been more vulnerable to job insecurity, layoffs/furloughs, as well as exposure to a deadly viral infection, but globally women have less access to social protections and are the majority of single-parent households (United Nations, 2020). Thus, for many women, like Adalia, their households are dependent on a single source of income *and* they provide financial support to more dependents on that singular income (Cohen, 2010). The intensified pressures compounded by already existing environmental stressors quickly impacted women in the beginning of the pandemic in the U.S. resulting in higher and worsening health-related socioeconomic risks, and corresponded with rates of depression and anxiety twice that of pre-pandemic benchmarks (Lindau et al., 2021).

Unpaid Care Work

While women's employment has been disproportionately impacted during the pandemic recession, or what some scholars refer to as the "shecession," many have also experienced increased pressure to perform the undervalued and invisible act of unpaid care work. Scholars have historically witnessed and posited that since women bear a larger responsibility for social reproduction, during times of crises they may experience pressure to substitute unpaid care work for lost income (ILO, 2018; Sayer, 2005). While women already out-performed men in unpaid care work globally prior to the pandemic (ILO, 2018), school and daycare closures, as well as increased numbers of those sick and in need of care have only increased the need for home-based care work (ILO, 2018; Bahn et al., 2020; Sayer, 2005).

Studies over the past year have revealed a couple of crucial phenomena with implications for women's vocational lives and therefore mental health. In a multi-country study, researchers found that over the past year, employed women, and especially mothers, spent more time on necessities such as childcare and chores – which was linked to lower reports of sub-jective well-being – than did employed men and fathers (Giurge et al., 2021). Within dual-earner heterosexual couples, mothers have reduced their work hours four to five times more than fathers, whose work has remained relatively stable and unchanged irrespective of the option for both parents to telecommute (Collins et al., 2021). Among academic researchers, productivity declined more among women than among men during the pandemic, with mothers of young children experiencing the largest productivity decline (Amano-Patino et al., 2020; Ribarovska et al., 2021; Barber et al., 2021).

Overall, the gender gap in work hours in the US during the first peak of the COVID-19 pandemic between February to April 2020 grew drastically (Collins et al., 2021). While some work flexibility, such as the option to tele-commute, have helped protect many women from job loss and have effectively helped to minimize the gender division of labor in that way, the results of these studies point to the disproportionate burden that women, and especially mothers, experience in terms of time spent on necessities, such as care work and chores (Collins et al., 2021; Alon et al., 2021).

Longitudinal Impacts

Not only have women been disproportionately impacted by job loss and the increased pressure in the face of unprecedented demand for unpaid care work, they also represent the population that has lagged the most in returning to the workforce – most notably Black and Hispanic women (Koeze, 2021). Women's labor supply is generally more elastic, or sensitive to change than that of men, suggesting that in the pandemic recession which is predominantly a "shecession," women's labor supply will take longer to bounce back (Alon et al., 2020b). A little over one year after the pandemic hit, it was clear that some groups were making faster progress than others in returning to the labor force. About seven percent fewer Black women and 7.2% fewer Hispanic women were employed in May 2021 compared to pre-pademic numbers in February 2020, representing the two largest gaps among other groups by a considerable margin (Koeze, 2021).

Economists have observed that losing employment during a recession is associated with persistent earnings losses for the affected workers (Stevens, 1997; Davis and von Wachter, 2011). Economic scholars speculate that because women have been disproportionately affected by employment losses during the pandemic recession, that the gender pay gap in the years after the recession will likely widen even further (Alon et al., 2021).

For many women who have been able to maintain employment throughout the pandemic while also facing the task of increased care work due to school or daycare closures, there may also be longer-term career implications. Even if the effects are not immediately prominent, scaling back work hours where men have not, or decreased productivity due to the challenge of juggling more responsibilities within the home will ultimately hinder career advancement and lower women and mothers' future merit-based opportunities (Collins et al., 2021; Alon et al., 2021; Blair-Loy, 2003; Stone, 2007). Thus, even among women whose workplaces have allowed for flexible telecommuting policies, they may still face long-term employment penalties as a consequence (Collins et al., 2021; Alon et al., 2021).

The realities of women's experiences, and namely minority women's experience in the labor market during the pandemic, represent real issues that have impacted the livelihood, physical health, mental health, and well-being of many and will undoubtedly have lasting effects. In these ways the human dignity of women has been disproportionately disregarded over the course of this pandemic insofar as women have not been afforded equal access to opportunities to apply their gifts to thrive.

To Let Go

To be amazed by these realities, or to practice amazement, is also, as Soelle puts it, "a beginning in leaving oneself.... In amazement we detrivialize ourselves and enter the second stage of the journey of resistance, that of letting go" (Soelle, 2001, 91). In radically opening oneself to be amazed by the suffering other—to truly descend into the particularities of the realities – we step outside of our ego selves and attempt to objectively interrogate as much as humanly possible, the negative dominant value systems, false desires promoted by consumerism and egotism, and interpersonal and systems-level barriers perpetuating exploitation. In other words, we attempt to faithfully reorient our fidelity to the reality of the suffering other. The process of letting go, therefore begins with questions that lead us to understand what needs to be un-formed before we can be transformed. This requires us to ask questions such as: *What have I been perceiving as a given of society or existence? What rules, norms or values (interpersonal or systemic) have I been accepting without examination and that have been perpetuating the suffering of the other?*

One of the notable reasons that women have been disproportionately impacted by the pandemic recession is due to the fact that the industries hardest hit were predominantly female-dominated sects such as hospitality and leisure. While this may be unavoidable, it is important to explore the particularities between regular "mancessions" versus "shecessions" and the ways that these differences need to be accounted for in the response to unprecedented job losses. Furthermore, women who dominate frontline and low-wage jobs have not been afforded adequate protections.

In their working paper, Alon et al. (2021) speculate that given that much of the pandemic recession is due to the response of the crisis rather than a direct consequence of disease, policy differences likely contributed to cross-country differences in the impact of the crisis. In their analysis of cross-country data, they point to the relevant use of furlough policies to protect employment during the pandemic. With little use of furlough policies, the United States experienced a much larger overall impact and increase in the gender gap in terms of employment (Alon et al., 2021). Other countries, such as Germany, which experienced no significant gender gap in employment, heavily utilized furlough policies that protected formal employment relationships while also providing flexibility for large adjustments of labor supply on the intensive margin (Alon et al., 2021). This is a particularly important factor to consider when understanding the fundamental differences between the pandemic recession and previous recessions. Since men's labor tends to be less elastic, and particularly so for married men, they are likely to stay in the labor force and return to full-time employment following employment loss in the recovery of a recession, which is not so for women (Alon et al., 2021). In contrast, women's labor supply is more elastic and when employment is lost, women are relatively more likely to drop out of the labor force or to only seek part-time work (Alon et al., 2021). Thus when job losses are concentrated on women in a recession, "decline in aggregate labor supply will be more persistent, and continue to be concentrated on women during the recovery" (Alon et al., 2020b). Therefore, utilizing intentional and informed policy responses are highly important and will have lasting implications in the process of recovery and beyond.

Another factor that is at play is societal reliance on women for care work. While this was explored earlier, it is important to note that while the pandemic provided an opportunity to disrupt traditionally held gender norms and expectations around care work, we saw instead that it served to reinforce these gender norms. This has proven costly for women across race, ethnicity, and socioeconomic status, albeit some women have felt this more heavily than others dependent on resources available.

Separate but intimately related to unhelpful gendered division in childcare responsibilities, is the unseen economy and phenomenon of *unpaid* care work. The perceived low value of paid and unpaid care work, and women's disproportionate representation and socially constructed responsibility in performing this work has been a long-standing issue in the field of feminist economics (Bahn et al., 2020). The pandemic has made visible the fact that the world's formal economies and the maintenance of our daily lives are built on the invisible and unpaid labor of women and girls (United Nations, 2020). While globally women were doing three times as much unpaid care work and domestic work as men before the pandemic, the increased demand for care work during the pandemic has only exacerbated already existing inequalities in the gender division in unpaid care labor (United Nations, 2020). The unpaid care and domestic work performed by women has always been critical to sustaining societies (United Nations, 2020; Bahn et al., 2020), and it has also been a direct link to wage inequality, lower income, poorer education outcomes, and physical and mental health stressors (United Nations, 2020). The immense economic value of unpaid care work needs to be recognized and supported by policies, not for the purpose of maintaining a gender division in this type of work, but precisely because it is a global reality.

To Resist

The third and final stage in Soelle's threefold process is one of healing and resistance (Soelle, 2001). In this stage, after having let go of those "givens" of society that promote consumerism and perpetuate inequality and suffering that we have comfortably left unexamined, Soelle suggests that we are to respond to these realizations with compassion and justice as our guides (Soelle, 2001). While this list is not exhaustive, some of the systemic and interpersonal barriers that have led to the disproportionate disregard of human dignity among women during the pandemic are: job precarity and lack of prudent policy action and employment protection, social norms placing undue responsibility for care work on women's shoulders, and the pervasive reality of unpaid care work.

To resist is to move towards institutionalizing human dignity by helping others to apply their gifts to thrive and provide equal access to opportunity. The pandemic recession has had clear gendered impacts, and ignoring such an impact will only serve to prolong the crisis and impede economic recovery (Özkazanç-Pan and Pullen, 2020). Decades of research has documented work as an essential aspect of optimal human functioning and wellness, and the pandemic provides an opportunity to engage in what the field knows in a new way to change the landscape of the labor market in a positive and lasting way (Autin et al., 2020).

While aid during this year such as the American Rescue Plan and the Child Tax Credit has provided some short-term relief, it is likely that the impacts, both economic and psychological, of the pandemic recession will most likely be long-lasting (Sharone, 2021; Autin et al., 2020; Alon et al., 2021). It's imperative for policy makers to adopt a feminist hermeneutic and understand the undue burden that has been placed on women who often experience already existing overlapping forms of inequality, and who dominate low-wage and frontline jobs.

Fighting for more permanent and flexible workplace policies such as the ability to telecommute could open the potential to reduce gender inequality in the labor market (Alon et al., 2021). Utilizing furlough policies more intentionally, especially if experiencing a recession predominantly felt by women could help mitigate future gender disparities in the labor market and expedite economic recovery for women (Alon et al., 2021). Furthermore, recommendations from leading thinkers in the field of vocational psychology are to encourage the public policy agenda to focus on efforts that provide work for all that is not only "decent, dignified, [and] safe, but that also affirms the importance of family and relationships as core aspects of life" (Autin et al., 2020). They also suggest putting efforts toward creating better working conditions – including physical and psychological safety – for essential workers, and supports for families that decouple financial stability from work such as basic income guarantees, guaranteed jobs, and financial and health care support for unpaid caregivers (Autin et al., 2020). Furthermore, encouraging more robust and lengthened unemployment insurance assistance is particularly important for minority women who have lagged the most in returning to work.

Outside of advocating for policies that boost the financial, psychological, and physical well-being of women and mothers, clinicians and career specialists can help in many ways. Among these are helping to develop critical consciousness in women at risk of internalizing shame around unemployment and financial hardships. Long-term unemployment, an experience laden with stigma, is one of the biggest barriers out-of-work individuals can face, and it may undermine well-being and lead to isolation (Sharone, 2021). While overall unemployment is down the spring of 2020 for some groups, long-term unemployment levels have trended up, and as of March 2021 was at over forty percent (Sharone, 2021). While women's labor is more elastic on the whole and it will take them longer as a group to re-enter the labor market, it is imperative that clinicians and career specialists are privy to the unique challenges for job-seekers who have been out of the labor force for longer periods of time. If the specific challenges that long term unemployment provides are ignored, clinicians may run the risk of providing irrelevant mental health care, or worse, they exacerbate the difficulties individuals are already experiencing by not being adequately attuned (Alon et al., 2021; Sharone, 2021). As women and mothers face unprecedented pressures to take on care work and necessary responsibilities, even while working full time, clinicians can facilitate conversations around shifting social norms and expectations that can lead to a more even gender split in responsibilities and care work within the home, or at the very least, bring a critical awareness to this reality for women. Furthermore, clinicians can help connect individuals with community-based support and encourage individuals who are in single-parent households, or who hold more communal value systems to seek support from others within their communities.

As policy and practice can benefit from a shift following the pandemic, research also holds an important role in resistance toward a cultural shift. As David Blustein writes, "working, at its essence, is about survival; however, working at its best, can encompass much more than survival" (Blustein, 2019, 3). Work has the potential to provide people with opportunities to create and contribute to the social and economic order, and to furthermore "determine the course of the overarching arc of one's life" (Blustein, 2019). Work has the potential to substantiate human dignity – to provide individuals the opportunity to apply their gifts to thrive. However, for this potential to be meaningful, it must be institutionalized. It is not enough to deconstruct harmful systems. We must at the same time build systems that free and liberate. This begins with research that can inform policy and practice suitable for the contemporary world. Shifting the field toward more inclusive theoretical models that account for the experiences of those on the margins and integrate historical, social, and contextual factors is imperative toward this end (Duffy et al., 2016). Therefore, frameworks such as the Psychology of Working Theory (Duffy et al., 2016) as well as Work as Calling Theory (Duffy et al., 2018), which place well-being and therefore human dignity as central, are particularly appropriate to guide the direction of the field and inform post-pandemic work-based policy.

Conclusion

The pandemic has exposed and exacerbated already existing inequities in the labor market (Autin et al., 2020). Historically marginalized communities are disproportionately vulnerable to precarious work, jobs that do not pay a living wage, and working environments that do not allow them to advocate for their needs, or provide access to basic benefits (Kalleberg, 2009; Blustein et al., 2020). When a global-wide crisis places an added layer of instability into the equation, these communities—the ones that have the least capacity to absorb the fallout—are the hardest hit by it.

Soelle's threefold theological framework of resistance provides an inductive approach to our way of proceeding and moving forward from the pandemic. This approach challenges us to remain faithful to the experience of those most afflicted and hold their dignity at the center in hopes of revealing the harmful systemic barriers, the limitations of our best intentions, and glimpses to caring for the whole person and the silenced suffering other, such as Adalia. Finding a way forward that places the realities of the most vulnerable at the center, and focusing on solutions that lead us towards upholding the value of human dignity – the fundamental agency of human beings to apply their gifts to thrive – allows us to imagine and work toward a future that is sustainable and safe for all.

References

Alon, T., Coskun, S., Doepke, M., Koll, D., and Tertilt, M. (2021, April) From man-cession to shecession: Women's employment in regular and pandemic recessions. National Bureau of Economic Research, Working Paper 28632. fromhttp://www.nber.org/papers/w28632.

Alon, T.M., Doepke, M., Olmstead-Rumsey, J., and Tertilt, M. (2020a, April) The impact of COVID-19 on gender equality. *Covid Economics: Vetted and Real-Time Papers*, 4, pp. 62–85. https://doi.org/10.3386/w26947.

Alon, T., Doepke, M., Olmstead-Rumsey, J., and Tertilt, M. (2020b) This time it's different: The role of women's employment in a pandemic recession. National Bureau of Economic Research, Working Paper 27660. https://www.nber.org/papers/w27660.

Amano-Patino, N., Faraglia, E., Giannitsarou, C., and Hasna, Z. (2020) The unequal effects of Covid-19 on economists' research productivity. Cambridge-INET Institute, Working Paper 22. Retrieved fromhttps://www.inet.econ.cam.ac.uk/working-paper-pdfs/wp2022.pdf.

Autin, K., Blustein, D., Ali, S.R., and Garriot, P.O. (2020) Career Development Impacts of COVID-19: Practice and Policy Recommendations. *Journal of Career Development*, 47(5), pp. 487–494. https://doi.org/10.1177/0894845320944486.

Averett, S., Argys, L. M., and Hoffman, S. D. (Eds.) (2018) *The Oxford handbook of women and the economy*. Oxford University Press. https://doi.org/10.1093/oxfordhb/9780190628963.001.0001.

Bahn, K., Cohen, J., and van der Meulen Rodgers, Y. (2020) A feminist perspective on COVID-19 and the value of care work globally. *Gender, Work & Organization*, 27, pp. 695–699. https://doi.org/10.1111/gwao.12459.

Barber, B.M., Jiang, W., Morse, A., Puri, M., Tookes, H., & Werner, I.M. (2021) What explains differences in finance research productivity during the pandemic? National Bureau of Economic Research, Working Paper 28493. https://www.nber.org/system/files/working_papers/w28493/w28493.pdf.

Blair-Loy, M. (2003) *Competing devotions: Career and family among women executives*. Harvard University Press.

Blustein, D. (2019) *The importance of work in an age of uncertainty: The eroding work experience in America*. Oxford University Press.

Blustein, D. L., Perera, H. N., Diamonti, A. J., Gutowski, E., Meerkins, T., Davila, A., Erby, W., & Konowitz, L. (2020) The uncertain state of work in the U.S.: Profiles of decent work and precarious work. *Journal of Vocational Behavior*, 122, 103481. https://doi.org/10.1016/j.jvb.2020.103481.

Cohen, J. (2010) How the global economic crisis reaches marginalised workers: The case of street traders in Johannesburg, South Africa. *Gender and Development*, 18 (2), pp. 277–289. https://doi.org/10.1080/13552074.2010.491345.

Collins, C., Landivar, L.C., Ruppanner, L., and Scarborough, W. J. (2021) COVID-19 and the gender gap in work hours. *Gender, Work & Organization*, 28, pp. 101–112. https://doi.org/10.1111/gwao.12506.

Constable, H. and Kushner, J. (2021) Stopping the next one: What could the next pandemic be? (ed. Ruggeri, A.) *BBC Future*. https://www.bbc.com/future/article/20210111-what-could-the-next-pandemic-be.

Davis, S. J., & von Wachter, T. (2011) Recessions and the costs of job loss. *Brookings Papers on Economic Activity*, 2, pp. 1–72. https://doi.org/10.1353/eca.2011.0016.

Duffy, R. D., Blustein, D.L., Diemer, M., & Autin, K. L. (2016) The Psychology of Working Theory. *Journal of Counseling Psychology*, 63(2), pp.127–148. http://dx.doi.org/10.1037/cou0000140.

Duffy, R. D., Dik, B. J., Douglass, P. R., England, J. W., and Velez, B. L. (2018) Work as a calling: A theoretical model. *Journal of Counseling Psychology*, 65(4), pp. 423–439. http://dx.doi.org/10.1037/cou0000276.

Giurge, L. M., Whillans, A. V., and Yemiscigil, A. (2021) A multicountry perspective on gender differences in time use during COVID-19. *Proceedings of the National Academy of Sciences*, 118(12). https://doi.org/10.1073/pnas.2018494118.

International Labour Organization (ILO) (2020, April 29) As job losses escalate, nearly half of global workforce at risk of losing livelihoods [Press release]. https://www.ilo.org/global/about-the-ilo/newsroom/news/WCMS_743036/lang–en/index.htm.

International Labour Organization (ILO) (2018, June 28) Care work and care jobs for the future of decent work [Report]. https://www.ilo.org/wcmsp5/groups/public/—dgreports/—dcomm/—publ/documents/publication/wcms_633135.pdf.

Kalleberg, A. L. (2009) Precarious work, insecure workers: Employment relations in transition. *American Sociological Review*, 74(1), pp. 1–22. https://doi.org/10.1177/000312240907400101.

Koeze, E. (2021, March 9) A year later, who is back to work and who is not? *New York Times*, U.S. Jobs. https://www.nytimes.com/interactive/2021/03/09/business/economy/covid-employment-demographics.html?searchResultPosition=1.

Lagon, M. P. and Arend, A. C. (2014) Human dignity in a Neomedieval world. In *Human dignity and the future of global institutions*. Georgetown University Press, pp. 1–22.

Laurencin, C. T. and McClinton, A. (2020) The COVID-19 pandemic: A call to action to identify and address racial and ethnic disparities. *Journal of Racial and Ethnic Health Disparities*, 7, pp. 398–402. https://doi.org/10.1007/s40615-020-00756-0.

Lindau, S. T., Makelanski, J. A., Boyd, K., Doyle, K. E., Haider, S., Kumar, S., Karnik, N., Pinkerton, E., Tobin, M., Vu, M., Wroblewski, K.E., and Lengyel, E. (2021) Change in health-related socioeconomic risk factors and mental health during the early phase of the COVID-19 pandemic: A national survey of U.S. women. *Journal of Women's Health*, 30(4), pp. 502–513. https://doi.org/0.1089/jwh.2020.8879.

Obinna, D. N. (2020) Essential and undervalued: Health disparities of African American women in the COVID-19 era. *Ethnicity & Health*, 26(1), pp. 68–79. https://doi.org/10.1080/13557858.2020.1843604.

Oliver, D. (2006) *Dorothee Soelle: Essential writings*. Orbis Books.

Özkazanç-Pan, B. and Pullen, A. (2020) Gendered labour and work, even in pandemic times. *Gender, Work & Organization*, 27, pp. 675–676. https://doi.org/10.1111/gwao.12516.

Ribarovska, A.K., Hutchinson, M.R., Pittman, Q.J., Pariante, C., and Spencer, S.J. (2021) Gender inequality in publishing during the COVID-19 Pandemic. *Brain Behavior and Immunity*, 91, pp. 1–3. https://doi.org/10.1016/j.bbi.2020.11.022.

Sayer, L. C. (2005) Gender, time and inequality: Trends in women's and men's paid work, unpaid work and free time. *Social Forces*, 84(1), pp. 285–303. https://doi.org/10.1353/sof.2005.0126.

Sharone, O. (2021, March 18) A crisis of long-term unemployment is looming in the U.S. *Harvard Business Review*. https://hbr.org/2021/03/a-crisis-of-long-term-unemployment-is-looming-in-the-u-s.

Soelle, D. (2001) *The silent cry: Mysticism and resistance*. Augsburg Fortress Press.

Stevens, A.H. (1997) Persistent effects of job displacement: The importance of multiple job losses. *Journal of Labor Economics*, 15(1), pp. 165–188. https://doi.org/10.1086/209851.

Stone, P. (2007). *Opting out? Why women really quit careers and head home*. University of California Press.

United Nations (2020, April 9). The impact of COVID-19 on women [Policy Brief]. https://www.un.org/sexualviolenceinconflict/wp-content/uploads/2020/06/report/policy-brief-the-impact-of-covid-19-on-women/policy-brief-the-impact-of-covid-19-on-women-en-1.pdf.

Chapter 14

Traumatic Racism

Homi Bhabha

The decolonizing movements of our times – be it Black Lives Matter or Rhodes Must Fall, or The Arab Spring – have all sought Frantz Fanon's witness. The Fanon that is restored to our political consciousness, today, is not the anti-colonial revolutionary of the mid-twentieth century struggling against the injustices of Empire while resisting the unrelenting winter of the Cold War. The significance of Fanon's work for the times in which we live – majoritarian, ethno-nationalist, populist— – is of another order. Today Fanon is the visual poet of public death and dislocation that stalks the black man on the highway, arrests him as he turns a corner, and fixes him with a deathly stare.

> "Look, a Negro!" The circle was drawing a bit tighter... I am being dissected under white eyes, the only real eyes. I am fixed. Having adjusted their microtomes, they objectively cut away slices of my reality. I am laid bare.
>
> (Fanon, Sardar & Bhabha, 2008)

Fanon's repeated references to the "fixity" of the racialized body – signified in tropes of fragmentation and dispersion and visualized in images of flayed skin and hemorrhaged organs – recall Michel Foucault's argument in *Society Must Be Defended,* that the violent aim of racial hierarchies is "to fragment, to create caesuras within the biological continuum addressed by bio-power" (Foucault, 2003, 255).

Bio-political fragmentations and caesurae are racial mechanisms of the Modern State that make it possible for state racism "to establish a relationship between my life and the death of the other that is not a military or warlike relationship of confrontation, but a biological type relationship" (Foucault, 2003, 255). Two decades before Foucault's seminar, Fanon's chapter, "The Lived Experience of the Black Man," enacts these "caesurae" as they occur in modern western postcolonial societies. Fanon stages a set of dramatic dialogues in which the black man ventriloquizes the violence of the white "gaze" while giving voice to the victim's agency and the witness's

DOI: 10.4324/9781003394327-15

testimony. Fanon's purpose carries the tone of Baldwin's resilience: "my whole effort is to try to bear witness to something which will have to be there when the storm is over. To help us get through the next storm" (Glaude, 2020, 137).

The speed of Fanon's prose catches the anxiety of racial trauma as if he were experiencing the encounter in this very moment, through the eye of the iPhone at thirty frames per second. And in that anxious temporality there lurks an invisible, impending risk not only to the end of black life, but a risk to the very means of black living. To be "fixed," in such circumstances, is not to be still or stationary; it is not to be a sitting target; fixity, in the Fanonian sense is to be tethered, like a moving target, to the contingent threat of impending racist risk that suddenly repeats, not everywhere but anywhere, not every time but anytime at all.

My desire to elaborate the idea of understanding "traumatic racism" as a significant, yet distinct, moment in the annals of "structural racism" critical for our times came to me as an echo of a few lines from W.E.B. Du Bois's finest work, *Darkwater*, that I could never fully understand, but could never forget. "My pale friend looks at me with disbelief and curling tongue," Du Bois writes when he confesses to his friend that, as a black man he lives each day with the anxiety of racial exclusion and insult. "Do you mean to sit there and tell me that this is what happens to you each day?", his pale friend asks with a touch of irony and disingenuity. At that moment, Du Bois, shoots back with a brief and brilliant answer:

> Not all each day, – surely not. But now and then – now seldom, now, sudden; now after a week, now in a chain of awful minutes; not every-where, but anywhere – in Boston, in Atlanta. That's the hell of it. Imagine spending your life looking for insults or for hiding places from them – shrinking (instinctively and despite desperate bolsterings of courage) from blows that are not always but ever; not each day, but each week, each month, each year. Just, perhaps, as you have choked back the craven fear and cried, "I am and will be the master of my – "
>
> (Du Bois, 2007, 223)

Suddenly, for me, the spatial divisions of physical segregation were translated (*not transcended*) into the temporal duration of discrimination. Time, as the trauma of racial indignity and bodily injury "in a chain of awful minutes... not everywhere but anywhere" has become the motif of my recent work. The reason for this is not hard to discern. Du Bois wrote his essay in 1920 and a century later, in 2020, a similar temporality of the "suddenness" of traumatic racism occurred "in a few awful minutes" – between 8:46 and 9 minutes in Minneapolis on May 25 2020 – and the world rose to protest the murder of George Floyd, as if the history of a hundred years had shrunk to a mere matter of awful minutes. In her essay, "The Trayvon Generation," Elizabeth

Alexander makes a tragic and graphic connection between Du Bois's insight and her own outrage:

> This one was shot in his grandmother's yard. This one was carrying a bag of Skittles. This one was playing with a toy gun in front of a gazebo. Black girl in bright bikini. Black boy holding cell phone. This one danced like a marionette as he was shot down in a Chicago intersection. The words, the names: Trayvon, Laquan, bikini, gazebo, loosies, Skittles, two seconds, I can't breathe, traffic stop, dashboard cam, sixteen times. His dead body lay in the street in the August heat for four hours.
>
> (Alexander, 2020)

To be racially tethered to the traumatic event – "fixed like a chemical solution is fixed by a dye...I burst apart (Fanon, 2008, 109) as Fanon describes it – is a form of trauma Freud associates with warlike circumstances that involve fatal risks. "The fixation to the moment of the traumatic accident lies at their root," Freud writes in the *Introductory Lectures On Psychoanalysis* (Freud, 1991, 314–315). The "affective coloring" (Freud's phrase) of a traumatic experience is excessively powerful, he explains. The temporal economy of the traumatic neuroses, Freud goes on to say "is an experience which within a short period of time presents the mind with an increase of stimulus too powerful to be dealt with or worked out in the normal way and this must result in permanent disturbances of the manner in which the energy operates...It is as though these patients had not finished with the traumatic situation, as though they were still faced with it as an immediate task which had not been dealt with, and we task this view quite seriously" (Freud, 1991, 315).

The temporal markers of the traumatic "moment" are short and sudden periods of time overwhelmed by the affective coloring of the anxious risk of everyday racial living – *not everywhere but anywhere*. The "moment" as a measure of traumatic time locates a quotidian, familiar place – his grandmother's yard, in front of her gazebo, at the corner of a Chicago intersection, Atlanta, Boston – which is then overcome by the traumatic, terrifying pace of imminent fear and fatality *in a matter of minutes*:

> This one was shot.... This one was shot... This one danced like a marionette as he was shot down in a Chicago intersection.... Eight minutes and forty-six seconds of a knee and full weight on his neck. "I can't breathe" and, then, "Mama!" George Floyd cried.
>
> (Alexandner, 2020)

This one, that one, the other one: these figures mount up, in time, to the indubitable statistical histories and practices of systemic racism: stop-and-frisk, police killings, and "qualified immunity" protections for law officers.

The rate of Black and Hispanic police killings are disproportionately twice the rate of White Americans, as reported in a Washington Post (2021) survey covering the years 2015–2021.

Ta-Nahesi Coates writes in *The Atlantic*:

> The deeper and more poignant charge is not simply that stop-and-frisk is a bad tool for recovering guns, but that it amounts to systemic discrimination against black and brown communities [who] are stopped twice as often after controlling for precincts.[1]

Black Lives Matter activists in 2020, alongside other activists protesting the police murder of George Floyd, took exception to the statute of "qualified immunity" that is built into the systemic legal protection of police violence. "One of the explicit and implicit demands of protesters on the streets today is that the law of the land be applied equally to all argues," writes Noah Feldman of the Harvard Law School. "The existence of the doctrine of qualified immunity sends the message that police should be protected from being sued under circumstances in which they have actually violated citizens' civil rights." And so a Section 1983 lawsuit against Derek Chauvin, the officer who is charged with murdering George Floyd, would have to show that clearly established federal law prohibited the placing of an officer's knee on an arrestee's neck (Feldman, 2020).

This one. this one…this one…this one – those who are part of what Elizabeth Alexander calls the Trayvon Martin generation are prone to becoming, over time, the "statistical lives" on which many policy-thinkers determine the cost-benefit calculation of racial risk. The metric of value that structures the utilitarian discourse that informs statistical lives is resistant to what statisticians recognize as "vividness." *What constitutes vividness?* The three qualities that convey "vividness" and are seen to disrupt the judicious balance of statistical rationality, according to Norman Daniels in his Hastings Center Report (Daniels, 2012), are the following: "that the story must be emotional, it must use visual images, and it must be unfolding in 'real time'." Affective identification, visual enactment, and narrative temporality are considered to be distractions to rational choice. There are, however, policy thinkers who justify vividness as foundational to moral decision-making, but they extend the range of emotionality or affectivity no further than *empathy* in their assessment of the risk to black lives and black living.

Scenarios of the traumatic "moment" of racial fixing are charged with affective stimuli that imprison the black subject in a spatial location – this street, this train, this city, this playground, this sidewalk – while the real-time narrative of traumatic racism puts its finger on the erratic pulse of ethical denigration and political dislocation which race through time in awful minutes. The emotional range of these traumatic moments far exceeds the moral and emotional norms of empathy: there is an overwhelming welter of projection, fear, introjection, inversion, anxiety, and the random repetition of time. Memory clashes with "real time" or is confused by it; an everyday custom suddenly becomes a carceral experience. You can *see* it in Fanon's visual scenes of black self-effacement that are also performances of the victim ventriloquizing the patronizing humiliation of white racists' savage civility:

> Understand, my dear boy, color prejudice is something I find utterly foreign... But of course, come in sir, there is no color prejudice among us... Quite the Negro is a man like ourselves...It is not because he is black that he is less intelligent than we are... I already knew that there were legends, stories, history, and above all historicity, which I had learned about from [Karl] Jaspers. Then, assailed at various points, the corporeal schema crumbled, its place taken by a racial epidermal schema.... I was battered down by tom-toms, cannibalism, intellectual deficiency, fetishism, racial defects, slave-ships...
>
> (Fanon, 2008, 112–113)

In a similar vein, The Trayvon Martin Generation is caught up in a Fanonian violence of vividness that extends beyond empathy. Here stories of black death accompany the very birth of a generation of black youth. Their voices and visions are primed by stories that, as Alexander writes, are "the ground soil of their rage;" traumatic "experiences whose affective coloring was excessive" – to use Freud's figure of speech – is everywhere to be seen and heard in Elizabeth Alexander's elegy for forlorn youth.

I call the young people who grew up in the past twenty-five years the Trayvon Generation. They always knew these stories. These stories formed their world view. These stories helped instruct young African-Americans about their embodiment and their vulnerability. The stories were primers in fear and futility. The stories were the ground soil of their rage. These stories instructed them that anti-black hatred and violence were never far...They watched these violations up close and on their cell phones, so many times over. They watched them in near-real time.

The political struggle against structural racism is crucial to the creation of a fair society. Statistical, data-driven knowledge is an essential aid in formulating reform strategies and evaluating their success; and statistical data is relevant whether we seek equity in the classroom, justice in the courtroom, or equal representation in the council-chamber. However, policy-driven "rationality" is fundamentally consequentialist: it is skeptical of the vividness of the storyline of racial trauma and instead privileges the cool calculation of the statistical graph; it is unconvinced of the efficacy of affective anomalies in emotional responses too vivid to be negotiated "reasonably"; and it is dubious of the validity of choices and judgments made in the pressure of real-time, in the heat of the moment. For these very reasons, the long arc of structural racism must be supplemented and interrogated by the vicissitudes of "vividness" – at once affective and narrative – as it shapes the imminent moment of the experience of traumatic racism.

Traumatic racism finds its most telling representational expression in the vivid urgency of the arts – in image, language, and movement – those very forms of life and language that depend on the "vividness" of embodied meanings and their phenomenological performance. There is a remarkable kinship between what Freud calls the affective economy of the traumatic effect, and what we might call the *affective temporality* of the traumatic arts. Like psychic trauma, poetic vividness provides an "experience whose *affective coloring* is excessively powerful"; and the power of the "coloring" of affect is less discernible in the original "content" of the trauma than it is visible or legible as repetitive, translational signification: traumatic coloring bleeds through time (Freud,1991).

Tropes of repetition in poetry and music iteratively and incrementally "work through" ideas and themes that are first introduced on the page or in the score, as surges of excessive meaning that *exceed* the sense and syntax of their originating insight and its containing moment. This process is similar to the "fixity" of trauma in the "short period of time" of its present, originating moment, which then requires another order of iterative and incremental time in which to work-through the traumatic affect "too powerful to be dealt with in the normal way." This "other" order of time that gives expression to the excessive affective coloring is not "normal time"; it is proleptic time. It is a form of time that represents something in the future as already done or existing.[2] Proleptic time is prognostic: it foreshadows the racial traumas of the future in the present as if it were the past poised for yet another attack not *everywhere but anywhere.* In addition, proleptic time does something more ethically and temporally compelling: it anticipates the present as if it had a foreknowledge of the impending traumatic violence occurring in real-time.

Racial profiling is just what it says it is: a profile of a racial body; a political silhouette in black and white; an outline of an Other emptied of his or her ontology. Racial profiling is not about a person or a citizen brought justly before the law where legal procedure protects human dignity and security. Stop-and-frisk, in disproportionate cases, is about a black body picked out like a shadow in the headlights of a police car; terrified by the "stretched out roar" of the siren, the body set against the horizon – fixed – like a cut-out figure. "*And you are not the guy and still you fit the description...*" "Our current politics tell you that should you fall victim to such an assault and lose your body, it somehow must be your fault," according to Ta-Nahesi Coates, "Travon Martyn's hoodie got him killed. Jordan Davis's loud music did the same" (Coates, 2015, 130).

Profiling goes beyond prejudice or discrimination; the outline of the black body or the minority figure, caught in the headlights of the police car, or the law-and order system, is a dismemberment of the black "person" – *limb by limb* – which is a more extreme form of psychic torture than "dehumaniza-tion" conveys. Fanon describes the traumatic moment of racial profiling as an unmerciful imprisonment: "On that day, completely dislocated…I took myself far from my own presence, far indeed and made myself an object. What else could it be for me but an amputation, an excision, a hemorrhage that spat-tered by whole body with black blood" (Fanon, 2008, 112).

Fanon's trauma of unbearable dislocation turns the black person into an "object" of visceral violence, hemorrhaging with the harms of profiling – tom-toms, cannibalism, intellectual deficiency, fetishism. Poetic justice has had its say in the spirit of vividness, but what of the letter of the Law? Let me turn, as I end, to Justice Sotomayor's dissenting judgment in *Utah vs. Strieff* from June of 2016 that follows almost seamlessly from Fanon. I am excerpting a few lines from her judgement on the police practice of "Pretextual stop" that she turns into a vivid phenomenological account of police harm and public humi-liation. As the black body is "broken down" for the purposes of evidence and examination, Sotomayor's narrative breaks down the police action into real-time "moments" – short, affective charges of traumatic racism—that provide a narrative of the black body caught in juxtaposed cinematic frames of alien postures: first you are told that you "look like" a criminal because *"because there is only one guy who is fitting the description"*; then your human dignity is soiled by an invasion of your bodily privacy; after that comes the curbside spectacle of public shaming; and finally the stripping of your rights as a citi-zen. Sotomayor writes a rare judgment in which the practical procedures of criminal justice – or criminal in-justice – are turned into narratives of extra-ordinary, extra-judicial "affective coloring" that speak up for the trials of traumatic racism that can change a life forever "in a matter of a few awful minutes."

> The indignity of the stop is not limited to an officer telling you that you look like a criminal…
>
> He may then "frisk" you for weapons…
>
> *This involves more than just a pat down. As onlookers pass by, the offi-cer may "feel with sensitive fingers every portion of [your] body. A thor-ough search [may] be made of [your] arms and armpits, waistline and back, the groin and area about the testicles, and entire surface of the legs down to the feet."*
>
> *Even if you are innocent, you will now join the 65 million Americans with an arrest record and experience the "civil death" of discrimination by employers, landlords, and whoever else conducts a background check.*
>
> *By legitimizing the conduct that produces this double consciousness, this case tells everyone, white and black, guilty and innocent, that an officer can verify your legal status at any time. It says that your body is subject to invasion while courts excuse the violation of your rights. It implies that you*

are not a citizen of a democracy but the subject of a carceral state, just waiting to be cataloged.
    I dissent. [3]

We are compelled to come to terms with freedom's possible futures as they fly past in present time, half-understood and never fully seen. How long will this protest last? How far will this movement go? These are absolutely the right questions to ask, so long as we don't believe that there is a right answer to them. In asking these questions we prepare ourselves for a political temporality of speech and action, for which we may as yet be unprepared, but which enables us to act beyond the "long-lasting" policies of evolutionary reform— health-care reform, police reform, criminal justice reform – that are, all too often, afflicted with short memories and broken promises. This intimation of the future's present is often an untimely moment; it disturbs our sense of historical duration and political direction; it bewilders us and renders us belated. At the same time, it is from within such disruption and disorientation that we move closer to Frantz Fanon's complex call to resistance, framed for his moment and ours in The Wretched of the Earth: "each generation must discover its mission, fulfill it or betray it, in relative opacity."

Notes

1 https://www.theatlantic.com/national/archive/2013/07/the-dubious-math-behind-stop-and-frisk/278065/.
2 OED defines prolepsis as such: "the representation of a thing as existing before it actually does or did so."
3 "Utah v. Strieff." Oyez. https://www.oyez.org/cases/2015/14-1373.

References

Alexander, Elizabeth (2020, June 22) The Trayvon Generation. *The New Yorker*.
Coates, Ta-Nehisi 2015 *Between the World and Me*. Random House Publishing Group.
Daniels, Norman (2012) Reasonable Disagreement About Identified Vs. Statistical Victims. *The Hastings Center Report*, 42(1), p. 37. https://doi.org/10.1002/hast.13.
Du Bois, W. E. B. (2007) *Darkwater : Voices from Within the Veil*. Oxford University Press.
Feldman, Noah (2020, June 9) Qualified Immunity. https://www.bloomberg.com/opinion/articles/2020-06-09/qualified-immunity-suggests-police-are-above-the-law.
Fanon, Frantz, Ziauddin Sardar, and Homi K. Bhabha (2008) *Black Skin, White Masks* (trans. Charles Lam Markmann). New edition. Get Political. Pluto Press.
Foucault, Michel, et al. (2003) *"Society Must Be Defended": Lectures at the Collège de France, 1975–76*. 1st ed., Picador.
Freud, Sigmund (1991) *Introductory lectures on Psychoanalysis*. Penguin.
Glaude, Eddie S. (2020) *Begin Again: James Baldwin's America and its Urgent Lessons for our Own*. Crown.

Index

Note: Page numbers followed by 'n' refer to notes.

For Product Safety Concerns and Information please contact our EU
representative GPSR@taylorandfrancis.com Taylor & Francis Verlag GmbH,
Kaufingerstraße 24, 80331 München, Germany

Printed and bound by CPI Group (UK) Ltd, Croydon, CR0 4YY
08/06/2025
01897008-0013